Accessing the E-book edition

Using the VitalSource® ebook

Access to the VitalBook™ ebook accompanying this book is via VitalSource® Bookshelf – an ebook reader which allows you to make and share notes and highlights on your ebooks and search across all of the ebooks that you hold on your VitalSource Bookshelf. You can access the ebook online or offline on your smartphone, tablet or PC/Mac and your notes and highlights will automatically stay in sync no matter where you make them.

1. **Create a VitalSource Bookshelf account at** *https://online.vitalsource.com/user/new* or log into your existing account if you already have one.

2. **Redeem the code provided in the panel below to get online access to the ebook.**
   Log in to Bookshelf and select **Redeem** at the top right of the screen. Enter the redemption code shown on the scratch-off panel below in the **Redeem Code** pop-up and press **Redeem**. Once the code has been redeemed your ebook will download and appear in your library.

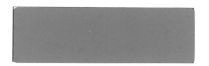

No returns if this code has been revealed.

DOWNLOAD AND READ OFFLINE

To use your ebook offline, download BookShelf to your PC, Mac, iOS device, Android device or Kindle Fire, and log in to your Bookshelf account to access your ebook:

On your PC/Mac

Go to *https://support.vitalsource.com/hc/en-us* and follow the instructions to download the free **VitalSource Bookshelf** app to your PC or Mac and log into your Bookshelf account.

On your iPhone/iPod Touch/iPad

Download the free **VitalSource Bookshelf** App available via the iTunes App Store and log into your Bookshelf account. You can find more information at *https://support. vitalsource.com/hc/en-us/categories/200134217-Bookshelf-for-iOS*

On your Android™ smartphone or tablet

Download the free **VitalSource Bookshelf** App available via Google Play and log into your Bookshelf account. You can find more information at *https://support.vitalsource.com/hc/en-us/categories/200139976-Bookshelf-for-Android-and-Kindle-Fire*

On your Kindle Fire

Download the free **VitalSource Bookshelf** App available from Amazon and log into your Bookshelf account. You can find more information at *https://support.vitalsource.com/hc/en-us/categories/200139976-Bookshelf-for-Android-and-Kindle-Fire*

N.B. The code in the scratch-off panel can only be used once. When you have created a Bookshelf account and redeemed the code you will be able to access the ebook online or offline on your smartphone, tablet or PC/Mac.

SUPPORT

If you have any questions about downloading Bookshelf, creating your account, or accessing and using your ebook edition, please visit *http://support.vitalsource.com/*

Botulinum Toxins in Clinical Aesthetic Practice

Third Edition

Volume Two: Functional Anatomy and Injection Techniques

Series in Cosmetic and Laser Therapy

Series Editors
Nicholas J. Gary P. Lask, and David J. Goldberg

Botulinum Toxins in Clinical Aesthetic Practice

Third Edition

Volume Two: Functional Anatomy and Injection Techniques

Edited by

Anthony V. Benedetto

Clinical Professor of Dermatology
Perelman School of Medicine
University of Pennsylvania
and
Medical Director
Dermatologic SurgiCenter
Philadelphia, Pennsylvania

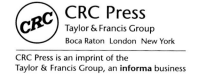

CRC Press
Taylor & Francis Group
Boca Raton London New York

CRC Press is an imprint of the
Taylor & Francis Group, an **informa** business

CRC Press
Taylor & Francis Group
6000 Broken Sound Parkway NW, Suite 300
Boca Raton, FL 33487-2742

© 2018 by Taylor & Francis Group, LLC
CRC Press is an imprint of Taylor & Francis Group, an Informa business

No claim to original U.S. Government works

Printed in the UK by Severn, Gloucester on responsibly sourced paper

 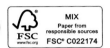

International Standard Book Number-13: 978-1-138-30480-2 (Pack- Hardback and eBook)

Library of Congress Cataloging-in-Publication Data

Names: Benedetto, Anthony V., editor.
Title: Botulinum toxins in clinical aesthetic practice / edited by Anthony V. Benedetto.
Description: Third edition. | Boca Raton, FL : CRC Press/Taylor & Francis Group, 2018. | Includes bibliographical references and index.
Identifiers: LCCN 2017024412| ISBN 9781138301849 (v. 1 : pack- hardback and ebook : alk. paper) | ISBN 9781138304802
(v. 2 : pack- hardback and ebook : alk. paper) | ISBN 9780203729847 (v. 1 : ebook) | ISBN 9780203729755 (v. 2 : ebook)
Subjects: | MESH: Botulinum Toxins, Type A--therapeutic use | Dermatologic Agents--therapeutic use | Skin--drug effects |
Cosmetic Techniques | Skin Diseases--drug therapy
Classification: LCC RL120.B66 | NLM QV 140 | DDC 615.9/5--dc23
LC record available at https://lccn.loc.gov/2017024412

Visit the Taylor & Francis Web site at
http://www.taylorandfrancis.com

and the CRC Press Web site at
http://www.crcpress.com

To Dianne, my loving wife of forty years, whose encouragement and support permitted me to accomplish that which seemed at times insurmountable and unattainable.

Contents

Preface

Because of the exponential developments in the clinical use of botulinum toxins (BoNTs), the need for a third edition quickly became a foregone conclusion. Maintaining the original mission of an instructional manual, this completely revamped and updated third edition attempts to record the phenomenal progress that has evolved in the use of BoNTs in clinical medicine over the past seven years. Updates of the literature, expanded indications, improved clinical photographs and illustrations, and newer and innovative ways to utilize the different BoNTs that are presently available worldwide are presented in this newly formatted third edition. It also has become strikingly obvious that BoNTs are injected in a variety of novel ways that differ from East to West. Therefore, a concerted effort has been made to include a profile of as many of the different BoNTs currently available around the world, including how they are utilized in a clinical aesthetic setting in both Western and Eastern cultures.

In the United States, glabellar and lateral canthal lines remain the only areas of the face that are approved by the FDA for the cosmetic use of onabotulinumtoxinA (OnaBTX-A) or BOTOX® Cosmetic. The other BoNTs available in the United States, abobotulinumtoxinA (AboBTX-A), incobotulinumtoxinA (IncoBTX-A), and rimabotulinumtoxinB (RimaBTX-B), have their own similar, but very specific, FDA indications. Consequently, except for glabellar and lateral canthal wrinkles, all the cosmetic injection techniques described in this third edition, as in the previous editions, apply to non-approved, off-label indications, which makes this book unlike most other textbooks in medicine.

It is sobering to realize that throughout human existence women and men have always sought ways to improve their appearance. To commence the in-depth and diverse discussions in this third edition on beautification and rejuvenation with BoNTs, Nina Jablonski, PhD, professor of anthropology at The Pennsylvania State University, and a world-renowned biological anthropologist and paleobiologist, provides us in her Prologue with a brief introduction to the evolutionary and anthropological perspectives on the importance of human facial attractiveness and expressivity. She cautions both patients and treating physicians in the over-use of face altering procedures that can effectively inhibit one's ability to express oneself accurately and in a completely natural manner.

Chapter 1 is written by Jean Carruthers, MD, to whom the world is indebted for her prescient identification of the cosmetic uses of the BoNTs. Dr. Jean Carruthers commences our venture through the fascinating evolving world of the BoNTs by presenting a historical account of the chronological events that led to the discovery, identification, isolation, and eventual synthesis of BoNTs for clinical use. Included is her seminal work in the development and advancement of the clinical uses of BoNT-A in ocular therapeutics, and her serendipitous discovery of its cosmetic properties. Jean describes the role she and her dermatologist husband, Dr. Alastair Carruthers, played in their provocatively sensitive introduction and promotion of the cosmetic uses of BoNT-A to the medical community.

Updates on the current advancements in the pharmacology and immunology of the different BoNTs are discussed by world-renowned scientists who are intimately involved in BoNT research and development. These include Chapter 2 by Mitchell F. Brin, MD, neurologist and one of the earliest clinical injectors of OnaBTX-A and now senior vice president of global drug development and chief scientific officer of BOTOX®, at Allergan Inc. (Irvine, CA). He presents an update on the pharmacology, immunology, recent developments, and future predictions on the use of BoNT-A. Chapter 3 by Juergen Frevert, PhD, head of botulinum toxin research at Merz Pharmaceuticals GmbH, (Potsdam, Germany), discusses the innovative pharmacology and immunology of a noncomplexed BoNT-A, and the advantages of its clinical uses.

Chapter 4 by the visionary dermatologist, Richard Glogau, MD, discusses the fascinating emerging science, development, and effective clinical uses of a new topically applied BoNT-A. Chapter 5 by Gary Monheit, MD, a dermatologist and leader in BoNT clinical research, and dermatologist James Highsmith, MD, elaborates on the recent advances of the different FDA approved BoNT-As and BoNT-B with updates on the pertinent literature and details on recent developments in their clinical use. Chapter 6 by Andy Pickett, PhD, Senior Program Leader & Scientific Expert, Neurotoxins for Galderma Aesthetic and Corrective, and Director and Founder of Toxin Science Limited, Wrexham, UK, identifies some of the different BoNTs used in clinical practice currently available in other parts of the world.

Chapter 7 by Alastair and Jean Carruthers, MD, presents updated and advanced clinical information on the adjunctive uses of the BoNTs in conjunction with injections of soft tissue fillers, and light- and energy-based devices for the aesthetic improvement of the face and body.

In Chapter 8, Arthur Swift, MD, an otorhinolaryngologist, Kent Remington, MD, a dermatologist, and Steve Fagien, MD, an ophthalmologist, add a new dimension to the aesthetic interpretation of how to use injectables when rejuvenating the face, change to including their explanation of facial proportions, geometrical Phi measurements, aesthetics, and beauty as they relate to the use of BoNTs.

For Chapter 9, dermatologists David Pariser, MD, and DeeAnna Glaser, MD, Secretary and President, respectively, of the International Hyperhidrosis Society, have comprehensively revised and updated the material on hyperhidrosis, discussing recent developments as well as new and different areas of treatment.

Chapter 10 by dermatologist Kevin C. Smith, MD, the master of novel injection techniques, along with dermatologists Irèn Kossintseva and Benjamin Barankin continues to enlighten us on unique ways to utilize BoNT-A for cosmetic and therapeutic purposes.

Chapter 11 by dermatologist and attorney David Goldberg, MD, JD, concludes the first volume with a revision and update of his chapter on the important medicolegal aspects of the cosmetic uses of BoNT.

Because of the ever-growing selection of the various BoNT products currently commercially available for clinical use in different parts of the world, the new Appendix 1 written by dermatologist Alica Sharova, MD, PhD, of Pirogov Russian National Research Medical University, Moscow, presents thought-provoking results of her meta-nalysis comparing consensus statements and recommendations for injecting different BoNT products in the United States, Russia, and different countries in Europe. She identifies and compares the fallacious recommendations of dose ratio equivalencies of the different available BoNTs injected, including number of injection points and dosaging for the different areas of the face and neck in males and females.

In the second volume, Sebastian Cotofana, PhD, a quintessential anatomist, has provided essential new material on functional facial anatomy in Chapter 12.

The nuclear Chapters 13, 14, and 15 on the cosmetic treatment of the face, neck, and chest with injections of BoNTs have been reorganized and expanded, assimilating many improved injection techniques by integrating updated information of recently published clinical and anatomical studies. All the anatomical figures and illustrations have been revised and enhanced throughout the text. The organization of these three chapters has remained the same. Each clinical topic is subdivided according to its facial and functional anatomy, and discussed in seven subheadings. The "Introduction" of each topic identifies the different anatomical changes acquired by men and women as they "age" and develop "wrinkles." Normal "Functional Anatomy" discusses the reasons these disconcerting changes and wrinkles occur so that a suitable plan of correction with a BoNT can be initiated. Functional anatomy is stressed and complemented by clinical photographs and detailed illustrations because the only way a physician injector can utilize any type of BoNT properly is to have an in-depth understanding of how to modify the normal and exaggerated movements of facial mimetic muscles and other potentially treatable muscles elsewhere in the body. When injections of a BoNT are appropriately performed, desirable and reproducible results without adverse sequelae are created. In the "Dilution" subheading, suggestions are given on how much diluent can be added to reconstitute a 100-unit vial of OnaBTX-A in order to arrive at various preferred concentrations per fluid volume dilutions when injecting certain muscles at different anatomical sites. The U.S. FDA-approved manufacturer's recommendation for the reconstitution of a 100-unit vial of OnaBTX-A is to add 2.5 mL of nonpreserved normal saline. This approved and recommended dilution is for injecting glabellar and lateral canthal frown lines only, since these areas on the face are the only approved indications for the cosmetic use of OnaBTX-A. However, when treating other areas of the face and body for cosmetic purposes, albeit in an off-label, unapproved manner, higher or lower dilutions of OnaBTX-A have proven to be more suitable and clinically more effective, depending on the muscles being treated. Options for "Dosing" are presented, with an emphasis placed on what to do and what not to do when injecting OnaBTX-A. Precise dosing and accurate injections of OnaBTX-A will diminish muscle movements of the face and body in a safe and reproducible way. Fastidious injection techniques are necessary to correct a particular aesthetic problem reliably, predictably, and for extended periods of time with any BoNT. "Outcomes" and results of different injection techniques are discussed to avoid "Complications" and adverse sequelae. Finally, how to inject a particular anatomical site and its projected results are summarized in the list of "Implications of Treatment".

Controversial and remarkable treatments for non-surgical breast augmentation for women and men are practiced by dermatologists Francisco Atamoros Perez and Olga Marcias Martinez and discussed in detail in Chapter 16. Their accumulated clinical evidence of the efficacy of BoNT-A injections of the pectoral area is clearly presented with an abundance of clinical illustrations.

Chapter 17, by a prominent and internationally well-known Korean dermatologist, Kyle Seo, MD, discusses the Asian perspective of the use of the different BoNTs currently available in his part of the world. Insight into the East and Southeast Asian cultural aesthetic needs and the Asian perception of aesthetics and beauty, is emphasized. He also presents a detailed description of the racial differences in the anatomy between Asians and Caucasians, which call for different indications and variations in appropriate dosing and injection points of BoNT-A treatments, necessary when treating Asian patients. He also provides some practical guidelines for the innovative use of BoNT-A in facial skin redraping and body muscle contouring injection techniques that are currently very popular in the East.

Many appendices supplying material for procedural reference conclude this second volume.

It is extremely fascinating and encouraging to understand that the cosmetic use of OnaBTX-A was initiated by the insight and convictions of two astute and courageous physicians, an ophthalmologist wife and her dermatologist husband. If it were not for the persistence of Jean and Alastair Carruthers in promoting their serendipitous observations, many other perceptive and insightful physicians would not have had the opportunity or the confidence to learn more about BoNT and its use in clinical aesthetic medicine. The challenge now being passed onto the reader is that with knowledge of how to inject a few drops of BoNT appropriately and safely, while treating patients with compassion and professionalism, additional innovative and ingenious uses of BoNT can be discovered, be they for cosmetic or therapeutic purposes.

We are all indebted to those physicians who have treated and continue to care for patients with BoNT for therapeutic and cosmetic purposes. Their commitment to the improvement of their patients' health and well-being through the advancement of sound and effective medical care is commendable and truly appreciated.

Finally, particular recognition and a special expression of gratitude is due to Kelly Heckler for her organizational skills and secretarial expertise that facilitated the completion of this book.

Anthony V. Benedetto, DO FACP
Philadelphia, PA

Acknowledgments

Many of the anatomical drawings not otherwise attributed (e.g., Figure 10.1) have base artwork from the Shutterstock archives and are reproduced with permission under licence; the annotations and overlays have been developed by the lead author of each chapter.

12 Functional facial anatomy, proportions of beauty, and neuromodulation
Sebastian Cotofana

DEVELOPMENT

The muscles of facial expression are derived from the second pharyngeal arch during embryologic development and thus receive their motor innervation from cranial nerve VII, the facial nerve. The primary function of these muscles is to protect the facial orifices and the organs located in their proximity from mechanical damage (orbicularis oculi), from ingestion of harmful substances (orbicularis oris), and to aid the uptake of food (levator anguli oris, levator labii superioris, depressor anguli oris, and depressor labii inferioris muscles) and air (nasalis, levator alaeque nasi, depressor septi nasi muscles). Previously important muscles for the movement of the ears, which were used, for example, during hunting or defense, can be still found as rudiments (e.g., the auricularis muscles).

During phylogenetic development, however, these muscles are progressively involved in the externalization of internal conditions and feelings (lat.: movere = emotions [= to move something out]), that is, for the expression of emotions. This was increasingly used for communication between individuals and for the coordination of social groups. A study in chimpanzees has shown[1] that the size of facial motor nucleus can be positively correlated to the group size and to the amount of time spent grooming, that is, social activity; indicating that the role of the facial muscles has been changed from rudimentary needs (food uptake and breathing) towards social interaction and group coordination. With the development of speech another important function of the muscles of facial expression was established: articulation. The perioral muscles are crucial in the formation of sounds due to their movement of the lips. These developments should be considered when trying to interfere with their primary function and effects of applied treatments should be also seen in the light of phylogenetic development. (See Prologue by N Jablonski in Volume 1.)

GENERAL FUNCTION

The muscles of facial expression are unique in their morphology as well as in their function. Regarding their macroscopic and histologic characteristics, muscles of facial expression do not contain an enveloping fascial layer, that is, epimysium, like most of the muscles in the human body. The absence of an epimysium enables these muscles to have a strong interaction with their surrounding tissues as no gliding plane is present, as opposed to having a gliding plane which reduces shear forces between neighboring structures for a frictionless and energy-efficient movement. Due to the strong interaction of the facial muscles with their surrounding tissues, distinct muscular contractions result in a minute movement of the neighboring tissues and most importantly the overlying skin. This is important for the delicate positioning of the skin during facial expressions and minute differences in contraction can result in an almost opposite effect, for example, smiling versus expression of disgust.

Another morphologic characteristic of these muscles is that they do not insert to bones, ligaments, or span joints to produce movements important for locomotion. They rather insert into the overlying skin or are of circular shape with origin and insertion being closely related. Therefore, the actions of the mimetic muscles cannot be described according to the general anatomic standards, that is, extension/flexion or abduction/adduction, but by elevation/depression with vertical, horizontal or diagonal movements resulting in facial expression on contraction.

Interestingly, histologic investigations have suggested that the muscles of facial expression have a reduced quantity of stretch receptors (as compared to regular skeletal muscles) and thus some authors have suggested that this is one of the reasons why the muscles of facial expression present with flaccid paralysis after a stroke rather than with spasticity. Recent studies revealed also that with aging the muscles of facial expression increase their muscular tone and have thus a reduced contractility. Facial exercises or the application of facial muscular training devices were less effective.[2]

ACTION MECHANISMS OF BOTULINUM TOXIN

The muscles of facial expression are classified as striated muscle fibers and are organized histologically by sequentially arranged subunits called the sarcomeres. Each sarcomere is formed by thin and thick myofilaments and receives its depolarizing signal from a cholinergic neuromuscular synapse. The ratio of recruited muscle fibers by one single lower motor neuron is 1: <100 whereas this ratio is 1: >1000 for thigh or back muscles. In regular neuromuscular transmission, an action potential is transmitted distally to the axon terminal, where neurotransmitter molecules (here acetylcholine) are stored in vesicles. On ion shift in the axon terminal, synaptic vesicles fuse with the presynaptic membrane and the vesicles' contents are released into the synaptic cleft. On the postsynaptic plate, specific receptors are present with the ability to bind the released neurotransmitter molecules and to generate a new postsynaptic potential which is then distributed across the muscle fiber and ultimately leads to muscle contraction.

The mechanism of vesicle fusion in the axon terminal requires the binding of SNARE (soluble N-ethylmaleimide-sensitive factor attachment protein receptor) proteins that are expressed on both the vesicle (V-SNARE) and on the inner side of the presynaptic membrane (T-SNARE). Binding of these proteins to one another induces their fusion and the release of the vesicles' content into the synaptic cleft. Without the binding of the V-SNARES to the T-SNARES, the vesicles will not fuse with the presynaptic membrane resulting in a persistent but reversible inhibition of neurotransmitter release.

Botulinum toxins (BoNT) are the most potent toxins known to humankind: the lethal dose for humans is 1 μg/kg by the oral, 10–13 ng/kg by inhalation, and 1–2 ng/kg by the intravenous or intramuscular routes. In detail, these toxins consist of a heavy chain and a light chain and there are seven known serotypes (A–G) of which toxin A (BoNT-A) is used in the majority of cosmetic procedures. The toxin light chain will cleave both the V-SNARES and the T-SNARES leading to a temporary flaccid paralysis as the incoming signal cannot be transmitted via the synaptic cleft to the muscle fiber.[3]

The application of BoNT-A in the proximity of a muscle will lead to the binding of the botulinum toxin to specific receptors at the presynaptic axon terminal of the supplying nerve, internalization of the toxin into the axon, and activation of its endopeptidase activity against the V- and T-SNARE proteins. Thus, BoNT-A applications have to be applied locally and in proximity to the intended muscle in order to induce the blockage of its neuromuscular transmission. After intramuscular injection, the dose-dependent paralytic effect of BoNT can be detected within 2–3 days. It reaches its maximal effect in less than 2 weeks, lasts somewhere between 3 and 6 months and gradually begins to decline in a few months due to the ongoing turnover of synapses at the neuromuscular junction.[4]

GENERAL FACIAL ANATOMY

The anatomy of the face can be best described as a layered concept. This concept is based on the fact that facial structures are arranged in specific layers, that is, in a specific depth within the face with the surrounding structures providing rigid or soft boundaries. From superficial to deep these layers are: skin (layer 1), superficial (subcutaneous) fat (layer 2), superficial musculo-aponeurotic system (SMAS) (layer 3), deep fat (layer 4), and deep fascia/periosteum (layer 5). Once this concept is taken into consideration the third dimension is accessible and the question: *"Where is the muscle?"* is not precise enough to target the respective muscle during treatment. Moreover, the additional question: *"In which layer is the muscle?"* must be answered to achieve the best possible outcome for botulinum toxin applications.

Having in mind that the facial musculature (like any other structure in the human body) is prone to variations in location, size, and course, individualized application patterns are of crucial importance. Rigid applications "according to the book" are outdated and individualized application schemes need to be applied. Facial wrinkles, independently if dynamic or static, are to be understood as muscular contractions of underlying muscles (accompanied by social, environmental, and demographic influences) and that the vector of contraction is perpendicular to the observed facial wrinkle.

MOTOR BRANCHES OF THE FACIAL NERVE

The motor component of the facial nerve emerges at the stylomastoid foramen at the base of the skull and enters the parotid gland from deep and posterior. Within the parotid gland the nerve divides into 3–7 branches and its divisions are called parotid plexus. At the anterior boundary of the parotid gland the nerve emerges between the superficial and the deep part of the parotid gland and its branches course toward the temple (temporal branches), in proximity to the zygomatic arch (zygomatic branches), horizontally across the cheek (buccal branches), along the inferior margin of the mandible (marginal mandibular branches) and inferiorly and anteriorly toward the neck (cervical branches) (Figure 12.1). The branches are deep to layer 5, that is, deep to the parotideomasseteric fascia at the level of the masseter muscle, but change planes toward superficial at the level of the anterior boundary of the masseter muscle. There the branches can be identified superficial to the facial vein and within the roof of the facial-vein canal. From there they distribute toward the respective muscles of facial expression and provide motor supply by entering into the muscles from inferior and posterior.

In the temporal region, the temporal branches can be located within layer 4, that is, deep to the superficial temporal fascia but superficial to the deep temporal fascia; superior to zygomatic arch and inferior to the inferior temporal septum.

In the midface, the branches are located deep to the superficial musculo-aponeurotic system (SMAS).

In the lower face, the marginal mandibular branch can be identified in 100% of the cases superficial to the facial artery and vein when crossing the mandible.

ARTERIES OF THE FACE

The face is primarily supplied by branches of the external carotid artery and only in minor parts (e.g., the upper face) by branches of the internal carotid artery. The major supplying arteries of the external carotid artery are: the facial artery, transverse facial artery, buccal artery, lingual artery, superficial and deep temporal arteries. Branches of the internal carotid artery are zygomaticofacial artery, zygomaticotemporal artery, dorsal nasal, supraorbital artery, supra- and infratrochlear artery, and medial and lateral palpebral arteries. One must be aware that the arteries display a huge variation in terms of course and presence as compared to facial veins (Figure 12.2).

The facial artery courses anterior to the facial vein and can be identified within the buccal space after crossing the mandible. At the angle of the mouth the artery is connected to the modiolus via muscular and ligamentous adhesions and lies deep to the muscles of facial expression but superficial to the buccinator muscle. After giving off the superior labial artery, the name of the vessel changes toward the angular artery. The angular artery gives off branches to anastomose within the SMAS with branches of the transverse facial artery which accesses the SMAS via the McGregor's patch. The angular artery courses in the depth of the nasolabial sulcus medially and superiorly within the deep pyriform space. Deep to the levator labii superioris alaequae nasi muscle it courses superiorly at the lateral margin of the nose, gives off connecting branches to the infraorbital arteries, and pierces in general the orbicularis oculi muscle around the medial canthus. There it connects with branches from the supratrochlear, dosal nasal, medial palpebral, and supraorbital arteries.

The upper lip is supplied by the superior labial artery whereas the inferior lip receives arterial blood supply from the inferior labial artery, the horizontal mental artery, and from the mental artery.

In the temporal region, an anterior and a posterior branch of the superficial temporal artery can be identified. The superficial temporal artery emerges from the depth 1 cm anterior and 1 cm superior from the tragus and courses imbedded within the superficial temporal fascial toward the temple.

VEINS OF THE FACE

The veins of the face are in course and variation much more stable than the facial arteries and thus can serve as excellent landmarks (Figure 12.2). The blood flow is in general directed as the facial venous vessels have valves with the exception of the angular vein. Here the blood flow is not directed and thus venous blood can drain both superiorly toward the superior ophthalmic and into the cavernous sinus or inferiorly toward the facial vein and into the external jugular vein. The facial vein crosses the mandible posteriorly to the facial artery and deep to the marginal mandibular branch. It enters the facial-vein canal, which is formed by the anterior and the posterior lamina of the parotideomasseteric fascia. The vein is found anterior to the masseter muscle where it gives off the inferior and superior labial vein and the deep facial vein, which drains into the pterygoid plexus. The vein can be identified anteriorly to the parotid duct, deep to the facial nerve branches, deep to the zygomaticus major muscle, and lateral to the infraorbital foramen. At this level, the vein courses more superficial and can be found superficial to the levator labii superioris alaeque nasi muscle and forms there the lateral boundary of the deep nasolabial fat compartment. It also has connections to the infraorbital veins at this level. The angular vein then courses medially and forms the medial boundary of the deep lateral cheek fat and of the suborbicularis oculi fat (SOOF). The distance between the inferior orbital rim and the vein was measured to be in mean 4 mm and this course corresponds to the nasojugal groove which represents the inferior boundary of the tear trough. It is important to note that the vein courses inferior to the tear trough and deep to the orbicularis oculi muscle and only at the level of the medial canthus does it change toward a more superficial position. There it connects with the dorsal nasal, the supra- and infratrochlear, the supraorbital and the central forehead veins.

FACIAL MUSCLES
Upper Face Region (Figure 12.3) (See Appendix 2)
Frontalis muscle
Origin: Epicranial aponeurosis
Insertion: Orbicularis oculi muscle complex

Innervation: Temporal branches of facial nerve

Vascularization: Supraorbital artery, supratrochlear artery, lacrimal artery, anterior branch of the superficial temporal artery

Function: Elevation of the supraorbital skin and eyebrow

Depth: Layer 3

Characteristics: The muscle is the anterior part of the occipitofrontalis muscle. Together with the temporoparietalis muscle, this muscle complex is also called epicranius muscle. Approximately 2–3 cm superior to the upper margin of the superior orbital rim the muscle is connected to the periosteum via the middle frontal septum. Movements of the overlying skin during muscle contraction converge toward this septum. Interestingly, the location of this septum correlates well with the location of the central forehead line, that is, the deepest horizontal forehead wrinkle. In some individuals, wavy (as opposed to straight) forehead lines can be observed. This is due to an increased muscle fascicle angle and due to the presence of a midline aponeurosis. Histological analyses have revealed that even in the midline aponeurosis muscle fibers can be identified, underscoring the importance of central neuromodulator applications.

(a)

(b)

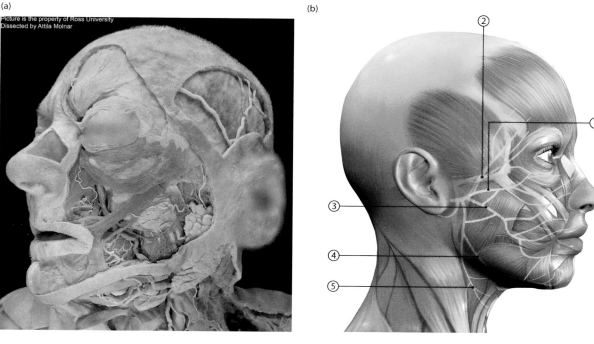

(c)

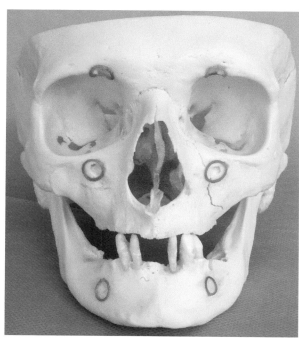

Figure 12.1 Nerves of the face. (a) Dissection. (b) The facial nerve, five motor branches: 1, zygomatic; 2, temporal; 3, buccal; 4, marginal mandibular; 5, cervical. (c) The trigeminal nerve, sensory branches (each emerging from the corresponding foramen): 1,supraorbital; 2,infraorbital; 3,mental. ([a] Courtesy of Ross University; dissection by Attila Molnar.)

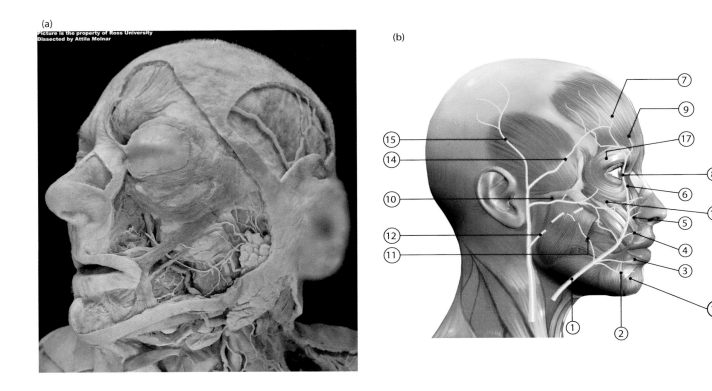

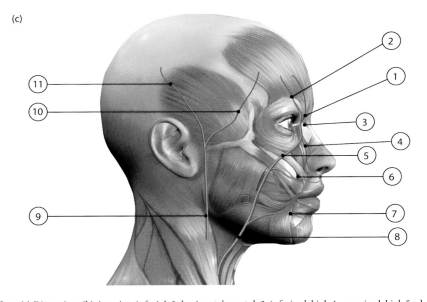

Figure 12.2 Arteries and veins of the face. (a) Dissection. (b) Arteries: 1, facial; 2, horizontal mental; 3, inferior labial; 4, superior labial; 5, alar branch of facial artery; 6, angular; 7, supraorbital artery; 8, dorsal nasal; 9, supratrochlear; 10, transverse facial; 11, lingual; 12, maxillary; 13, infraorbital; 14, anterior branch of superficial temporal artery; 15, posterior branch of superficial temporal artery; 16, mental; 17, infratrochlear. (c) Veins: 1, central forehead; 2, supraorbital; 3, dorsal nasal; 4, lateral nasal; 5, angular vein; 6, superior labral; 7, inferior labial; 8, facial; 9, retromandibular; 10, anterior branch of superficial temporal vein; 11, posterior branch of superficial temporal vein. ([a] Courtesy of Ross University; dissection by Attila Molnar.)

Orbicularis Oculi Muscle

Origin: Frontal process of the maxilla, anterior lacrimal crest, medial palpebral ligament

Insertion: Lateral palpebral ligament, lateral palpebral raphe

Innervation: Temporal branch of facial nerve, zygomatic branch of facial nerve

Vascularization: Facial artery, anterior branch of superficial temporal artery, supraorbital artery, lacrimal artery, supra- and infratrochlear artery, infraorbital artery

Function: Closure of the eye lids, depression of the eyebrow, drainage of lacrimal fluid

Depth: Layer 3 (Change of layer in the medial canthus—described as Horner's muscle at this point)

Characteristics: The orbicularis oculi muscle consists of an orbital part, septal part and a presepal part. The latter is described as Horner's muscle at the medial canthus and facilitates the drainage of the lacrimal sack. The differentiation between the orbital and septal part is represented by the orbital margin and the separating

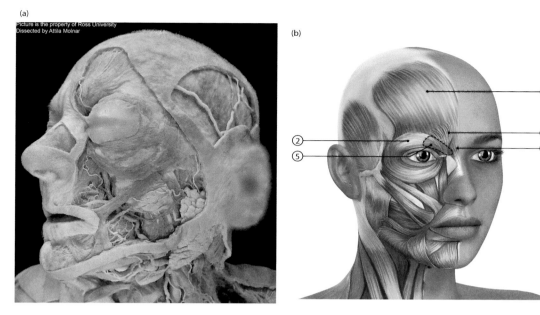

Figure 12.3 Muscles of the upper face. (a) Dissection; (b) muscles: 1, frontalis; 2, orbicularis oculi; 3, depressor supercilii; 4, procerus; 5, corrugator supercilii (deep to orbicularis oculi). ([a] Courtesy of Ross University; dissection by Attila Molnar.)

structure there is the orbicularis retaining ligament. The orbital part, however, can reach laterally and inferiorly into the midface and in dedicated cases muscular distentions (Figure 12.3) are identified, where fat from deeper structures can protrude. The laterally observed contraction at the level of the lateral canthus—also called "Crow's feet"—are arranged in perpendicular orientation to the muscular contractions in this area.

Depressor Supercilii Muscle
Origin: Frontal process of the maxilla
Insertion: Skin in the medial third of the eyebrow and into the orbicularis oculi muscle complex
Innervation: Temporal branch of facial nerve
Vascularization: Supra- and infratrochlear artery, supraorbital artery
Function: Medial and inferior movement of the eyebrow
Depth: Layer 3 (moving superficially from the medial third of the eyebrow and radiating into the skin [Layer 1])
Characteristics: The depressor supercilii muscle can be regarded as the fourth part of the orbicularis oculi muscle. This muscle is located in the same plane as the orbicularis oculi muscle and a clear separation between these two is almost impossible during gross dissections.

Corrugator Supercilii Muscle
Origin: Superciliary arch of the frontal bone
Insertion: Skin in the medial third of the eyebrow and into the orbicularis oculi muscle complex
Innervation: Temporal branch of facial nerve
Vascularization: Supra- and infratrochlear artery, supraorbital artery
Function: Medial movement of the eyebrow
Depth: Layer 5 (emerging from the bone and inserting into skin in the medial third of the eyebrow)
Characteristics: The corrugator supercilii muscle originates from the bone medial to the supraorbital foramen. However, its innervation reaches from the lateral side the muscle.

Procerus Muscle
Origin: Nasal bone, transverse part of the nasalis muscle
Insertion: Skin between the eyebrows (glabella), frontalis muscle

Innervation: Zygomatic branch of the facial nerve
Vascularization: Dorsal nasal artery, supra- and infratrochlear artery, anterior ethmoidal artery
Function: Depression of the skin superficial to the glabella between the eyebrows
Depth: Layer 5 (originating from bone and moving superficially toward the area of the glabella and radiating into the skin [Layer 1])
Characteristics: The procerus muscle originates from the bone and crosses all layers. In the central part of the muscle the dorsal nasal artery and vein can be identified, whereas in its lateral part branches of the angular vein, as well as of the supra- and infratrochlear artery, and supraorbital artery are coursing in a vertical direction. Its fibers are radiating into the superficial fatty tissue, that is, the glabellar fat body, and are anchored there. The most cranial fibers connect with the central part of the frontalis muscle and can pull the central part of the forehead inferiorly.

The interaction of the frontalis muscle, orbicularis oculi muscle, procerus, depressor, and corrugator supercilii muscle can be classified as the orbicularis occuli muscle complex in the periorbital region. All muscles show their effect on the movement of the eyebrows as well as the skin movement in this area. Also, the orbicularis oculi muscle complex must be balanced against the cranial pull of the frontalis muscle, which in turn is the only elevator of the eyebrow.

Midface Region (Figure 12.4): Nose (See Appendix 2)
Nasalis Muscle
Origin: Alveolar canine jugum, canine fossa
Insertion: Aponeurosis of the dorsal nose, skin of the nasal wing
Innervation: Zygomatic branch of facial nerve
Vascularization: Internal carotid: dorsal nasal artery, external nasal artery, anterior ethmoid artery; external carotid artery: facial artery, maxillary artery, lateral nasal artery, superior labial artery, septal artery, alar artery
Function: Elevation of the nasal wings and nasal tip, opening of nasal nares
Layer: Dorsal nose (layer 3, part of the superficial musculo-aponeurotic system)

(a)

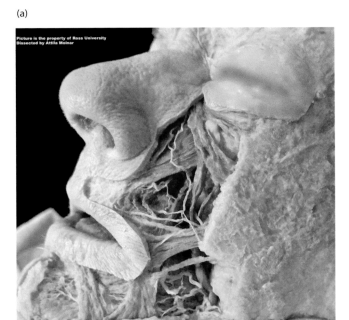

(b)

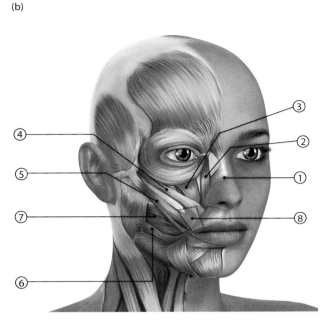

Figure 12.4 Muscles of the midface. (a) Dissection; (b) muscles: 1, nasalis; 2, nasal part of the levator labii superioris alaeque nasi; 3, labial part of levator labii superioris alaeque nasi; 4, zygomaticus minor; 5, zygomaticus major; 6, risorius; 7, buccinator; 8, levator anguli oris (deep to all others except buccinator). ([a] Courtesy of Ross University; dissection by Attila Molnar.)

Characteristics: The nasalis muscle is composed of a transverse and an alar part. Contraction of the nasalis muscle leads to the formation of nasal lines, also called "bunny lines."

Depressor Septi Nasi Muscle
Origin: Processus alveolaris incisivus
Insertion: Nasal septum
Innervation: Zygomatic branch of facial nerve, buccal branch of facial nerve
Vascularization: Superior labial artery, septal artery, alar artery
Function: Depression of the wings and nasal tip
Depth: Layer 5 (variation: layer 3)
Characteristics: The depressor septi nasi muscle originates in certain cases from the orbicularis oris muscle. On contraction, the muscle reduces the lip-nose distance and thus creates the impression of a short upper lip.

Levator Labii Superioris Alaeque Nasi Muscle
Alternative name: Angular head of the quadratus labii superioris muscle
Origin: Frontal process of the maxilla, medial infraorbital margin
Insertion: Skin of the nasal wings, lateral part of the nasolabial sulcus, medial part of the modiolus
Vascularization: Infraorbital artery, superior labial artery, external nasal artery, angular artery
Function: Elevation of nasal wings and upper lip
Innervation: Zygomatic branch of facial nerve
Depth: At its origin layer 5, the further caudally the more superficial (layer 1)
Characteristics: The muscle can be subdivided into a labial part (alternative name: infraorbital head of the quadratus labii superioris muscle) and an alaequae nasi part. The latter is located more medially toward the nose whereas the labial part is located more laterally with its fibers inserting into the modiolus. The angular vein

can be identified superfial to this muscle whereas the infraorbital foramen is located deep to this muscle.

Zygomaticus Major Muscle
Origin: Zygomatic bone (anterior to the zygomaticotemporal suture)
Insertion: Modiolus, orbicularis oris muscle, skin of the nasolabial sulcus
Innervation: Zygomatic branch of facial nerve
Vascularization: Zygomaticofacial artery, anterior branch of superficial temporal artery, angular artery, infraorbital artery
Function: Supero-lateral movement of the lip, causes a deepening of the nasolabial sulcus
Depth: At its origin layer 5, the further inferomedial the more superficial (layer 1)
Characteristics: The origin of the zygomaticus major can be found in close proximity to the McGregor's patch, which also represents the beginning of the zygomatic ligament. The zygomaticus major muscle forms with its broad-based origin the lateral boundary of the deep lateral cheek fat compartment. In its medial third the muscle can be identified superficial to the facial vein and may thus cause compression during contraction. Its terminal muscle fibers radiate into the skin of the nasolabial sulcus and form the floor of the superficial (subcutaneous) nasolabial fat compartment.

Zygomaticus Minor Muscle
Alternative name: Zygomatic head of the quadratus labii superioris muscle
Origin: Zygomatic bone, medial to the zygomaticus major muscle
Insertion: Modiolus, orbicularis oris muscle, nasolabial sulcus
Innervation: Zyomatic branch of facial nerve
Vascularization: Zygomaticofacial artery, anterior branch of superficial temporal artery, angular artery, infraorbital artery
Function: Supero-lateral movement of the lip, causes a deepening of the nasolabial sulcus

Depth: At its origin layer 5, the further inferomedial the more superficial (layer 1)

Characteristics: The zygomaticus minor muscle originates from the zygomatic bone and its fibers intermingle with the fibers of the orbital part of the orbicularis oculi muscle, which can be found in layer 3. As the orbicularis oculi muscle is discontinuous in some anatomical variations, the zygomaticus minor muscle can be listed as a part of the orbicularis oculi muscle or even as a part of the levator labii superioris muscle.

Levator Anguli Oris Muscle
Alternative name: Caninus muscle
Origin: Canine fossa, inferior to the infraorbital foramen
Insertion: Modiolus, orbicularis oris muscle
Innervation: Zygomatic branch of facial nerve
Vascularization: Infraorbital artery, angular artery, superior labial artery
Function: Supero-medial movement of the lip and of the labial angle
Depth: At its origin layer 5, the further inferomedial the more superficial (layer 1)
Characteristics: The levator anguli oris muscle originates inferior to the infraorbital foramen and forms the floor of the deep medial cheek fat compartment and the deep pyriform space.

Risorius Muscle
Origin: Masseteric fascia, SMAS, skin (very variable)
Insertion: Modiolus
Innervation: Buccal branch of facial nerve
Vascularization: Facial artery
Function: Lateral movement of the labial angle
Depth: Layer 5 (when originating from the parotideomasseteric fascia), layer 3 (when originating from the SMAS), layer 2 (when originating from the subcutaneous tissue)
Characteristics: The risorius muscle displays a high variation regarding origin and course and in some dedicated cases, it is absent during gross dissections.

Buccinator Muscle
Origin: Alveolar process of the maxilla, buccinator crest, pterygomandibular raphe

Insertion: Modiolus, orbicularis oris muscle
Innervation: Buccal branch of facial nerve
Vascularization: Buccal artery, lingual artery, facial artery
Function: Assisting during chewing via creating tension of the cheeks
Depth: Layer 6 (muscle is covered by extension of buccopharyngeal fascia, which can be regarded as deep fascia)
Characteristics: The buccinator muscle can be subdivided into three main muscle fascicle bundles: upper, medial, and lower, which crisscross each other at the modiolus and thus form the deep component (layer) of the orbicularis oris muscle. The parotid duct pierces the muscle anterior to the masseter muscle, but posterior to the facial vein. In its covering fascia, the juxtaoral organ is embedded, which is postulated to have a function either as a stretch receptor or as a neuroendocrine organ.

Masseter Muscle
Origin: Deep aspect of zygomatic bone (deep part) and inferior aspect of zygomatic bone (superficial part)
Insertion: Lateral aspect of the ramus of the mandible (deep part) and mandibular angle (superficial part)
Innervation: Masseteric nerve of mandibular nerve of trigeminal nerve
Vascularization: Maxillary artery
Function: Elevation and protrusion of the mandible
Depth: Layer 6 (deep to the parotideomasseteric fascia, which is considered layer 5)
Characteristics: The masseter muscle plays an important role in the lateral shaping of the face and its volume contributes significantly to the overall facial appearance. The branches of the facial nerve run on its surface medially.

Lower Face (Figure 12.5) (See Appendix 2)
Orbicularis Oris Muscle
Alternative name: Incisivus labii superioris muscle/incisivus labii inferioris muscle for its part originating at the upper and lower jaw
Origin: Alveolar jugum caninus of the maxilla (superiorly) and of the mandible (inferiorly)
Insertion: Same as origin and skin of the upper and lower lip
Innervation: Zygomatic branch of facial nerve, buccal branch of facial nerve, marginal mandibular branch of the facial nerve

(a)

(b)

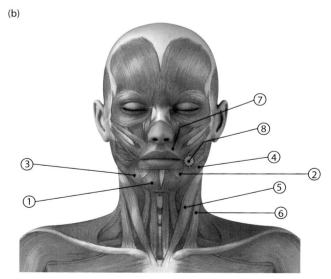

Figure 12.5 Muscles of the lower face. (a) Dissection; (b) muscles: 1, mentalis; 2, depressor labii inferioris; 3, depressor anguli oris; 4, platysma; 5, sternal part of the sterno-cleidomastoid muscle; 6, clavicular part of the sternocleidomastoid muscle; 7, orbicularis oris; 8, modiolus. ([a] Courtesy of Ross University; dissection by Attila Molnar.)

111

Vascularization: Superior labial artery, inferior labial artery, horizontal mental artery

Function: Closure of the oral cavity, internal torsion of the vermilion

Depth: Layer 3

Characteristics: The orbicularis oris muscle consists of a superficial and a deep part. The deep part is formed by the fibers of the buccinator muscle, whereas the superficial part is formed by the fibers of the muscles of facial expression. The modiolus is the hypomochlion of the peri-oral musculature as here a total of three layers of muscles merge together to form a muscular pillar of $1 \times 1 \times 2$ cm in extent. The modiolus can be found 0.7–1.5 cm laterally to the labial angle and spans from layer 2–6. The facial artery is firmly attached to the modiolus, but can vary in its course along the upper and lower lips with three potential positions: subcutaneous, intramuscular, and submucosal.

Depressor Anguli Oris Muscle

Alternative name: Triangularis muscle

Origin: Inferior mandibular margin

Insertion: Modiolus, lower lip (lateral end)

Innervation: Marginal mandibular branch of facial nerve, buccal branch of facial nerve

Vascularization: Inferior labial artery, horizontal mental artery, mental artery

Function: Depression of the lower lip and labial angle

Depth: Layer 3

Characteristics: The depressor anguli oris muscle originates from the bone in layer 5 but becomes more superficial toward its course to the modiolus. The muscle can be identified superficial to the depressor labii inferioris muscle and its lateral fibers merge with those of the platysma (layer 3).

Depressor Labii Inferioris Muscle

Alternative name: Quadratus inferioris muscle

Origin: Inferior mandibular margin, but cranial to the depressor anguli oris muscle and inferior to the mental foramen

Insertion: Modiolus, lower lip (lateral third)

Innervation: Marginal mandibular branch of facial nerve

Vascularization: Inferior labial artery, horizontal mental artery, mental artery

Function: Depression of the lower lip

Depth: Layer 3

Characteristics: The depressor labii inferioris muscle can be identified deep to the depressor anguli oris muscle having a fiber direction perpendicular to the orientation of those of the depressor anguli oris muscle. Medial to a vertical line passing through the angle of the mouth the depressor labii inferioris muscle and lateral to this imaginary line, the depressor anguli oris muscle can be identified.

Mentalis Muscle

Origin: Alveolar jugum of the mandible inferior to the transverse mental septum

Insertion: Skin of the chin

Innervation: Marginal mandibular branch of facial nerve

Vascularization: Inferior labial artery, horizontal mental artery, mental artery

Function: Cranial movement of the skin of the chin, creating a prominent labiomental sulcus

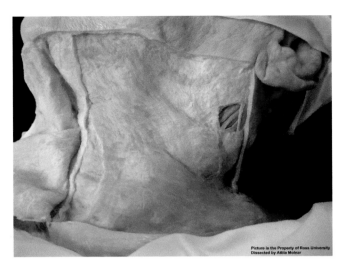

Figure 12.6 Platysma: dissection. (By courtesy of Ross University; dissection by Attila Molnar).

Depth: Layer 5 to layer 1

Characteristics: The mentalis muscle can originate as a two-headed or one-headed muscle from the mandibule, and the difference in the muscle morphology can be inspected by the presence of a mental fovea, which is more prominent if a two-headed variation is present.

Platysma (Figure 12.6)

Origin: Modiolus, subcutaneous plane with adhesions at the level of the inferior mandibular margin

Insertion: Skin of the neck

Innervation: Cervical branch of facial nerve

Vascularization: Superficial branch of transverse cervical artery, mental artery

Function: Depression of the labial angle, movement of the skin of the neck

Depth: Layer 3

Characteristics: The platysma is continuous with the SMAS in the midface and with the superficial temporal fascia in the upper face. It is discontinuous in the midline which can be observed in the aging neck or during forced muscular contractions. The longitudinal bands of the neck result from adhesions to the overlying skin but also from projections of the mandibular ligament and from the submental septum.

REFERENCES

1. Burrows AM, Li L, Waller BM, Micheletta J. Social variables exert selective pressures in the evolution and form of primate mimetic musculature. *J Anat* 2016; 228(4): 595–607.
2. Cotofana S, Fratila AA, Schenck TL, Redka-Swoboda W, Zilinsky I, Pavicic T. The anatomy of the aging face: A review. *Facial Plast Surg* 2016; 32(3): 253–60.
3. Kumar R, Dhaliwal HP, Kukreja RV, Singh BR. The Botulinum toxin as a therapeutic agent: Molecular structure and mechanism of action in motor and sensory systems. *Semin Neurol* 2016; 36(1): 10–9. https://www.ncbi.nlm.nih.gov/pubmed/26866491
4. Dressler D, Benecke R. Pharmacology of therapeutic botulinum toxin preparations. *Disabil Rehabil* 2007; 29(23): 1761–8.

13   Cosmetic uses of botulinum toxin A in the upper face
Anthony V. Benedetto

INTRODUCTION

In the United States, injections of botulinum neurotoxin (BoNT) to diminish horizontal forehead wrinkle lines, glabellar (central brow) frown lines and lateral canthal rhytides (crow's feet) are the only cosmetic and aesthetic indications approved by the Food and Drug Administration (FDA) in the United States of America (USA).[1-3] Injecting BoNT for cosmetic purposes in any other part of the face or body is not approved in the United States (US) by the FDA and therefore is considered off label use.[1-3] It remains to be seen whether the FDA and other governmental regulatory agencies of other countries will ever approve every single indication for which the BoNTs have proven to be effective in clinical practice. The fact remains that BoNTs are extremely reliable, nontoxic, and safe.[1-6] BoNTs provide reproducible results when administered as prescribed. Consequently, BoNTs have now become a major component of the armamentarium of any physician who practices aesthetic medicine in any capacity and who wants to produce the best cosmetic results for their patients.

In the early 1980s, botulinum neurotoxin serotype A (BoNT-A), known at that time as Oculinum™, was found to be effective for the treatment of strabismus in humans as an alternative to surgery.[7] Soon thereafter, Oculinum™ was acquired by Allergan, Inc. and renamed BOTOX®. In 1989, BOTOX® was approved by the FDA for the therapeutic treatment of strabismus and blepharospasm.[7] By 2000, BOTOX® was approved by the FDA for the therapeutic treatment of cervical dystonia. In April 2002, the FDA approved BOTOX® for the cosmetic treatment of glabellar frown lines. This resulted in the manufacturer's redesignation of the additional brand name of BOTOX® Cosmetic.[1] Both BOTOX® and BOTOX® Cosmetic are exactly the same product: they contain the same active ingredient in the same formulation, are manufactured by identical methods, and are only distributed under different names for different labeled indications and usage. BOTOX® is to be used for therapeutic purposes, whereas BOTOX® Cosmetic is to be used for cosmetic purposes.[1,8]

Subsequently, new and different formulations of BoNT-A other than BOTOX® and BOTOX® Cosmetic were approved for use in the US for both therapeutic and cosmetic purposes. The first of these was DYSPORT®,[2,9-11] which was approved by the FDA in May 2009 (see Chapter 5 by Monheit and Highsmith). In July 2011, XEOMIN®, a non-complexed BoNT-A was approved by the FDA for therapeutic and cosmetic purposes[3,12-14] (see Chapter 3 by Juergen Frevert).

To distinguish the current and future different formulations of BoNT from one another without mentioning their trade names, the FDA has assigned nonproprietary names, a type of "generic" name, to the different formulations of the currently approved BoNTs. (OnaBTX-A) was assigned to BOTOX® and BOTOX® Cosmetic, also known as Vistabel® in certain countries in Europe, and Vistabex® in Italy. AbobotulinumtoxinA (AboBTX-A) was assigned to DYSPORT®, also known as Azzalure® in Europe and Reloxin® elsewhere. IncobotulinumtoxinA (IncoBTX-A) was assigned to XEOMIN®, otherwise known as XEOMEEN® in Belgium and Bocouture® in Europe and elsewhere. Botulinum neurotoxin type B (BoNT-B) known as Myobloc® in the United States and Neurobloc® in Europe was given the designation of RimabotulinumtoxinB (RimaBTX-B) (see Chapter 5). Other BoNTs currently available for use in other parts of the world are discussed in Chapter 6 by Andy Pickett.

Chapters 13 through 15 discuss cosmetic injections of BoNT for the face and body. It is of particular importance to understand that in order to avoid ambiguity and confusion with the injection of appropriate and effective doses of BoNT, any reference to BoNT-A in these three chapters will indicate specifically BOTOX® Cosmetic and explicitly onabotulinumtoxinA or OnaBTX-A. The reason for this is not preferential usage by the author, but because OnaBTX-A was the first BoNT-A to be used for cosmetic purposes worldwide, and for many years a multitude of patients have been treated with OnaBTX-A before any of the other BoNT-As were available. Consequently, most of the patients illustrated in these next three chapters were treated with OnaBTX-A with the preferred dosages indicated. Therefore, for the sake of clarity and uniformity, all dosage units specified throughout Chapters 13 through 15 are expressed in units of OnaBTX-A.

Some may criticize the "cookbook" approach to Chapters 13 through 15. This systematic detailing of why, where, and how much OnaBTX-A to inject in a particular area of the face and body, however, is necessary to understand when correcting a certain aesthetic problem, and, therefore, was done intentionally. Moreover, it is important to note that the face is the only area of the body where there is no deep subcutaneous membranous fascia beneath the skin, thus allowing slips of muscle fibers that are attached to the facial skeleton at their origin to insert directly into the undersurface of the skin. But not all facial muscles have their origins attached to bone. Some arise from aponeuroses, but then they still insert onto the undersurface of the skin. Consequently, when these muscles contract, they move the skin of the face, producing folds and wrinkles always in a perpendicular orientation to the direction of muscle contraction. Nowhere else in the body are there similar types of muscles that contract voluntarily or involuntarily, pulling on the skin and expressing an emotion.

The face can be divided topographically into three segments using anatomical and cosmetic unit boundaries: the upper, mid, and lower part of the face. In these segments of the face there are either single or multiple muscles, that when contracted, move mostly in one direction. Depending on their location on the face and the anatomic position of their fibers, these mimetic muscles can move the skin in an upward, oblique, or downward direction. For example, this allows one to either raise or lower the eyebrows, smile or frown, open or shut the eyes, and so on. This difference in the direction of skin movement is done by muscles in a complementary, opposing fashion, that is, by elevating (levator) or lowering (depressor) muscles. These competing movements by agonistic or antagonistic muscles contracting intentionally or unintentionally cause horizontal, radial, or vertical wrinkling of the face. Consequently, nonverbal communication can be expressed with the slightest contraction of one or a combination of facial muscles (hence the designation "mimetic facial muscles").

The reader must never lose sight of the fact that every single individual patient is different and he or she should never be treated in an identical fashion without justification. These Chapters 13 through 15 strive to provide both the learning and experienced physician injector, the rationale for why and how a patient should be treated with a particular dose of OnaBTX-A in one area or another for a distinct and reproducible outcome. The reader also must understand that the explicit injection techniques, described with their indicated preferred dosages of OnaBTX-A, are only the author's perception of a given aesthetic problem. The reason for the particular pattern of wrinkles and the interpretation of a potential solution is this author's approach to the management of that specific problem for that particular patient, who may or may not present again in the future in exactly the same way. Therefore, when a physician is evaluating a patient prior to a treatment with a BoNT, it does not matter if the patient has or has never been treated previously with BoNT. The physician should approach that patient as if he or she were receiving BoNT for the very first time. Prior to commencing with injections of a BoNT, the physician must evaluate the patient's current aesthetic problem completely and have a comprehensive understanding of the patient's current concerns. The physician injector should not necessarily rely on past treatment dosing or on instructional photographs that address injection techniques and dosing for similar problems. With a substantial understanding of functional anatomy, the physician injector should be flexible enough to evaluate correctly and treat appropriately the patient's concerns and specific offending changes which are visible at the time of presentation. An expert injector utilizes BoNT to improve a patient's excessively dynamic muscle movements—thus treating the patient, not a picture.

The "before and after" clinical photographs of patients treated with OnaBTX-A presented in Chapters 13 through 15 are pictures not of study subjects, but of actual patients treated on a regular basis with effective and different doses of OnaBTX-A in a long-standing dermatologic clinical aesthetic practice. Hence, the reason for the lack of standardization in the quality of the photographs. These before-and-after clinical photographs are presented here only as examples of reasonably acceptable clinical outcomes. The reader in turn, after some personal experience with treating patients, should be able to use these examples of injection techniques and treatment outcomes to develop a preferred approach with his or her own personal injection techniques and produce comparable results when treating patients with similar clinical problems.

It is extremely important to understand that the specific units and dosages of BoNT-A discussed in Chapters 13 through 15 are only for OnaBTX-A (i.e., BOTOX® Cosmetic) unless explicitly stated otherwise. The same number of units specified in detail in these chapters for OnaBTX-A should absolutely not be used with an identical unit dose of another source or manufacturer, to treat patients with BoNT-A, even if a dose ratio of equivalency is provided as being 1:1.[1] The confusion with dose equivalencies using OnaBTX-A as the standard to which, regardless of serotype, all other BoNTs are measured, will only become more apparent and less reliable when different formulations of BoNT-A or other BoNT serotypes are utilized in the future.[15,16] The reason for this interchangeable indecipherability of dosing of the different brands of BoNTs is because currently the proprietary cell-based potency assay used by Allergan is different from other manufacturers' proprietary potency assays of their own BoNT and varies according to vehicle, dilution scheme, and laboratory protocols. Therefore, when using any type of BoNT including OnaBTX-A (i.e., BOTOX® Cosmetic), it is imperative that one learns how to administer that particular brand of BoNT independently of any conversion ratio because individual muscles may respond in a distinctly different manner to certain formulations and specific serotypes of BoNT (see Appendix 1).[15] Understanding the pharmacokinetics and pharmacodynamics of BoNT is still only in its early stages, and the possibilities for future developments are limitless[17–19] (see Chapter 2 by Mitchell Brin).

In 2002, the muscles of the central brow or "glabellar complex" were the first muscles of the face or body into which OnaBTX-A could be injected for cosmetic purposes that were approved in the United States (US) by the FDA.[1] Then in 2013, the FDA approved injections of OnaBTX-A for the cosmetic reduction of lateral canthal wrinkles or "crow's feet."[1] In 2017, OnaBTX-A was approved by the FDA for the temporary reduction of moderate to severe forehead wrinkles lines. Treatment of all other muscles in any other part of the face or body with injections of OnaBTX-A or any other BoNT for cosmetic reasons is done solely and expressly in an off-label, non-approved manner.

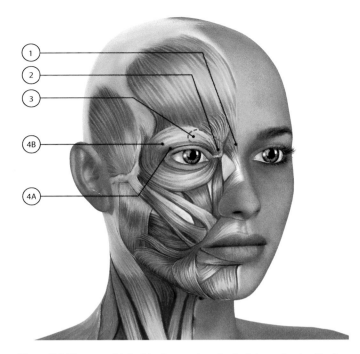

Figure 13.1 The upper third of the face consists of a single brow elevator (the frontalis) and four brow depressors: 1, procerus; 2, depressor supercilii; 3, corrugator supercilii (its path underlying orbicularis oculi is shown here); 4A palpebral and 4B orbital fibers of orbicularis oculi. (See Appendix 2—muscle attachments.)

CENTRAL BROW (GLABELLAR) FROWN LINES
Introduction: Problem Assessment and Patient Selection

The area most frequently treated with BoNT is the central brow or glabella and its frown lines.[20–26] On the skin surface, the glabella is the space between the eyebrows. There are four depressor muscles of the brow that cause the horizontal and vertical creases of the glabella (Figure 13.1). These muscles allow one to squint to protect the eyes from projectiles, gusts of air, and the elements (i.e., glaring light, wind, dust, sand) by lowering the eyebrows and adducting them medially. However, resting hyperkinesis of these depressor muscles can cause persistent, unintentional adduction and lowering of the medial aspect of the eyebrows, causing vertical and horizontal wrinkles between the eyes. This central brow frowning during moments of intense concentration, for example, can be misinterpreted by others as a veritable frown, which usually expresses negative feelings of concern, fatigue, disappointment, frustration, anger, pain, suffering, advanced age, and so on. (Figure 13.2a). Weakening the four depressors of the glabella with injections of BoNT can raise and slightly abduct the eyebrows and virtually eliminate the frown lines of the glabella. This allows a person to appear more relaxed, expressing a positive demeanor, even when in reality one might be frowning and attempting to convey a negative sentiment (see the Prologue from Nina Jablonski) (Figure 13.2b and c). An elevated brow generally expresses a positive attitude, whereas a depressed brow is indicative of a negative one. In addition, low-set eyebrows that progressively appear with age, eventuate in the formation of upper eyelid and lateral canthal hooding (Figure 13.3). Arched or peaked eyebrows usually are more attractive in women (Figure 13.2c), whereas men in general possess more horizontal eyebrows (Figures 13.4 and 13.5). However, be aware of women who pluck or have had permanent tattooing of their eyebrows, because the natural position of their brows may be altered (see Figure 13.42).

The brow has both static qualities of beauty and dynamic quantities of expressiveness that change with advancing age. As one ages,

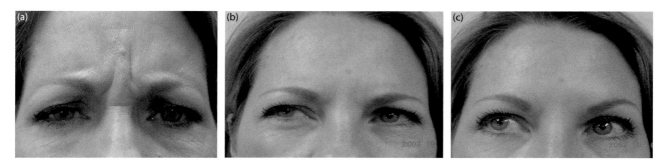

Figure 13.2 (a) A 53-year-old patient with unintentional frowning during intense concentration. An OnaBTX-A treatment was subsequently given. (b, c) 3 weeks after OnaBTX-A injections in the forehead and glabellar area seen here (b) with and (c) without frowning.

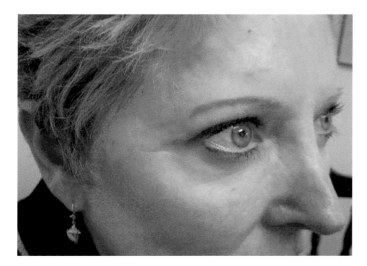

Figure 13.3 Low set eyebrows and upper eyelid and lateral canthal hooding in a 59-year-old patient.

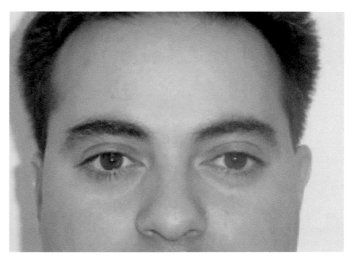

Figure 13.4 The ideal eyebrows for a man are less arched and lower set than a woman's.

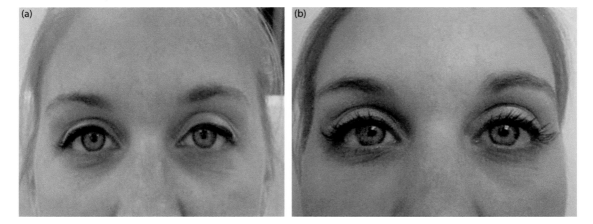

Figure 13.5 (a) A 28-year-old patient with relatively flat eyebrow arches before treatment. (b) After treatment with strategically placed OnaBTX-A, the eyebrows are elevated and arched. Note the right eyebrow also is slightly lifted and more symmetrical with the left.

the skin of the face and the rest of the body become inelastic and redundant. In the periorbital area, the skin of the eyebrows and forehead becomes lax and can drop inferiorly to lie over the superciliary bony ridge of the brows. This is recognized as brow ptosis of varying degrees of severity. Brow ptosis can alter the shape and position of the eyebrows, thereby compromising a person's youthful appearance and aesthetic attractiveness.

Trindade de Almeida et al. have classified glabellar frown lines into five distinct patterns[27] (see Figures 13.20 through 13.24). Although the muscular anatomy is by and large alike in most patients, individual skeletal morphology and idiosyncratic muscular movements can produce unique variations in the pattern of wrinkles in the glabellar area during intentional animation and spontaneous expression. The same is true anywhere else on the face for exactly the same reasons. The differences in glabellar wrinkle patterns indicate that the strength of each of the four glabellar muscles are not identical or uniform in size and strength in every patient and one set of muscles may be stronger or weaker than its codepressor set of muscles. Their response to neurostimulation also is uniquely different in every individual. Therefore, the pattern of glabellar frowning is dependent on which muscles are idiosyncratically stronger or weaker, and the injected dose of OnaBTX-A must vary accordingly. Some glabellar wrinkle patterns are observed more frequently than others according to Trindade de Almeida et al.[27]

Functional Anatomy of the Central Brow (Glabella)
(See Appendix 2)
On the skin surface, the center of the brow, that is, the space between the eyebrows is referred to as the glabella. In the area of the central brow or glabella in some individuals, both vertical and horizontal lines may develop, which frequently can project unintended negative social cues when one frowns. The bony glabella is the smooth, flat, triangular elevation of the frontal bone superior to the nasal radix positioned between the two superciliary ridges or arches. Contracting any of the mimetic muscles of the face will cause wrinkling of the skin perpendicular to the orientation of those muscle fibers and in the direction of their movement. The muscles that produce the *vertical* lines of the glabella do so because their fibers are oriented more or less horizontally and they move in a horizontal direction when contracted. They are the corrugator supercilii and the adjacent medial horizontal fibers of the upper eyelid orbicularis oculi.[28–30] The horizontal lines between the eyebrows across the root and bridge of the nose result from the contraction of the vertical fibers of the "medial" brow depressors, which move in a vertical direction when contracted. They are the procerus, depressor supercilii, and the adjacent medial vertical fibers of the orbicularis oculi (Figure 13.1). All four brow depressor muscles, corrugator supercilii, orbicularis oculi, depressor supercilii, and procerus oppose the contractions of the single brow levator muscle, the frontalis, in an agonistic/antagonistic fashion which is functionally characteristic of all the mimetic muscles of the face and anterior aspect of the neck (Figure 13.1).

The corrugator supercilii is a small, pyramidal, deeply situated paired muscle that arises from the frontal bone just inferior to the medial aspect of the bony superciliary arch approximately 4 mm lateral to the nasion[31,32] (Figure 13.6). The nasion is the point of juncture of the nasofrontal bony sutures with the internasal bony sutures (Figure 13.7). Clinically, the nasion can be palpated as the center of the concavity at the nasal radix (or root). The corrugator supercilii lies directly against the frontal bone just beneath the interdigitating muscle fibers of the superior orbicularis oculi, procerus, depressor supercilii, and frontalis medially and travels upwardly and laterally at an oblique angle of approximately 30°, to emerge from beneath the interdigitating fibers of the frontalis and superior orbicularis oculi and inserts underneath the skin into the soft tissue and dermis above the middle of the eyebrow in the vicinity of the midpupillary line and the supraorbital notch. The insertion point of the corrugator is approximately 4.2–4.5 cm lateral to the midline and is often seen as a dimple in the skin just above the medial brow ("corrugator dimple") (see Figure 13.8).

In anatomical dissections, the medial aspect of the corrugator can be seen partially interdigitating with the frontalis superiorly, procerus medially, and orbicularis oculi inferiorly.[29,33] The bulk of the corrugator supercilii usually is found overlying the inferior aspect of the superciliary arch (Figure 13.7).[31] Anatomic studies have demonstrated that the thickest portion of the belly of the corrugator is at or just above a horizontal plane drawn through the middle of the eyebrow and approximately 2.0–4.0 cm from the nasion (Figures 13.6 and 13.7).[28,29,31–35] In some individuals the corrugator can be shorter and more oblique or even bifid with a *transverse* and an *oblique* head,[33] which is one of the reasons why there are different patterns of glabellar frown lines[27] (see the frown lines in Figures 13.20 through 13.26). The supratrochlear neurovascular bundle passes through the corrugator supercilii, while the supraorbital nerve runs underneath the muscle and divides into two upward running branches: the medial *superficial* and the lateral *deep* nerve branches.

(a)

(b)

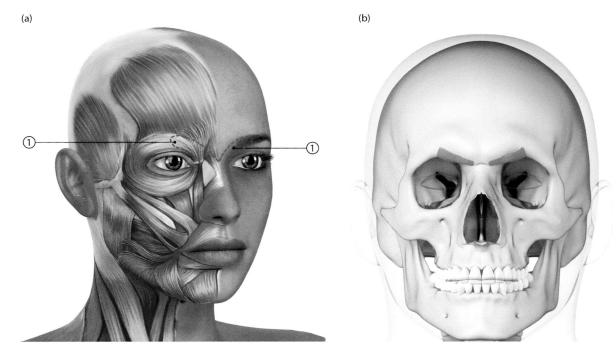

Figure 13.6 (a) The corrugator supercilii lies on the bone and deep beneath the other glabellar muscles; its course is shown here. (See Appendix 2—muscle attachments.) (b) The origin and insertion of the corrugators.

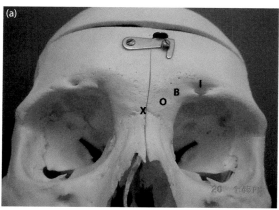
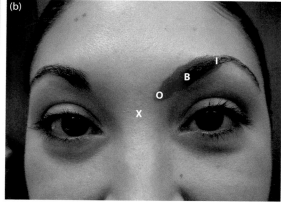

Figure 13.7 The corrugator supercilii. (a) Skull with view of the corrugator supercilii superimposed with letters. The thickest part of the belly of the muscle is approximately 2.0 cm from the nasion. (b) A patient with representation of corrugator supercilii drawn in red with superimposed lettering. *Abbreviations*: X, naison; O, origin; B, belly; I, insertion of corrugator supercilii.

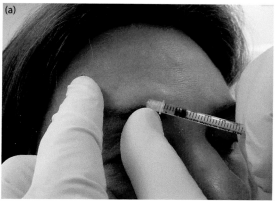
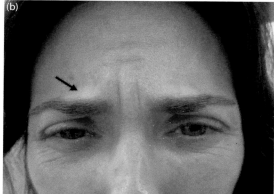

Figure 13.8 (a) Injection just above the middle of the eyebrow where the lateral aspect of the corrugators insert into the undersurface of the midbrow, just medial to the supraorbital notch or midpupillary line. (b) Note the obvious dimpling of the skin as the patient forcibly frowns.

The supraorbital artery and vein travel alongside the deep branch of the supraorbital nerve.[29]

The orbicularis oculi is a thin, broad, flat muscle whose fibers form a concentric ring over the eyelids and around the orbit. This sphincteric muscle can be divided into three parts. The outermost fibers of the orbicularis oculi are called the *orbital* portion of the orbicularis oculi. The orbital orbicularis oculi arises from the bony structures of the lateral nose and medial orbit, including the medial canthal ligament. Its fibers then run superiorly and inferiorly, forming a wide sphincteric ring surrounding and extending beyond the edges of the bony orbital rim and also into the eyelids (Figure 13.9).[28-30] A portion of the medial aspect of the orbital orbicularis oculi, whose fibers have a more distinctly vertical orientation, is occasionally referred to as the "depressor supercilii" by some authors (Figure 13.10).[33,36] Contraction of the medial aspect of the orbital orbicularis oculi lowers the eyebrow downward and medially and slightly depresses the lateral aspect of the brow. The inner portion of the orbicularis oculi which overlies the eyelids is identified as the *palpebral* portion of the muscle. The palpebral orbicularis oculi is further subdivided into the *preseptal* and *pretarsal* portions (Figure 13.10).[28-30] Contraction of the palpebral orbicularis oculi approximates the upper with the lower eyelids, either deliberately or involuntarily.

The horizontal lines of the glabella and nasal root are produced by the contraction of the vertically oriented fibers of the procerus, depressor supercilii, and the medial vertical fibers of the orbital orbicularis oculi. These three muscles also are referred to as the "medial brow depressors."[33]

The procerus is a thin ($\leq$1 mm thick), paired muscle, pyramidal in shape and centrally located in the midline of the glabella between the two eyebrows. It overlies the nasion and the bony origin of the corrugator supercilii. Inferiorly at its origin, the paired muscle bellies of the procerus are joined together but can separate in the form of a V superiorly at their attachments into the skin.[29] The shape, size, and strength of the procerus will determine the different types of frown lines that are created across the nasal radix (see de Almeida's glabellar frown lines, Figures 13.20 through 13.26). Its location 2–4 mm beneath the surface of the skin makes it an easy target for injections of BoNT[32] (Figure 13.10). The procerus arises from the fascial aponeurosis attached to the periosteum covering the lower caudal part of the nasal bridge (i.e., the upper portion of the nose overlying the nasal bone), the perichondrium covering the upper cephalic part of the upper lateral nasal cartilages, and the aponeurosis of the transverse part of the nasalis. It inserts superiorly into the skin and subcutaneous tissue at the nasal radix and lower part of the forehead between the two eyebrows. Superiorly, muscle fibers of the upper border of the procerus also interdigitate with muscle fibers of the lower central frontalis. Inferiorly, muscle fibers of the procerus interdigitate with fibers of the transverse nasalis. Laterally, the procerus interdigitates with the corrugator supercilii, depressor supercilii, and the medial fibers of the orbital orbicularis oculi. Contraction of the procerus pulls the medial aspect of the eyebrows downward, creating the horizontal

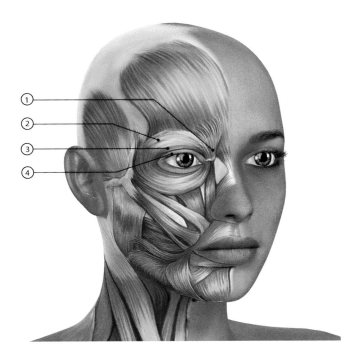

Figure 13.9 The orbicularis oculi has different subdivisions and interdigitates with the other depressors and elevator of the glabella: 1, depressor supercilii; 2, orbicularis oculi, *orbital* portion; 3, orbicularis oculi, *palpebral* portion *preseptal*; 4, orbicularis oculi, *palpebral* portion, *pretarsal*. (See Appendix 2—muscle attachments)

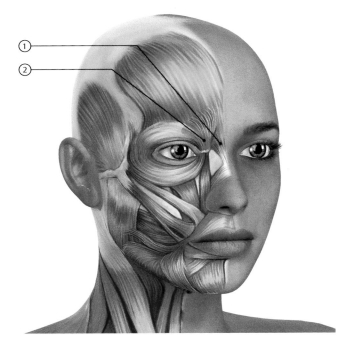

Figure 13.10 The depressor supercilii is the diminutive muscle of the glabella. The procerus is the midline, deep muscle of the glabella. 1, procerus; 2, depressor supercilii. (See Appendix 2—muscle attachments)

frown lines across the root and bridge of the nose. Anatomic studies also have demonstrated that the procerus can be longer in women than in men and, at times, bifid similar to the frontalis.[29,34]

The depressor supercilii is considered by many a component part of the medial, vertical fibers of the orbital orbicularis oculi (Figure 13.10).[28–30,34] Yet others consider it a separate and distinct muscle from the orbicularis oculi and corrugator supercilii.[33,36] The depressor supercilii is a small, vertically oriented muscle that has been found to originate directly from bone as one or two distinct muscle heads from the frontal process of the maxilla roughly 2–5 mm below the fronto-maxillary suture line, and the nasal process of the frontal bone slightly posterior and superior to the posterior lacrimal crest. Clinically, the depressor supercilii can be located approximately 10–15 mm above the medial canthal tendon.[36] In cadaver dissections where the depressor supercilii originated as two separate heads, the angular vessels passed in between the two bundles of muscles. In cadavers where there was only one muscle head originating at the medial canthus, the angular vessels were found coursing anteriorly to the muscle before traveling deeper into the glabellar area.[29] The depressor supercilii then passed vertically upward and over the origin of the corrugators to insert into the undersurface of the skin at the medial aspect of the eyebrow, approximately 13–16 mm superior to the medial canthal tendon. It overlies the corrugator supercilii and the medial aspect of the orbital orbicularis oculi, but interdigitates with some of the more superficial fibers of the orbital orbicularis oculi.[28,31,34] Not only does it help move the eyebrow downward and close the eyelid, but the depressor supercilii also participates in the functioning of the physiological lacrimal pump by compressing the lacrimal sac (see page 174).

Opening and shutting the eyes is partially accomplished by the contraction of the accessory muscles of the upper eyelid: one is a cholinergic, striated muscle, the levator palpebrae superioris; the other is an adrenergic, nonstriated, smooth muscle called the superior tarsal muscle of Müller. The levator palpebrae superioris is the main retractor of the upper eyelid. It is a thin, flat, triangular sheet

of striated muscle originating at the apex of the bony orbit at the common tendinous ring or annulus of Zinn on the lesser wing of the sphenoid behind the globe and just above the origin of the superior rectus (Figure 13.11a).[28,30] The levator palpebrae superioris is positioned above the superior rectus as they both pass over the superior aspect of the eyeball within the bony orbit. Approximately at the level of Whitnall's transverse suspensory ligaments, the superior rectus attaches to the superior aspect of the globe at the level of the superior-conjunctival fornix, while the levator palpebrae superioris continues anteriorly as a wide aponeurosis. As the aponeurosis continues forward, some of its tendinous fibers attach to the anterior surface of the tarsus, and the rest of the fibers pass in between the muscle fibers of the pretarsal orbicularis oculi and attach to the undersurface of the eyelid skin.[28,30] Its tendinous attachments in the upper eyelid are responsible for the formation of the superior eyelid crease (Figure 13.11a).

Dilution for Injecting the Central Brow (Glabella) (See Appendix 3)

Different clinicians have their favorite patterns of injecting the glabella with varying doses of different concentrations of OnaBTX-A. The manufacturer's package insert recommends reconstituting the 100 U vial of OnaBTX-A with 2.5 mL of unpreserved normal saline, thus yielding 4 U of OnaBTX-A for each 0.1 mL of solution.[1] However, since the brow depressors interdigitate with each other in close proximity in a very small and confined area, it is extremely important to inject accurately precise amounts of OnaBTX-A in this area. Therefore, many seasoned injectors still reconstitute the 100 U vial of OnaBTX-A with only 1 mL of normal saline. This provides 1 U of OnaBTX-A in every 0.01 mL of solution, which is easily injected using a 0.3 mL Becton-Dickinson insulin U-100 syringe with a 31-gauge needle directly attached (Becton, Dickinson and Company, Franklin Lakes, NJ).[37] The advantage of using an insulin syringe is that the needle is directly swaged onto the hub of the syringe barrel, so there is little or no additional wastage of product in the hub of the needle or in the neck of the syringe (Figure 13.12). In addition, each

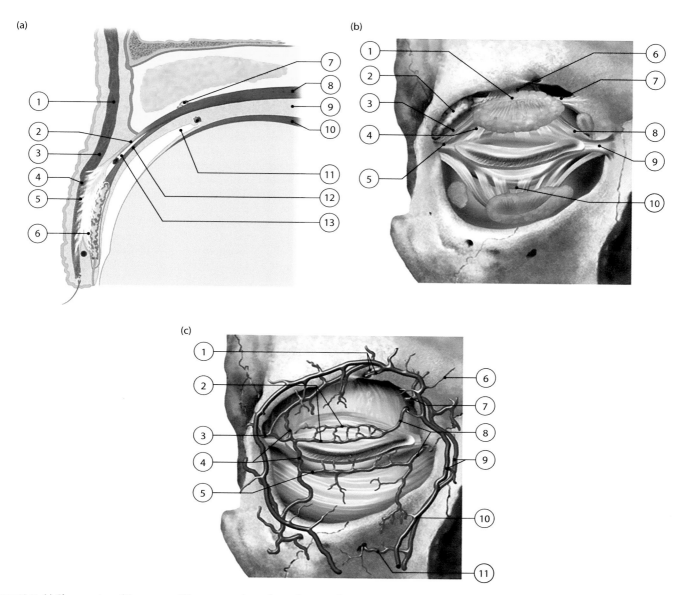

Figure 13.11 (a) Close-up view of the upper eyelid anatomy and muscle attachments. The levator palpebrae superioris is the main retractor of the upper eyelid; it is a striated muscle. Mueller's superior tarsal muscle is not striated, but a smooth muscle. 1, orbicularis oculi (orbital); 2, levator aponeurosis; 3, orbicularis oculi (preseptal); 4, orbicularis oculi (pretarsal); 5, levator aponeurotic insertion into orbicularis; 6, levator aponeurotic insertion into superior tarsus; 7, Whitnall's ligament; 8, levator palpebrae superioris; 9, common sheath; 10, superior rectus; 11, superior conjunctival fornix; 12, superior tarsal muscle; 13, post-aponeurotic space. (b) Anterior view of the upper orbit with the attachments of the levator aponeurosis and lower lid retractors. 1, pre-aponeurotic fat pad; 2, lacrimal gland; 3, lateral horn of levator aponeurosis; 4, levator aponeurosis inserting into superior tarsus; 5, lateral canthal tendon; 6, levator muscle; 7, Whitnall's ligament; 8, medial horn of levator aponeurosis; 9, medial canthal tendon; 10, lower lid retractors inserting into inferior tarsus. (c) Anterior view of the orbit showing the complexity of the vascular arcades and other vascular structures. 1, supra-orbital artery and vein; 2, tarsal arcade upper lid; 3, lacrimal artery; 4, lateral palpebral artery; 5, tarsal arcade lower lid; 6, frontal vein; 7, supratrochlear artery; 8, medial palpebral artery; 9, angular artery and vein; 10, facial artery and vein; 11, infraorbital artery and vein.

unit line marked on the syringe barrel corresponds to 0.01 mL or 1 U of OnaBTX-A when a 100 U vial of OnaBTX-A is reconstituted with 1 mL of saline. In this way, only minimal volumes of OnaBTX-A will be needed to produce the desired cosmetic results. Moreover, most practitioners now have switched to using preserved saline with 0.9% benzyl alcohol.[38–41]

Dosing: How to Correct the Problem (See Appendix 4) (What to Do and What Not to Do) When Treating the Central Brow (Glabella)

The pretreatment evaluation should include examining the patient at rest and in full motion. Lightly palpate the muscles of the glabellar area with the palmar surface of the fingertips of the nondominant hand as the patient squints and frowns. This will help determine the location, size, and strength of the individual muscles of the glabella (Figure 13.1). A frequently used and standardized technique for treating the glabella is to inject OnaBTX-A into five different sites with doses that range anywhere from 4 to 10 U or more at each site (Figure 13.13).[16,41–43] Electromyographic guidance in this area has not particularly improved treatment outcomes because these facial muscles are superficial and easily localized by palpation and topographical landmarks.[3,21,34,44]

Patients who possess thinner, less sebaceous skin with finer wrinkles and shallower skin furrows and folds that can be spread apart and reduced with the fingers ("glabellar spread test") seem to have better, longer-lasting results.[45] There are, however, some patients who are

119

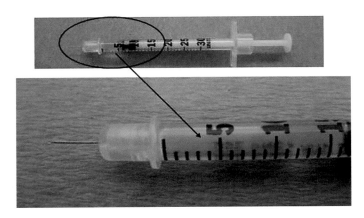

Figure 13.12 A 3/10 mL Becton-Dickinson insulin U-100 syringe with a 31-gauge needle swaged directly onto the syringe barrel. Note the absence of any dead space between the hub of the needle and the neck of the syringe. Each unit notch on the barrel corresponds to 0.01 mL or 1 U.

more difficult to treat because they are less responsive to the effects of OnaBTX-A. In this group of patients who are more difficult to treat, there is one type of patient who possesses thick sebaceous skin with deep, intractable wrinkles whose furrows are difficult to pull apart with the fingers. Usually these turn out to be men and sometimes women who spend a lot of time outdoors or constantly in front of a computer screen. The other type of patient is the one who possesses the inelastic, redundant skin seen with dermatochalasis and whose furrows also are deep but very easy to pull apart. These patients characteristically are older (>65–70 years old) and unfortunately are not ideal candidates for glabellar chemodenervation. Typically, in these patients, after having OnaBTX-A injected with impeccable technique, the resultant relaxation of the glabellar muscles causes a drop in the brow and infolding of the inelastic, redundant glabellar skin. Consequently, brow ptosis and persistent frown lines and wrinkles are the only outcome, even if higher doses of OnaBTX-A are subsequently injected.

Generally, glabellar frown lines in women can be satisfactorily treated with a total dose of about 20–30 U of OnaBTX-A injected into the standard five injection sites (Figure 13.14).[46–48] Men, on the other hand, usually require a significantly higher dose of OnaBTX-A (40–80 U) injected at seven or more sites across the glabella and medial brow to produce a reasonable effect that lasts at least 3–4 months (Figure 13.15).[49–53] When glabellar lines are deeper, longer, or thicker on one side of the midline, that set of medial brow depressor muscles (e.g., procerus, depressor supercilii, and medial aspect of the orbital orbicularis oculi) should receive a slightly higher dose of OnaBTX-A than the medial brow depressors on the contralateral side. Especially when treating men and those patients who have the "V" and deep "parallel lines" patterns of glabellar wrinkles (see Figure 13.21), the two additional injection points can be given along with the standard five injection points to reduce these deep glabellar lines effectively (Figure 13.13). The two additional injections usually are given *superficially* as one injection over the midpupillary line, bilaterally, which is in the vicinity where the lateral fibers of the corrugator supercilii pass upward and through the interdigitating fibers of the frontalis and orbicularis oculi and attach to the undersurface of the skin. Superficial injections avoid weakening the interdigitating fibers of the frontalis and orbital orbicularis oculi thereby avoiding brow ptosis, while injections given at least 3–4 cm above the bony orbital rim or 2–3 cm superior to the superciliary arch or ridge at the midpupillary line prevent, blepharoptosis (Figure 13.14).

At one time, there were some injectors who preferred treating the glabella separately in one session first, before injecting the frontalis in a different, later session, especially with first-time patients.[41,54] This concern might have been justified in the earlier years when injection techniques were just being developed, especially since high doses of

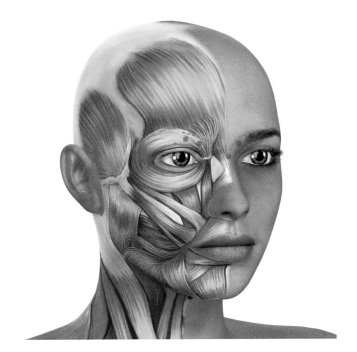

Figure 13.13 Standard five injection points for treating glabellar frown lines.

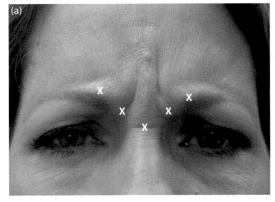
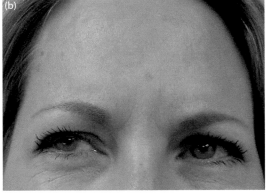

Figure 13.14 Standard five injection points for treating glabellar lines in a female frowning (a) before and frowning (b) 3 weeks after an OnaBTX-A treatment.

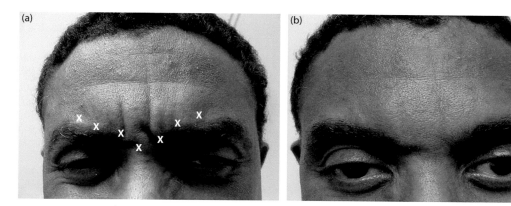

Figure 13.15 Standard seven injection points for treating stronger glabellar muscles causing deeper furrows and frown lines in a 51-year-old male (a) before and (b) 1 month after an OnaBTX-A treatment in a forced frown.

OnaBTX-A were being injected into the forehead. By injecting both the glabellar depressor muscles at the same time as the one brow elevator muscle, overdosing with total immobility of the forehead and glabella frequently was seen. At times, even brow ptosis was inevitable with those previously recommended doses.[41] With the evolving aesthetics and appeal of a "less frozen" look to the forehead, along with the recent FDA approval of injecting OnaBTX-A into the frontalis to reduce the appearance of horizontal forehead lines and into the lateral orbital orbicularis oculi to reduce the appearance of crow's feet, most injectors are now treating the entire upper one-third of the face during the same session effectively and safely (Figure 13.1).[42,55,56]

Treating glabellar lines with OnaBTX-A and producing optimal results are not simple tasks. There have been many injection patterns reported in the literature over the years, and they all produce optimal results when the ideal patient is treated appropriately with a given injection pattern. This leads one to believe erroneously that any injection pattern will work and so injecting OnaBTX-A is easy. However, this is not quite the case (see the glabellar patterns in Figures 13.20 through 13.26).

What is most important for a successful treatment outcome is for the physician injector to evaluate the patient comprehensively prior to treatment and to understand why certain wrinkles are formed and which muscles are creating them. Once a sound assessment is made and a justifiable treatment approach is designed, it does not matter which of the injection patterns one uses. Patients should be treated individually according to their idiosyncratic pattern of muscle movements

and the resultant wrinkles they produce. A three, five, seven, or even more injection-point pattern can be used if it is appropriate for that particular patient.[57,58] However, the novice injector needs a point of reference; a standard of injection patterns to guide him or her during their initial treatment sessions. As the neophyte injector acquires a better understanding of the functional anatomy and its responses to different patterns of injections with OnaBTX-A, then a more directed and personalized approach to OnaBTX-A injections will automatically develop. The physician injector should also not forget to identify, photograph, and indicate to the patient prior to all OnaBTX-A injections any variation in the anatomy that might be present and cause the patient's eyebrows to be asymmetric. It appears that as much as 45%–65% of the general female and male population has some form of brow asymmetry prior to ever being treated with a BoNT (author's personal observation). The patient's permanent clinical record should contain photographic documentation along with a written summary of the physician's clinical assessment and conversation with the patient addressing any idiosyncrasies and asymmetries the patient may possess. It is absolutely necessary to include in the record, the patient's response to the conversation, including acknowledgment of any particular anatomical differences, in addition to a written and signed consent for treatment before initiating treatment with any BoNT.

The pretreatment position and symmetry or asymmetry of the eyebrows and eyelids will dictate the technique with which one will need to treat the glabellar frown lines (Figure 13.16). In women whose eyebrows

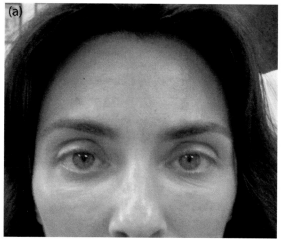
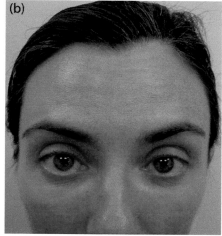

Figure 13.16 Woman with eyebrows barely arched (a) before strategically placed injections of OnaBTX-A were placed into the brow depressors. Same patient (b) after treatment with eyebrows more highly arched.

are barely arched, strategically placed injections of OnaBTX-A into the brow depressors can elevate the eyebrows by allowing the untreated lower fibers of the frontalis to raise the eyebrows unopposed by the weakened interdigitating fibers of the corrugator supercilii, procerus, orbicularis oculi, and depressor supercilii (Figures 13.17 and 13.18).

To treat the glabellar frown lines with optimal, reproducible results and the least amount of complications, precise injections of relatively concentrated doses and low volumes of OnaBTX-A must be used on both sides of the midline whether the doses are equal. With the patient sitting up or in the semireclined position, gently palpate the medial aspect of the eyebrows as the patient squints and frowns. After locating the belly of the corrugator supercilii with the second and third fingertip pads of the nondominant hand, ask the patient to raise the eyebrows as high as possible, while keeping the tip of the index finger positioned over the thickest part of the belly of the corrugator supercilii (Figure 13.17). Prior to inserting the needle, the index finger of the nondominant hand should be advanced slightly cephalad and above the point of maximal muscle thickness. This usually is just above the eyebrow. The thumb is placed at the margin of the supraorbital bony

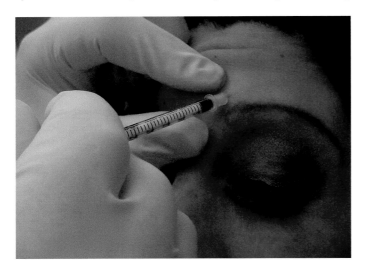

Figure 13.17 Technique of injecting the medial corrugator supercilii (note the position of the thumb and index finger of the nondominant hand).

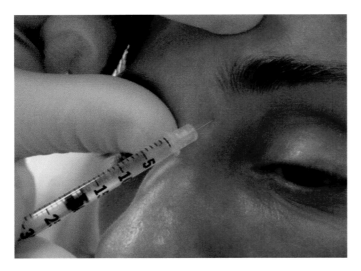

Figure 13.18 Technique of injecting the medial aspect of the orbicularis oculi and depressor supercilii starting at the most infero-medial aspect of the superciliary arch. Note the 60° angle and superficial placement of the needle, approximately 2 cm directly above the ocular caruncle.

rim. The bore of the needle tip should be pointed upward and away from the globe. The needle is inserted into the skin at a 60°–90° angle and allowed to glide over the upper edge of the thumb between it and the index finger. The needle is slowly advanced into the belly of the corrugator supercilii in an oblique direction, slightly upward and lateral, until penetration into the belly of the corrugator can be felt. Entry into a muscle usually is detected when, after passing through the dermis and subcutaneous tissue, an abrupt release of resistance is felt as the needle penetrates fascia and muscle fibers. At this point, the needle may or may not impinge on the bone. If it strikes a bone, the patient will sense sharp pain. The needle should then be withdrawn gently enough to move away from the bone, but not far enough to exit the belly of the corrugator. The needle should always remain deep within the muscle, medial to the supraorbital notch and approximately 2–2.5 cm superior to the supraorbital bony margin during injections of the BoNT. The physician injector must refrain from striking the frontal bone with the needle tip, so as not to inflict any additional pain to the patient, which occurs when the periosteum is pierced. However, this may not be avoidable when first learning how to find the deeply seated corrugators and effectively inject them at the proper depth.

Placing the nondominant index finger and thumb on the brow just above and below the eyebrow prior to injecting OnaBTX-A serves many purposes. It prevents injecting OnaBTX-A too low and close to the orbital rim. When direct pressure is applied with the thumb inferior to the border of the supraorbital bony rim, Binder et al. felt they could reduce the migration of OnaBTX-A behind the orbital septum and avoid blepharoptosis.[59] This maneuver also helps identify the location and position of the corrugator supercilii because the muscle can be felt between the index finger and thumb with light palpation. *Slow, deliberate,* and *gentle* injections prevent OnaBTX-A from dispersing into surrounding, nontargeted muscle fibers. While in position, inject 4–10 U of OnaBTX-A into the strongest portion of the muscle, which is located approximately 10–15 mm superior and 15–20 mm lateral to the nasion or the center of the concavity at the nasal radix.[31–35,57–59]

Next, watch as the patient frowns again, and notice to what extent the midbrow adducts toward the glabella. Stronger corrugators will visibly pull the skin medially toward the midline just above the eyebrows in the vicinity of the mid-pupillary line. In some patients, additional vertical corrugations along the brow parallel to the central vertical glabellar lines also will be formed (see Trindade de Almeida's glabellar "converging lines" in Figures 13.24 through 13.27). These corrugations can be reduced by injecting 2–4 U of OnaBTX-A *intradermally* into the skin just above the middle of the eyebrow where the corrugators insert into the undersurface of the midbrow, which is just medial to the supraorbital notch or midpupillary line. This point is identified by an obvious dimpling (corrugator dimple) of the skin as the patient forcibly frowns (Figure 13.8b). These more lateral injections over the midbrow should be applied first by asking the patient to raise their eyebrows and then physically raising the center of the eyebrow with the thumb of the nondominant hand. Then approach the skin at a 45°–60° angle and injecting *superficially*, confirmed by raising a wheal. The fibers of the corrugators in this location are superficial and insert into the under surface of the skin. These injections should reduce the adduction of the brow and eliminate brow corrugations adjacent to glabellar frown lines and along the central brow (see Figures 13.25, 13.26a and b). If the injections are too deep, then fibers of the frontalis also will be affected and brow ptosis can result. If the injections are too low and close to the bony orbital rim, blepharoptosis will result.

Next withdraw the needle out of the skin and redirect the tip of the needle medially in the direction of the head of the eyebrow. Insert the needle 60°–90° to the skin surface at, or adjacent to the most medial aspect of the superciliary arch and eyebrow, approximately 2 cm directly superior to the ocular caruncle at the inner canthus (Figure 13.18). Injections should be given superficially, and confirmed by raising a wheal. Approximately 2–6 U of OnaBTX-A at this point of maximum muscle contraction will treat the vertical muscle fibers of the medial orbital orbicularis oculi and the depressor supercilii. Because the fibers of the orbicularis oculi and depressor supercilii are closely adherent to the overlying skin at this location, injections can be given either intradermally or in the superficial subcutaneous plane. Superficial injections at this location also avoid puncturing the supratrochlear vessels and nerve. A pleasing vertically upward lift to the medial brow can be accomplished by this technique, if fibers of the frontalis are not inadvertently affected.[60,61] Gentle massage in an upward and lateral direction for a few seconds immediately after the injection helps relieve the typical acute pain of a transcutaneous injection. Heavy-handed massage will definitely disperse the OnaBTX-A beyond the target area and into muscle fibers not intended for treatment, that is, into the fibers of the lower frontalis, which can result in brow ptosis.

Next, treat the procerus with an injection of approximately 4–10 U of OnaBTX-A given between the eyebrows at the nasal root into the belly of the procerus (Figure 13.19). Some spread of the onaBTX-A into the interdigitating fibers of the depressor supercilii and medial fibers of the orbital orbicularis oculi often occurs, potentiating the weakening effect on all three muscles. The dose needed for this injection of OnaBTX-A will depend on the overall muscle strength and depth of the horizontal glabellar wrinkles that are present. The strength of the procerus can be determined by gently palpating the mid-glabellar area with the pads of the second and third fingertips of the nondominant hand, while the patient repeatedly squints and frowns. Glabellar wrinkles can be deeply fixed in the skin, especially the horizontal ones. Those that are more resistant to treatment with OnaBTX-A commonly are found in men and women who spend a lot of time outdoors or in front of a computer screen, because their glabellar muscles are significantly hypertrophied from frequent squinting. Intramuscular instead of subcutaneous injections of OnaBTX-A into the procerus should be performed by gently grasping the skin and soft tissue of the root of the nose between the thumb and the index finger of the nondominant hand. Then elevate the skin and muscle before placing the needle between the two fingers and injecting OnaBTX-A into one or two sites in the center of the nasal radix. This maneuver also will avoid the needle puncturing the nasal bone and causing additional unwarranted pain on the patient. The site of injection should be anywhere from 1 to 3 mm above or below

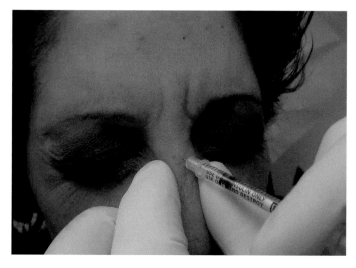

Figure 13.19 Technique of injecting the procerus (note the position of the index finger and the thumb of the nondominant hand).

the center of the nasion. The weaker muscle fibers of the procerus are injected with at least 2 U of OnaBTX-A, while the stronger ones usually can be injected with up to 10 U and possibly even more in one, two, or more injection points. The depressor supercilii already will have been partially treated by the injections given at the medial aspect of the superciliary arch and eyebrows when the medial orbital orbicularis oculi and the depressor supercilii are treated. Likewise, gentle massage performed in and around the nasal radix immediately after injecting the procerus also will result in some spread of the OnaBTX-A into the interdigitating fibers of the depressor supercilii and medial orbital orbicularis oculi.

Some patterns of glabellar frowning are seen more frequently than others.[27] The most common pattern observed by Trindade de Almeida and colleagues were those produced by the simultaneous adduction and depression of the skin of the glabella (64%). This occurs when the corrugators contract and parallel vertical lines are formed in the center of the glabella as the skin of the brow moves toward the midline. At the same time, the procerus pulls the skin of the brow inferiorly, forming horizontal lines across the root of the nose. There are two distinct variations of this most commonly seen pattern of glabellar frowning. The less frequently observed pattern (27%) of the two is what Trindade de Almeida et al. call the "U" pattern (Figure 13.20).[27] In these patients, the 5-point injection technique is corrective with 4–10 U of OnaBTX-A given at each injection point.[27] Stronger, more hyperkinetic corrugators and procerus produce a similar pattern of glabellar frown lines but they are deeper and more acute, resulting in a pattern that better resembles a "V." This was seen in 37% of the patients studied (Figure 13.21). Higher doses of OnaBTX-A in the 7-point injection pattern are usually necessary to diminish these lines.[27]

Another, less frequently observed pattern, named the omega pattern, was seen in only (10%) of patients. When these individuals frown, their eyebrows initially adduct centrally and glabellar skin drops slightly forming deep parallel vertical lines. Then with continued forceful frowning the upper part of the center of the glabella will slide upward toward the frontal hairline, forming deep horizontal furrows and folds. The medial end of the brows continues to move inferiorly producing slight horizontal lines along the lateral sides of the nasal radix to create an overall wrinkle pattern that outlines the Greek letter omega (Ω) (Figure 13.22).[27] In these individuals the corrugators and fibers of the medial brow depressors seem to contract in unison with the muscle fibers of the lower to mid central frontalis. Injections of 4–8 U or more of OnaBTX-A at multiple sites into the corrugators and medial brow depressors, while 2–6 U of OnaBTX-A into the procerus and 2–6 U into the lower medial frontalis in divided doses at multiple sites will diminish the omega pattern of glabellar frowning.[27]

The "inverted omega" pattern was the least encountered (6%) of all the five patterns identified by the Trindade de Almeida group and was attributed to individuals with a flat nasal radix, which is commonly found in the Asian population (Figure 13.23).[27] When these individuals frown the center of their glabella drops inferiorly along with their eyebrows, creating deep horizontal wrinkle lines across the nasal radix but minimal to no vertical glabellar lines.[27,62] In such individuals, treat the procerus with 6–10 U of OnaBTX-A and the depressor supercilii and medial orbital orbicularis oculi with 4–8 U of OnaBTX-A and the corrugators with 4–8 U of OnaBTX-A.

Another less commonly seen glabellar frown pattern (20%) is the one where there is just adduction of the mid-to-lateral brow toward the center of the glabella. There is minimal vertical movement of the glabella either inferiorly or superiorly because there seems to be a neutralizing balance of movements between the procerus and the frontalis that produces barely perceptible or no horizontal glabellar frown lines in this "converging arrows" (or "parallel lines," the author's preferred term) pattern (Figure 13.24).[27] In these individuals, the extent and depth of the lateral-to-medial brow corrugations are dependent on the

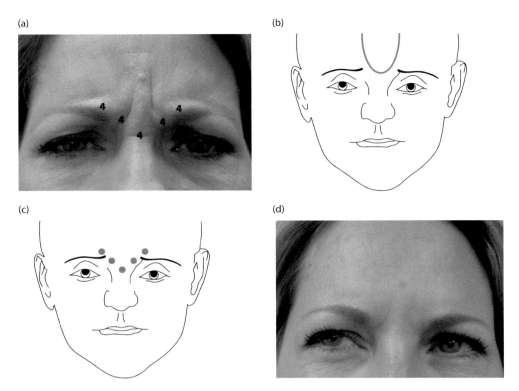

Figure 13.20 (a) Mild to moderate approximation and depression of the medial brow forming the typical and one of the most commonly seen patterns of glabellar frown lines (the "U" pattern). (b) Commonly seen "U" type of glabellar contraction and resulting pattern of frown lines. Muscles involved: predominantly the corrugators and procerus (see Reference 26). (c) Five-point pattern of injection for this commonly encountered glabellar "U" pattern (see Reference 26). (d) Same patient frowning 2 weeks after an OnaBTX-A treatment.

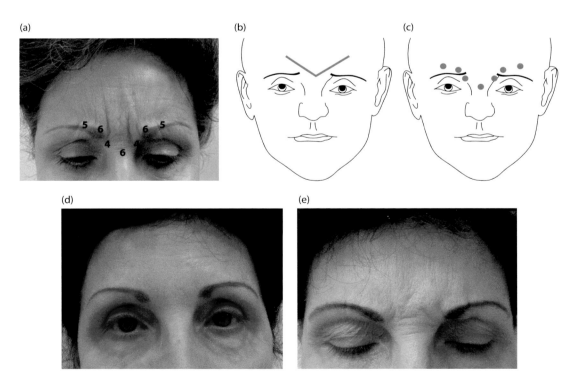

Figure 13.21 (a) Moderate to severe approximation and depression of the medial brow forming the more commonly seen pattern variation identified by very deep glabellar frown lines (the "V" pattern) in a 62-year-old woman. (b) Vigorous glabellar contraction and resulting "V" pattern of frown lines. Muscles involved: strong corrugators, procerus, and medial aspect of the orbicularis oculi (see Reference 26). (c) Seven-point pattern of injection for this exaggerated glabellar "V" pattern. Higher doses of OnaBTX-A are usually needed for treatment (see Reference 26). (d) Same patient at rest and (e) frowning 2 weeks after an OnaBTX-A treatment.

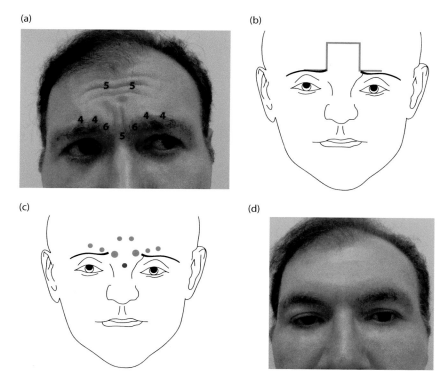

Figure 13.22 (a) Adduction of the medial eyebrows and elevation of the center of the glabella along with depression of the mid and lateral brow forms the "omega" pattern of glabellar frowning. (b) This type of glabellar contraction results in the "omega" pattern of frown lines. Muscles involved: corrugators and lower central frontalis (see Reference 26). (c) This eight-point pattern of injection is used for the glabellar "omega" pattern. Higher doses of OnaBTX-A are needed for the corrugators and lower central frontalis and usually none for the procerus (blue, author's modification). (d) Same patient frowning 2 weeks after an OnaBTX-A treatment. ([c] From Trindade de Almeida AR et al. *Dermatol Surg* 2012; 38(9): 1506–15.)

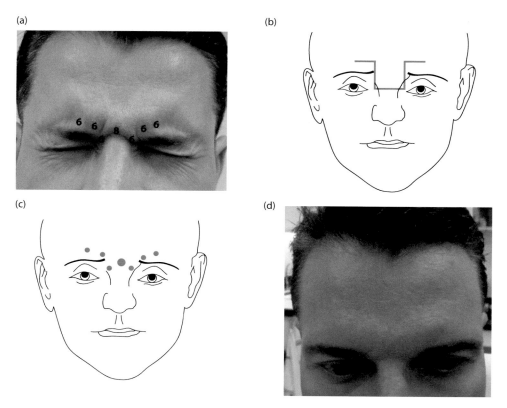

Figure 13.23 (a) More depression than adduction of the medial brow forms the "inverted omega" pattern of glabellar frowning. Note the deep horizontal line at the root of the nose. (b) Less frequently seen type of glabellar adduction producing an "inverted omega" pattern of frown lines. Muscles involved: mostly the procerus and depressor supercilii (see Reference 26). (c) A different seven-point pattern of injection for this uncommon glabellar "inverted omega" pattern. Higher doses of OnaBTX-A are needed for the procerus (see Reference 26). (d) Same patient frowning 2 weeks after an OnaBTX-A treatment.

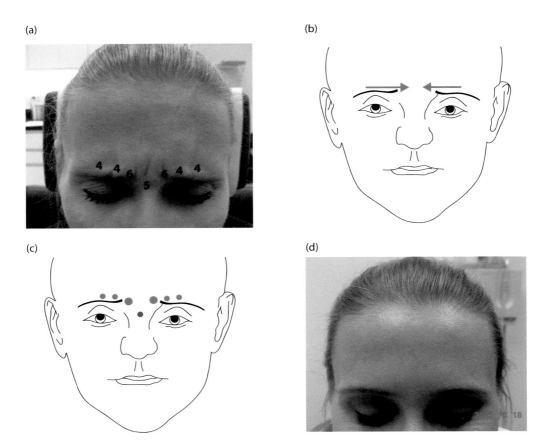

Figure 13.24 (a) Adduction and approximation mainly of the eyebrows form this "converging arrows" pattern of glabellar "corrugated" frowning. There is little to no depression or elevation of the medial brow. (b) This is an uncommon type of glabellar contraction resulting in a "converging arrows" or "parallel lines" (author) pattern of frown lines. Muscles involved: mainly the corrugators and the upper mid horizontal *orbital* orbicularis oculi. (see Reference 26). (c) This six-point pattern of OnaBTX-A injections targets mainly the corrugators and the mid-section of the upper orbital orbicularis oculi (blue, author's modification). (d) Same patient frowning 3 weeks after an OnaBTX-A treatment. ([c] From Trindade de Almeida AR et al. *Dermatol Surg* 2012; 38(9): 1506–15.)

person's age and the amount of skin laxity present. Increased skin laxity promotes an increased number of vertical corrugations along the medial brow. Injections of a higher than usual dose (6–10 U or more) of OnaBTX-A into the belly of the corrugator supercilii, along its body and into the tail, will nicely relax the excess wrinkling across the brow (Figures 13.25 and 13.26). The medial horizontal muscle fibers of the upper orbital orbicularis oculi also may play a role in the brow corrugations, which would then require one or more *intradermal* injections of 2–6 U of OnaBTX-A, approximately 2–3 cm above the supraorbital bony rim at the midpupillary line and medially along the superciliary arch if corrugations persist after treatment. The procerus also can be treated with 4–10 or even more U of OnaBTX-A when indicated (author's preferred technique) (see Figures 13.22 and 13.24).[27]

Outcomes (Results) When Treating the Central Brow (Glabella) (See Appendix 4)

A clear and accurate record of all the units and where they were injected must be maintained of each treatment session on all patients. Meticulously detailed clinical records facilitate reproducible results. Consequently, when proper injection techniques are followed, results are predictable and reproducible. The vertical lines between the eyebrows and the horizontal ones across the root of the nose will diminish and eventually disappear. Glabellar and midbrow corrugations if treated appropriately also will be reduced and temporarily eliminated.

There can be a noticeably high arching of the eyebrows of approximately 2–3 mm, caused by the levator action of the frontalis in those patients whose glabellar depressors have been substantially

weakened, when the interdigitating muscle fibers of the frontalis immediately above the brow have not (Figure 13.27).[60–64] There also can be an increase in the horizontal distance between the eyebrows along with an elevation of the medial aspect of the eyebrows when glabellar frown

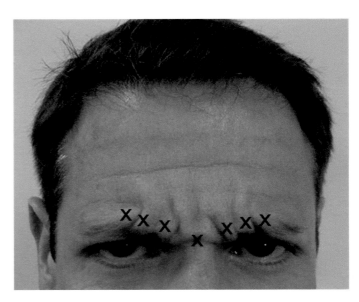

Figure 13.25 Converging arrows or parallel lines pattern of glabellar wrinkling before treatment in a 48-year-old male. Note the strong procerus contraction producing the deep horizontal line across the nasal radix.

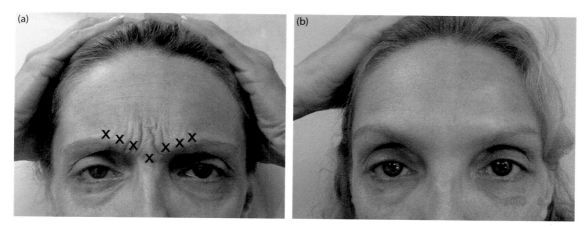

Figure 13.26 (a) Converging arrows or parallel lines pattern of glabellar wrinkling before treatment in a 61-year-old female. Note the absence of procerus contraction and horizontal line across the nasal radix. (b) Same patient 2 weeks after treatment with OnaBTX-A.

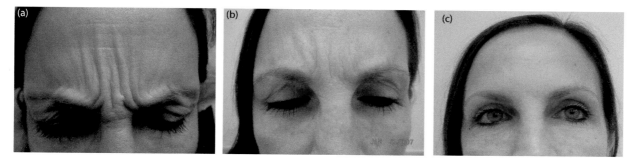

Figure 13.27 Arching of the eyebrows while frowning (a) before and (b) after OnaBTX-A treatment in a 52-year-old woman with a converging arrows pattern of glabellar wrinkling. (c) Same patient at rest. Note the nicely arched eyebrows.

lines are treated with OnaBTX-A because of the dynamic relationship between the brow depressors (corrugator supercilii, depressor supercilii, orbicularis oculi, and procerus) and their brow elevator (frontalis), (Figure 13.28).[60,62] Accentuated high arching eyebrows may be attractive in most women, but usually not in men. To avoid a high arching brow in men, an additional 2–6 U of OnaBTX-A can be injected intradermally or intramuscularly into the frontalis 2.5–4.0 cm above the supraorbital ridge at the midpupillary line. This maneuver should straighten a high arching eyebrow without provoking a low-lying brow ptosis, (see section on "horizontal forehead lines").

Usually, one can expect the effect of an OnaBTX-A treatment of glabellar frown lines to last at least 3–4 months. Patients who are treated for the very first time with OnaBTX-A may experience some asymmetry and therefore should return for an evaluation and possible touch-up injections within 2–3 weeks after a treatment. Frequently, the effects of OnaBTX-A may last longer with each subsequent treatment session. Therefore, after the first 2–3 years of regularly scheduled treatment sessions every 3–4 months, some patients may prefer to return for their next retreatment at 5- or 6-month intervals (see Appendix 3).

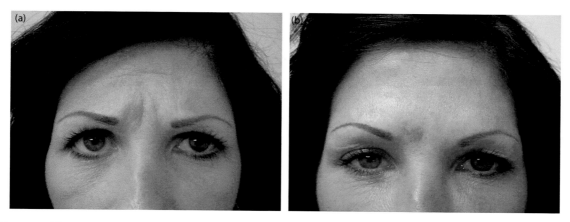

Figure 13.28 This 37-year-old patient had both the glabella and the forehead frown lines treated during the same session. (a) Frowning before OnaBTX-A treatment. (b) Same patient frowning 2 weeks after treatment. Note the increase in interbrow distance after treatment and elevation of the medial brow.

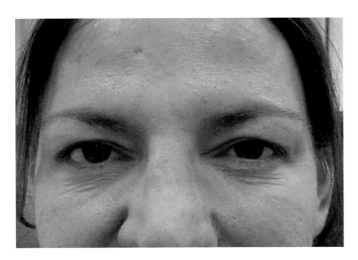

Figure 13.29 Eyelid ptosis in a 49-year-old patient. Note a drop of 1–2 mm of the left upper eyelid that occurred approximately 10 days after an OnaBTX-A treatment.

Complications (Adverse Sequelae) When Treating the Central Brow (Glabella) (See Appendix 6)

Ptosis of the upper eyelid is one of the most significant and frequently occurring complications seen when injecting OnaBTX-A in and around the glabella (Figure 13.29).[8,54,64] It is felt by many that blepharoptosis is caused by the migration of injected OnaBTX-A through the orbital septum, weakening the levator palpebrae superioris (Figures 13.10 and 13.30). This can occur more frequently in older patients in whom the barrier function of the orbital septum is attenuated, or when large volumes of highly diluted OnaBTX-A are injected quickly, deeply, low down and close to the bony supraorbital margin at the midpupillary line. Occasionally at this location, some actual muscle fibers of the levator palpebrae superioris can extend anteriorly into the levator aponeurosis, allowing for easy access of the OnaBTX-A that has diffused through the barrier of the orbital septum to weaken some of the muscle fibers of the levator palpebrae superioris, and produce ptosis of the upper eyelid (Figure 13.10). Unexpected blepharoptosis in a younger patient is usually the result of forceful injections of OnaBTX-A placed too deeply in the area of the midbrow, particularly with high volumes of highly diluted OnaBTX-A. Another reason for inadvertent blepharoptosis is when OnaBTX-A is routinely injected at a fixed distance of 2 cm from the upper border of the *eyebrows* instead of 2 cm from the bony superciliary arch or ridge. In most men and some women, their eyebrows are situated low on the brow and directly over the bony orbital rim (see brow positions below). Injecting OnaBTX-A just above the eyebrows in these individuals puts their levator aponeurosis at risk of contact with the BoNT as the aponeurosis exits the superior margin of the bony orbit (Figure 13.10). OnaBTX-A then can easily weaken any exposed levator muscle fibers contiguous with the aponeurosis, reducing the levator action of the upper eyelid and causing blepharoptosis.

Ramey and Woodward demonstrated by their cadaveric study using injectable blue methylene dye that deep and forceful injections of OnaBTX-A in the vicinity of the supraorbital foramen potentially could allow the toxin to penetrate into the superior aspect of the bony orbit, presumably through the foramen, and affect the levator palpebrae superioris.[65] After injecting 1% methylene blue deep into the corrugator supercilii just above the supraorbital foramen, they found, by an anterior dissection approach, the anterior orbital septum and anterior surface of the levator aponeurosis stained blue. They also found by a posterior dissection approach the intraorbital surface of the periosteum and the periorbita stained with the blue dye. There also was blue dye staining the superior surface of the levator palpebrae superioris

and adjacent tissues, including the superior ophthalmic vein and some of its tributaries. From this study, they hypothesized two mechanisms of blepharoptosis. First, BoNT may reach the levator palpebrae superioris as it traverses the pre-periosteal plane anteriorly after a forceful injection. Second, BoNT may track along tributaries of the superior ophthalmic vein, which travels along the levator palpebrae superioris for part of its course. Consequently, blepharoptosis may be avoided by carefully positioning the injection needle far away from the supraorbital foramen and using a gentle, slow injection technique with highly concentrated, low volume BoNT. Deep injections, particularly those overlying the bulk of the supraorbital nerve or near branches of the superior ophthalmic vein, should be avoided to prevent perineural or perivascular infiltration around the levator palpebrae superioris.[65,66]

To avoid injecting OnaBTX-A too close to the bony orbital rim, one should inject superficially and at a point at least 3–4 cm superior to the bony orbital rim or 2–3 cm superior to the superciliary ridge or arch. Any injection less than 3 cm away from the bony orbital rim, regardless of where the eyebrow sits over the superciliary ridge, will allow OnaBTX-A to reach the levator aponeurosis directly or indirectly and weaken its proximal muscle fibers and cause blepharoptosis.

In female patients, the eyebrows commonly sit approximately 5 cm above the upper eyelid crease. On the other hand, men's eyebrows usually grow directly over or below the superciliary ridge. There are some women, however, whose eyebrows rest just as low as men's, that is, at or below the superciliary ridge. Instead of using the eyebrows as a point of reference from where to inject, the upper orbital bony margin or rim should be the reference point. Therefore, injections should be placed no lower than 3–4 cm above the upper margin of the bony orbit.

Blepharoptosis, when it occurs, is seen as a 1–2 mm or more drop in the upper eyelid, obscuring the upper border of the iris (Figure 13.30).[64] Ptosis can appear as early as 48 hours and up to 7–10 days after an OnaBTX-A injection and usually can last 2–4 weeks or even longer. The margin to reflex distance (MRD) is a way to measure and diagnose upper lid blepharoptosis. MRD is defined as the distance from the mid-pupil corneal light reflex to the lower cutaneous margin of the upper eyelid with the eyes in forward primary gaze. A normal MRD should equal approximately 4 mm in vertical height. Blepharoptosis is present when an MRD is measured less than 2 mm. Moreover, an asymmetrical comparative height of more than 1-2 mm between both eyes indicates a certain degree of unilateral compensatory brow elevation[67] (Figure 13.31b).

An antidote for blepharoptosis is apraclonidine 0.5% eye drops (Iopidine®, Alcon Laboratories, Inc., Fort Worth, TX). The ocular instillation of apraclonidine, an alpha-2-adrenergic agonist with mild alpha-1 activity, causes Müller's muscle (a nonstriated, smooth, sympathomimetic levator muscle of the upper eyelid) to contract, temporarily raising the upper eyelid approximately 1–2 mm (Figures 13.10 and 13.30). One or two drops should be instilled into the affected eye. If ptosis persists after 15–20 minutes, intraocular instillation of an additional one or two drops may be required before the affected eyelid will elevate. This procedure can be repeated three to four times a day. It is advisable to use apraclonidine eye drops only when absolutely necessary because approximately 20% of patients can develop a contact conjunctivitis with frequent use. The mydriatic and vasoconstrictor phenylephrine (Mydfrin 2.5%, Alcon Laboratories, Inc., Fort Worth, TX, or Neo-Synephrine® HCl, 2.5% Ophthalmic Solution, USP, Paragon BioTeck, distributed by Bausch & Lomb [a division of Valeant, Laval, Quebec, Canada] also known by other brand names: AK-Dilate, AK-Nefrin, Isopto Frin, Neofrin) is an alpha-1 agonist that also can be used when apraclonidine is not available.[41] However, there are more potential side effects associated with the use of phenylephrine than with apraclonidine. Specifically, even when only the 2.5% ophthalmic solution is used, phenylephrine can increase intraocular pressure, cause systemic allergic and urticarial reactions,

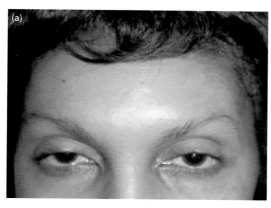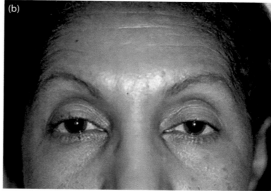

Figure 13.30 (a) Eyelid ptosis in a 67-year-old patient. Note a drop of 1–2 mm of the right upper eyelid that occurred approximately 7 days after OnaBTX-A was used to treat forehead and glabellar wrinkles. Patient is actively blinking. (b) Same patient 30 minutes after the instillation of 2 drops of apraclonidine into the right eye.

local contact and irritant dermatitis and acutely exacerbate narrow angle glaucoma, cardiac arrhythmias, and hypertension. Because it also is a mydriatic, even one drop of phenylephrine will prevent the patient from accommodating as usual and visual acuity can be compromised. Naphazoline (Naphcon-A®, Alcon Laboratories, Inc., Fort Worth, TX) is another ophthalmic decongestant containing adrenergic properties that can be used to stimulate Müller's muscle to contract, temporarily lifting a ptotic upper eyelid.[64] The different brands of naphazoline (e.g., Vasocon-A®, [naphazoline HCl 0.05%, antazoline phosphate 0.5%,], Novartis Ophthalmics, East Hanover, NJ) also contain different antihistaminic additives, and because of their multiple side effects profile, should be used infrequently and with caution, strictly on an as-needed basis when utilizing them just to elevate blepharoptosis. When a patient cannot tolerate any of the topical anti-blepharoptosis medications, then additional injections of OnaBTX-A into the palpebral orbicularis oculi, can be attempted to reduce the remaining strength of the upper eyelid depressor (Figure 13.31a).[64] For the expert, well-seasoned injector, subdermal injections of low-dose, low-volume OnaBTX-A into the pretarsal orbicularis oculi, the antagonist to the upper lid levator (levator palpebrae superioris) can be performed. Similar injections are used to treat various blepharospastic disorders. Depending on the severity of the blepharoptosis, inject 0.5 unit and no more than 1.5 units of OnaBTX-A subdermally into the extreme medial and lateral aspects of the pretarsal orbicularis oculi just above the lid/lash margin, so as to avoid any further exposure of the centrally located muscle fibers of the levator palpebrae superioris with additional onaBTX-A. (Figure 13.31a).[64] An obvious wheal should be produced with these injections.

Blepharoptosis also can be induced secondarily when the lower fibers of the frontalis are weakened, producing a drop in the height of the brow. The weight of the ptotic brow then impinges on the upper eyelid and causes it to drop, narrowing the vertical palpebral aperture or fissure. This secondary blepharoptosis seems to occur more frequently in older patients who possess dermatochalasis of the skin of the eyelids and brow. To compensate for a heavy, lax brow, some individuals, regardless of age, involuntarily use the lower fibers of their frontalis to lift the soft tissue of the brow, which also maintains their upper eyelids in a constantly raised position.[64] When this compensatory brow lifting of the frontalis is weakened by BoNT, a secondary blepharoptosis results.

Careful examination of the upper eyelids for the presence of a separation or weakness of the levator palpebrae superioris can be a preinjection method to identify individuals at risk for true blepharoptosis and to avoid its occurrence after a treatment with any BoNT. The functional strength of the levator palpebrae superioris is determined by measuring the distance of the excursion of the upper eyelid margin from far downward gaze to upward gaze while the frontalis muscle is held still with

the injector's hand. A normal excursion is approximately 14 mm or more.[68] When the excursion is less than 14 mm, some degree of blepharoptosis after any BoNT treatment of the glabella mostly likely will occur (Figure 13.31c). Another way to predict the risk for unmasking and intensifying the potential for blepharoptosis is to identify someone with lash ptosis (LP). Individuals with either congenital or acquired blepharoptosis can manifest LP, which is a generalized declination or downward pointing of the eyelash follicles of their upper eyelids. The presence of LP suggests laxity of the terminal fibers of the levator aponeurosis which weave through orbicularis oculi to insert into the subcutaneous tissue and skin of the upper eyelid[69] (Figure 13.31d).

In younger patients with taut skin and no compensatory brow lifting, brow ptosis often can occur medially when there is an overzealous injection of a BoNT in the center of the forehead. Medial brow ptosis is exhibited by the medial head of the eyebrows appearing excessively lower than the lateral tail of the eyebrows. A bulge of skin in the center of the glabella also can accompany this "medial brow dip" of the eyebrows. This occurs because the lower central fibers of the frontalis are overly weakened and there is some activity of the fibers of the medial brow depressors, that is, the procerus, depressor supercilii, and medial orbital orbicularis oculi, pulling down on the center of the forehead and glabella (Figure 13.32).

Lagophthalmos or incomplete eyelid closure is another potential complication that can occur particularly when overzealous injections of a BoNT are given in the periorbital area. Lagophthalmos results when there is a loss of the normal sphincteric function of the orbicularis oculi, and the upper eyelid does not close and approximate firmly against the lower eyelid. Loss of the sphincteric function of the orbicularis oculi either with involuntary blinking or with deliberate forced eyelid closure can occur when BoNT diffuses into the *palpebral* portion of the orbicularis oculi, causing undue eyelid weakness. Lagophthalmos is seen more frequently in patients treated for strabismus when extraocular muscles are injected with higher doses of OnaBTX-A instead of the usual lower doses given for cosmetic purposes in the periocular area. On the other hand, patients who have an attenuated orbital septum because of age or other reasons may be more prone to this adverse sequela. If incomplete eyelid approximation is present for extended periods of time, exposure of the cornea can result in symptomatic dry eyes or exposure keratitis.[70] There is no antidote for lagophthalmos which can persist as long as the effects of the OnaBTX-A are present. So, protecting the patient from developing secondary dry eyes is extremely important because excessive corneal exposure will lead to desiccation of the cornea and superficial punctate keratitis. Immediate consultation with an ophthalmologist at the first sign of lagophthalmos will prevent any additional injury to the eye.

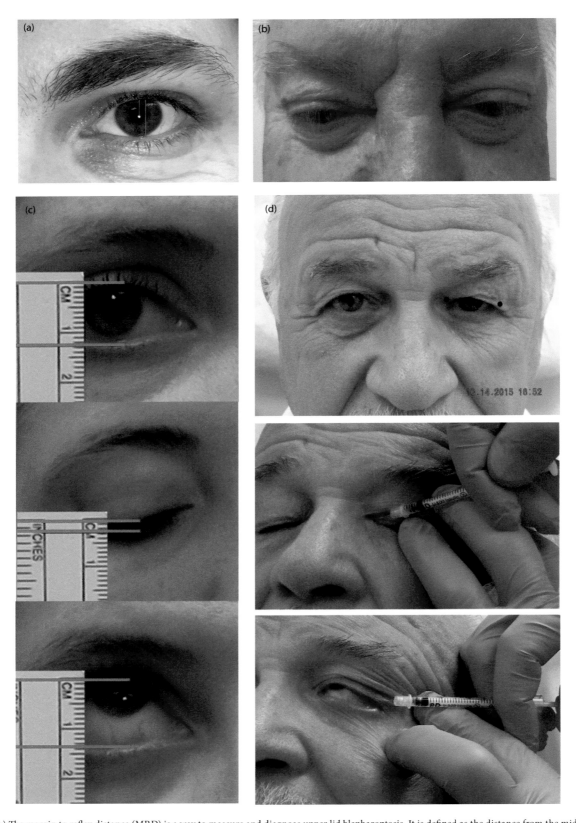

Figure 13.31 (a) The margin to reflex distance (MRD) is a way to measure and diagnose upper lid blepharoptosis. It is defined as the distance from the mid-pupil corneal light reflex to the lower cutaneous margin of the upper eyelid with the eyes in forward primary gaze. A normal MRD, shown here in red, should equal approximately 4 mm in vertical height. The palpebral fissure, shown here in green, is the distance between the upper and lower lid margins and normally measures between 7 and 12 mm. (b) A 69 year old male with lash ptosis and acquired blepharoptosis. Note the generalized declination or downward pointing of the upper eyelashes. (c) The functional strength of the levator palpebrae superioris is determined by measuring the distance of the excursion of the upper eyelid margin from far downward gaze to upward gaze while the frontalis muscle is held still with the injector's hand. A normal excursion is approximately 14 mm or more. When the excursion is less than 14 mm, some degree of blepharoptosis after any BoNT treatment of the glabella mostly likely will occur. (d) To treat mild upper lid blepharoptosis OnaBTX-A is injected into the (far) medial and lateral *pretarsal* orbicularis muscle fibers in the subdermal plane. (See further Reference 64.)

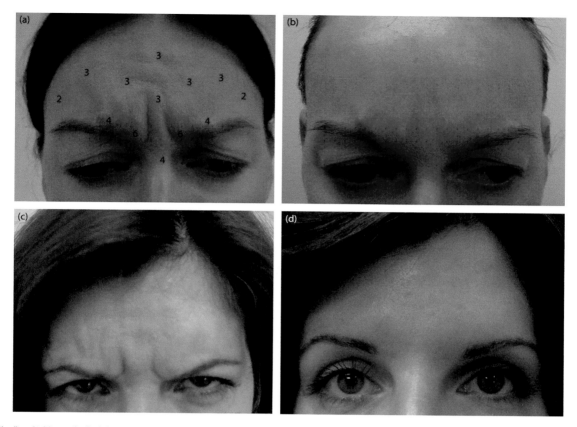

Figure 13.32 The "medial brow dip" of the central glabella and eyebrows of this 40-year-old occurred after OnaBTX-A injections because the lower central frontalis was overly treated. Patient is frowning (a) before and (b) after OnaBTX-A. Note the fullness of the medial brow skin after treatment. (c and d) The "medial brow dip" of the central glabella of this other 45-year-old patient was avoided after OnaBTX-A injections because the central frontalis was not treated.

Asymmetry is a minor adverse sequela that sometimes is unavoidable, particularly when a patient is treated for the first time with a BoNT (Figure 13.33). There are three types of asymmetry that can be corrected with injections of OnaBTX-A: iatrogenic, idiosyncratic, and incidental or acquired. An example of incidental or acquired asymmetry is Bell's or facial (7th cranial) nerve palsy. Additional examples are when one side of the face acquires a weakness because of an event (e.g., cerebral vascular accident), or an accidental, traumatic, or surgical denervation injury. Idiosyncratic asymmetry occurs when a person is born with the inability to control or move a facial muscle to its fullest extent, while its counterpart muscle on the contralateral side of the face is unaffected. This can result, for example, in one eyebrow or one eyelid being higher than the other (Figures 13.34 and 13.35) or in a crooked asymmetric smile (see Chapter 15).

Iatrogenic asymmetry arises when an injection of OnaBTX-A causes one side of the face to become weaker than the other (see Figure 13.34 and 13.39a). There are many reasons for this. The primary reason is because the stronger side is not injected with an equivalent dose of OnaBTX-A as the contralateral side. This could be the result of the OnaBTX-A not diffusing as equally and completely through all the fibers of a muscle or group of muscles. Another reason could be that some of the fibers might have been physically resistant to the OnaBTX-A, because those particular fibers were idiosyncratically thicker or stronger than the rest of the area and may have required a higher dose of OnaBTX-A. Another possibility is that the injections were not given precisely symmetrically or in the thickest and strongest part of the muscle, causing a particular section of muscle to retain most or some of its strength. Iatrogenic asymmetry is probably the easiest type of asymmetry to rectify. Generally, with a few additional units

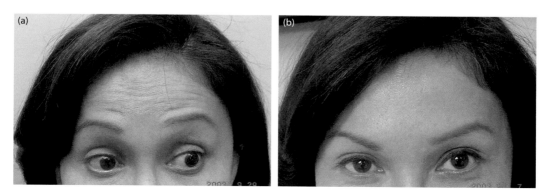

Figure 13.33 (a) Note the left eyebrow is higher than the right before and after treatment with OnaBTX-A. (b) Note the medial brow dip after treatment.

of OnaBTX-A injected into the appropriate area, iatrogenic asymmetry can be expeditiously ameliorated (Figure 13.39b).

Another type of asymmetry is pseudoblepharoptosis. Many individuals regardless of age possess, unbeknownst to them, an idiosyncratic lower lying asymmetric brow on one side. They commonly will also possess a lower lying upper eyelid on the same side and a smaller vertical palpebral aperture causing a narrower eyelid fissure (i.e., a secondary blepharoptosis, see Figure 13.35). With age, compensatory brow lifting will raise the affected lower lying brow and upper eyelid to maintain unobstructed vision (Figure 13.36a).

When the frontalis of these patients is treated with injections of OnaBTX-A, the patient's compensatory brow lifting can be unintentionally weakened. This inadvertent diminution of compensatory brow lifting can occur even when only the higher upper fibers of the frontalis are weakened with injections of OnaBTX-A. The lower fibers of the frontalis do not necessarily have to be treated directly with injections of OnaBTX-A to drop the brow a few millimeters. With a drop in brow height comes a concomitant drop in upper eyelid height and a narrowing of the palpebral fissure. Those patients who already have an asymmetrically lower upper eyelid

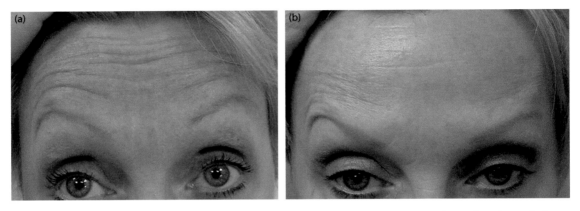

Figure 13.34 Patient is shown (a) before and (b) 2 weeks after OnaBTX-A treatment. Note the slightly higher elevation of the right eyebrow, which is seen as the patient raises her eyebrows before and after treatment. Note also the medial brow dip and right "Mephisto" brow after treatment.

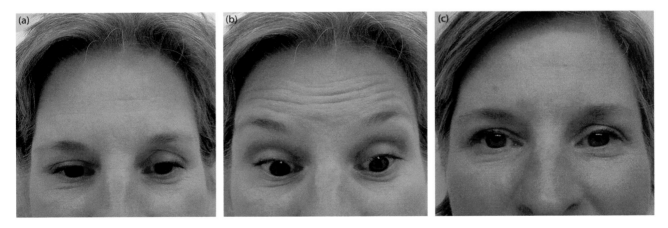

Figure 13.35 (a) This 53-year-old woman at rest did not know that she had a naturally occurring brow ptosis on the right with an accompanying secondary blepharoptosis of the right eyelid. (b) Same patient with an asymmetrical left brow elevation found with forced raising of the eyebrows before a treatment of OnaBTX-A. (c) Same patient at rest and gazing forward, 8 weeks after an OnaBTX-A treatment.

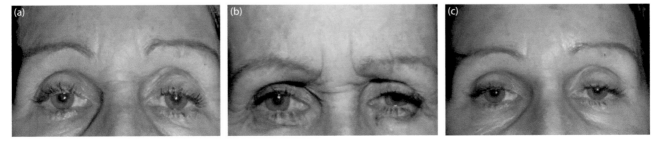

Figure 13.36 A 70-year-old with compensatory brow lifting and an undetected left eyelid ptosis (a) at rest and (b) frowning before OnaBTX-A treatment. (c) Blepharoptosis is seen at rest 1 month after OnaBTX-A. The patient and treating physician assumed the blepharoptosis was caused by OnaBTX-A until the before and after treatment pictures were compared, which then prompted the diagnosis of "pseudoblepharoptosis".

on one side now appear to have developed blepharoptosis from the OnaBTX-A injections (Figure 13.36). In reality, these patients more accurately have pseudoblepharoptosis, which is simply an unmasking of the secondary blepharoptosis they already possessed prior to any BoNT treatment. At times, this can be enhanced because of an age-related attenuation of the strength of the upper lid levator of that eye (Figure 13.37). When the patient first realizes that one upper eyelid is lower than the other, blame on the injector and OnaBTX-A is a foregone conclusion.[71] However, the astute physician will evaluate the patient carefully prior to any treatment and document the asymmetric clinical findings with pretreatment photographs. This will enable the physician to discuss the actual problem with the patient and graphically demonstrate the presence of the compensatory brow lifting before embarking on a perilous course of inevitable treatment failure (Figure 13.38). So, instead of the physician being led to believe that the patient developed blepharoptosis because of a poor injection technique, the physician will be able to identify that the patient always had an idiosyncratic asymmetry and subclinical upper eyelid ptosis that can be unmasked and even exaggerated with injections of OnaBTX-A (Figure 13.39). This manifestation of

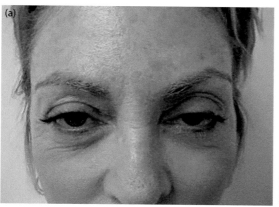 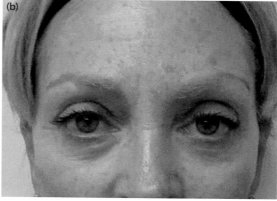

Figure 13.37 (a) A 57-year-old patient with a compensatory left brow lift before treatment with OnaBTX-A injections. (b) Same patient 2 weeks after OnaBTX-A demonstrates a slight pseudoblepharoptosis on the left.

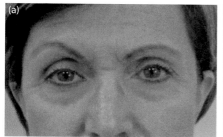 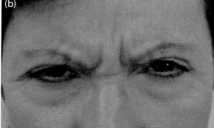 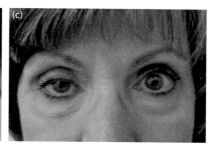

Figure 13.38 (a) Compensatory brow lifting raises the right eyebrow in this 60-year-old patient to correct a ptotic right eyelid. (b) Same patient, brows are fairly symmetrical with frowning, but the right upper lid is still ptotic before injections of OnaBTX-A. (c) Same patient, 1 week after injections of OnaBTX-A. The left brow was lifted with OnaBTX-A and both eyebrows appeared fairly symmetrical. This paradoxically makes the upper eyelid appear ptotic even though the right brow was not treated with OnaBTX-A.

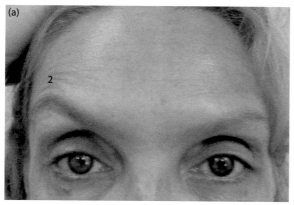 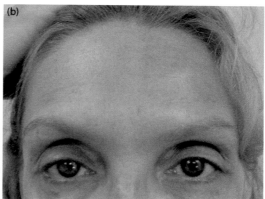

Figure 13.39 An example of iatrogenic asymmetry. (a) A 42-year-old patient is seen at rest with a higher right eyebrow 2 weeks after OnaBTX-A injections of the glabella and forehead and just before an additional 2 U of OnaBTX-A were given. (b) Same patient at rest 3 weeks after the additional 2 U of OnaBTX-A were given and 5 weeks after her initial treatment with OnaBTX-A. Notice the relative symmetry of both eyebrows.

pseudoblepharoptosis frequently occurs in patients over the age of 60 years who are treated for forehead wrinkles and glabellar frown lines with injections of BoNT. Correction of pseudoblepharoptosis is not always completely successful but can be attempted by injecting intradermally the extreme lateral and medial pretarsal orbicularis oculi of the upper eyelid on the affected side with low doses (0.5–1.0 units) of concentrated low volume OnaBTX-A.[64,71]

The best way to avoid additional difficulties with patient rapport and confidence is to keep carefully documented written clinical notes and before and after treatment photographs (see Appendix 4). Discuss the physical findings with the patient and point out existing idiosyncratic asymmetries, anatomical differences, and potential adverse outcomes prior to treatment. Informing the patient of any atypical findings before commencing with a treatment always is regarded by the patient as an accurate diagnosis of a unique situation. Explaining the circumstances and reasons for a particularly poor outcome after treatment always, is considered by the patient as an excuse for an improperly executed procedure.

Other untoward sequelae of more limited significance and duration can occur. These are the same adverse sequelae as those experienced with any type of subcutaneous or intramuscular injection. They include ecchymoses, edema, and erythema at the injection sites (Figure 13.40), headache, and flu-like malaise. Rarely, if ever, do any of these side effects last beyond the day of treatment, except for ecchymoses which can last up to 10 days or more.

For some patients, a dull and transient headache with or without general body malaise occurs after injections of OnaBTX-A that can last beyond 24–72 hours.[72] The occurrence of headache immediately after an OnaBTX-A injection seems paradoxical since OnaBTX-A injections are now FDA approved for treating tension and migraine headaches.[1,73] Headaches seem to occur more frequently in patients after their first and subsequent 2 or 3 treatment sessions. They usually cease to occur with repeat treatments. Studies have documented the incidence of patients who develop headaches after a treatment of OnaBTX-A were similar to those receiving placebo.[45] This seems to indicate that the transient headaches which occur after a treatment of BTX-A are due more likely to the physical act of injection rather than to the actual BoNT-A itself.[45] Other studies have found that patients are more prone to headaches when the volume of the injected BoNT-A is higher than usual. This also seems to support the opinion that headaches after injections of OnaBTX-A are probably due to the trauma of the injection rather than to the actual BoNT product.[74]

For the first-time recipient of a periorbital treatment of OnaBTX-A, the presence of periorbital edema lasting a few hours to days may occur. This can be attributed to lymph stasis, possibly produced by a nondetectable attenuation of the sphincteric pumping action of the inferior preseptal orbicularis oculi, reducing the efficiency of lymph fluid clearance from the surrounding soft tissue.[64] Moreover, when there is a blatant reduction in lower eyelid tone, eversion of the punctum and reduced blinking can compromise the action and efficacy of the "lacrimal pump," resulting in transient epiphora, until the lower eyelid tone returns (see Figure 13.132).

For some women, habitual squinting and scowling are the result of spending a lot of time outdoors, in front of a computer screen, or suffering from constant and persistent headaches, or being plagued with poor vision and refusing to wear corrective eyeglasses, among many other things. Incessant contraction of the corrugator supercilii and orbicularis oculi, manifested by habitual scowling, causes the medial end of the eyebrows to approach the midline. Sclafani and Jung measured the difference in interbrow distance from maximum elevation to maximum contraction of the brow, and it was slightly greater than 4 mm. The average distance traversed by the medial brow from frowning to repose was 3.26 mm in women and 3.76 mm in men.[75] Many women will pluck and shorten the transverse length of their eyebrows by removing eyebrow hair from the medial end of their brow. This will widen the glabellar interbrow space, so they do not look like they are habitually scowling, when they actually are (Figures 13.39 and 13.41). After injections of OnaBTX-A are given to reduce the number and extent of glabellar frown lines, the corrugators are no longer constantly contracting and adducting the eyebrows toward each other. Consequently, the transverse width of the glabella returns to its normal anatomical position because the corrugators now are more relaxed and less hyperkinetic when they are in repose. However, those women who have plucked the medial portion of their eyebrows now complain after injections of OnaBTX-A that they look practically hyperteloric because their eyebrows appear widely separated. However, it is only because the medial aspects of their eyebrows have been excessively plucked that causes them to appear this way and not the injections of OnaBTX-A. Such an adverse sequela is difficult to predict, but warning patients who pluck their eyebrows of such a potential side effect will prevent further disappointment on the part of the patient and additional frustration on the part of the physician. Also, be aware of the patients without any eyebrow hair who need to color in, the shape of their eyebrows. The shape that is chosen on the day of an OnaBTX-A treatment may not necessarily correspond to the natural anatomical position of that person's brow. Injections of OnaBTX-A may return the area to its natural anatomical position, which paradoxically may appear to be distorting the glabellar area, when in reality it is not. Patients with permanent eyebrow tattooing may present with similar challenges and post-treatment confounding disappointments (Figure 13.42).

Serious reactions, particularly those of immediate hypersensitivity such as anaphylaxis, urticaria, soft tissue edema, and dyspnea have been extremely rare. When they occur, appropriate medical treatment must be instituted immediately (see Appendix 6).[76] However, there has not been a confirmed serious case of spread of toxin effect away from the injection site when OnaBTX-A has been used at the recommended dose to treat glabellar frown lines.[1]

Figures 13.43 through 13.51 are some examples of different patients treated with OnaBTX-A for glabellar frown lines. Note also those who have had their forehead frown lines treated during the same treatment session.

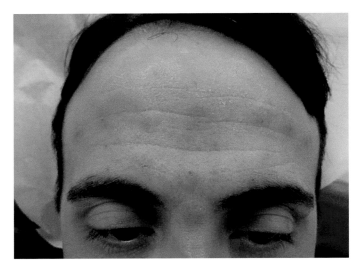

Figure 13.40 Note the erythema and edema in the pattern of the injections 10 minutes after a treatment of OnaBTX-A of the forehead and glabella.

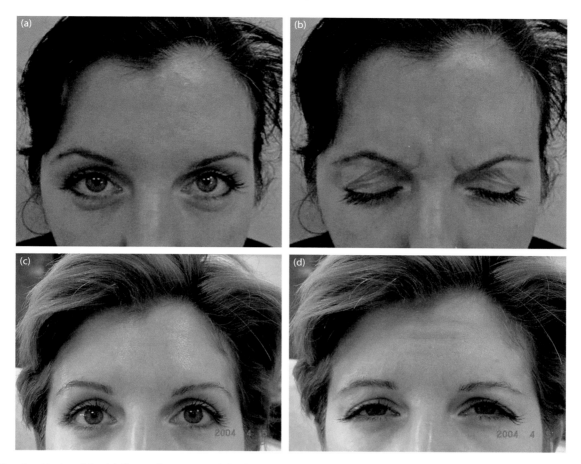

Figure 13.41 Note the widening of the glabellar interbrow space and the shortening of the transverse length of the brow (a) at rest and (b) frowning due to excessive plucking of the eyebrows. Same patient at rest (c) and frowning (d) after a treatment with OnaBTX-A. Note additionally the change in hair color after treatment.

Treatment Implications When Injecting the Glabella

1. Precise amounts of accurately placed injections of minimal volume OnaBTX-A reduce the incidence of brow and eyelid ptosis.
2. Men may need higher doses of OnaBTX-A than women for comparable results.

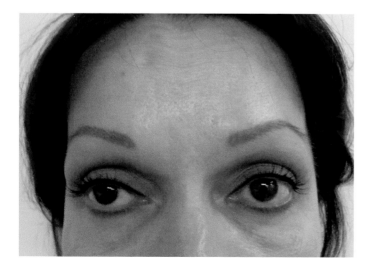

Figure 13.42 This 58-year-old patient had her eyebrows permanently tattooed prior to any OnaBTX-A treatments. Many years later, after regularly scheduled OnaBTX-A treatments, her eyebrows are now permanently and widely spaced lateral to the medial canthus.

3. Women prefer arched eyebrows; most men prefer straighter, non-arched eyebrows.
4. When injecting the corrugator supercilii with OnaBTX-A, remain medial to the midpupillary line and 3–4 cm above the supraorbital bony margin, and deep within the belly of the muscle.
5. Blepharoptosis can be transiently reversed with alpha-adrenergic agonist eye drops, but brow ptosis cannot be reduced and remits only when the effects of OnaBTX-A diminish.
6. Preexisting asymmetry of the brow and eyelids should be identified and discussed with the patient before treatment, and might be corrected by accurately injecting appropriate doses of OnaBTX-A on both the affected and non-affected sides.
7. Patients with inelastic, redundant skin of the brow who have compensatory brow lifting because of a preexisting subclinical secondary blepharoptosis can easily develop pseudoblepharoptosis when injections of OnaBTX-A decompensate their brow lifting on the affected side.

HORIZONTAL FOREHEAD LINES

Introduction: Problem Assessment and Patient Selection

One of the easiest areas of the face to treat with injections of OnaBTX-A is the forehead.[57] Many individuals contract their frontalis constantly for various and sundry reasons, and, in so doing, the skin buckles, creating parallel furrows and folds transversely across their foreheads. On the other hand, the presence of horizontal forehead lines seems to be directly proportional to one's age or time spent in the sun. Older individuals generally have many forehead lines that become deeper

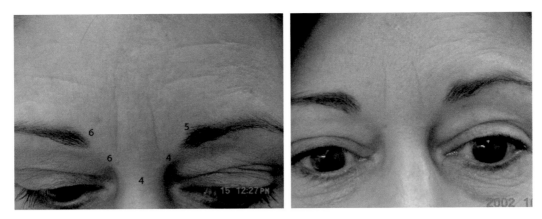

Figure 13.43 A 56-year-old patient at rest (a) before and (b) 1 month after OnaBTX-A treatment of the glabellar frown lines. Note the different dosages for areas of stronger muscle contraction.

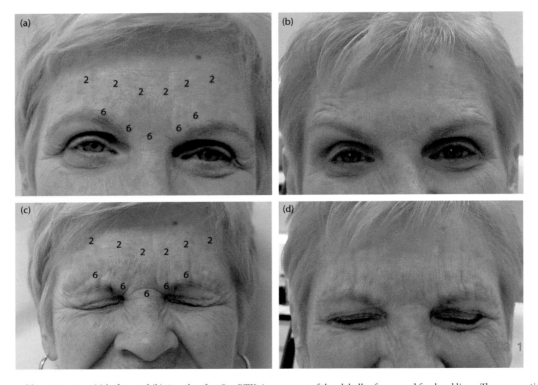

Figure 13.44 A 66-year-old patient at rest (a) before and (b) 4 weeks after OnaBTX-A treatment of the glabellar frown and forehead lines. The same patient is shown frowning (c) before and (d) 4 weeks after OnaBTX-A treatment of the glabellar frown lines.

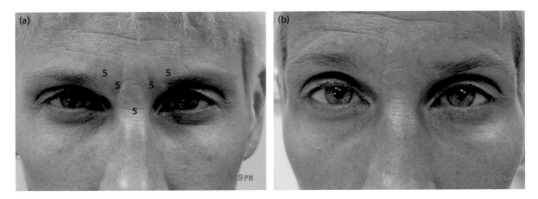

Figure 13.45 A 43-year-old patient at rest (a) before and (b) 2 weeks after an OnaBTX-A treatment of the glabellar frown lines.

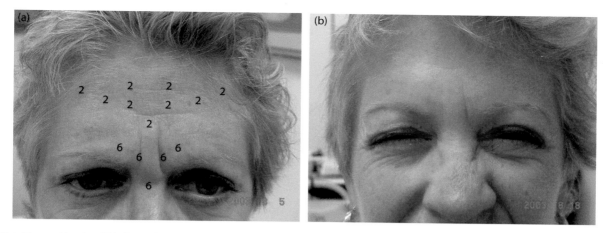

Figure 13.46 A 57-year-old patient (a) before and (b) frowning 2 weeks after an OnaBTX-A treatment of the glabellar frown and forehead lines.

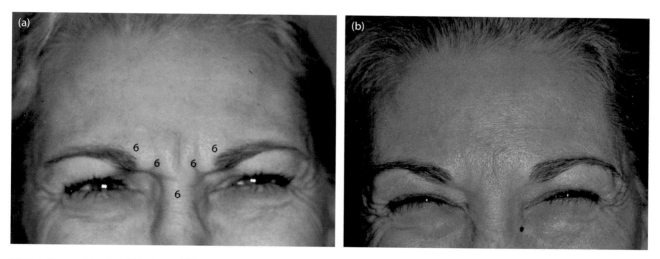

Figure 13.47 A 52-year-old patient (a) before and (b) 2 weeks after an OnaBTX-A treatment of glabellar frown lines.

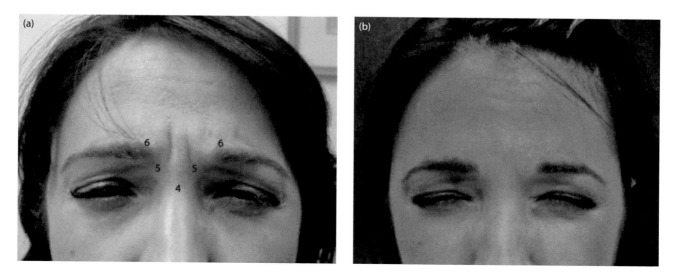

Figure 13.48 A 43-year-old patient frowning (a) before and (b) 2 weeks after OnaBTX-A treatment of glabellar frown lines.

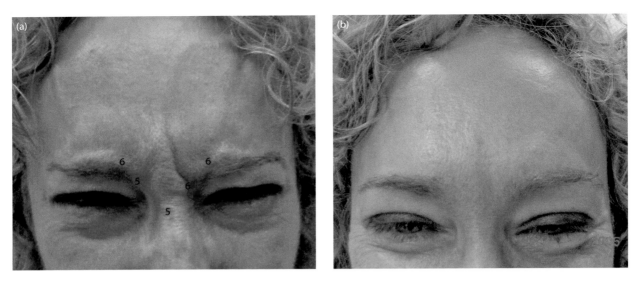

Figure 13.49 A 59-year-old patient frowning (a) before and (b) 2 weeks after an OnaBTX-A treatment of glabellar frown lines.

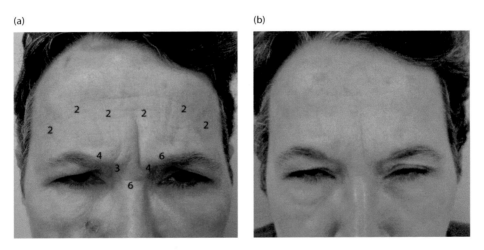

Figure 13.50 A 71-year-old patient frowning (a) before and (b) 2 weeks after an OnaBTX-A treatment of glabellar frown and forehead lines.

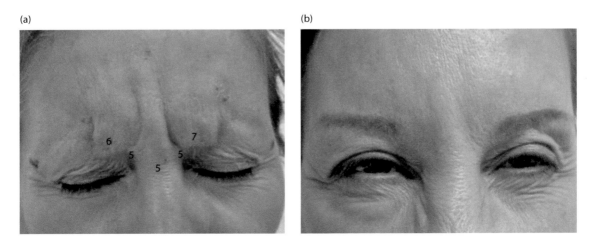

Figure 13.51 A 49-year-old patient frowning (a) before and (b) 2 weeks after an OnaBTX-A treatment of glabellar frown lines.

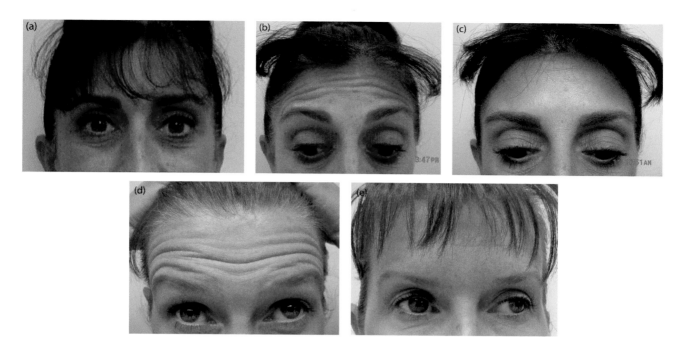

Figure 13.52 (a) Note the fringe of hair concealing the forehead in a 52-year-old with deep forehead lines (b) before and (c) 2 weeks after a treatment with OnaBTX-A. (d) A patient before and (e) 3 weeks after a treatment with OnaBTX-A. The bangs were pulled back to show the forehead rhytides.

with time. As one ages, the skin of the face, along with that of the rest of the body, typically becomes more inelastic and redundant. When this occurs in the upper face, not only do horizontal forehead lines appear, but there also is a characteristic hooding of the brow that frequently develops. Age-related brow hooding first develops commonly over the lateral aspect of the brow, whereby brow skin extends over the lateral aspect of the upper eyelids. This usually occurs in the sixth or seventh decade in those individuals so predisposed (Figure 13.2). For these individuals, a properly functioning frontalis is essential in maintaining a normal unobstructed field of vision. It is the frontalis that will keep the brow from dropping and causing the skin to drape over the upper eyelids, which can interfere with their forward and upward gaze.

Younger women who have horizontal forehead lines commonly attempt to conceal their obtrusiveness by wearing their frontal hair with a fringe or in bangs (Figure 13.52). Generally, the presence of horizontal forehead lines causes one to appear stressed, worried, tired, or old. Abruptly raising the eyebrows by acutely contracting the frontalis also can express an emotion of surprise or even fear; a social cue that one usually may not want to express too readily in certain situations (Figure 13.53). When done properly, injections of OnaBTX-A can diminish forehead wrinkling and replace one's unintended negative expressions with those that are more positive.

All too often it is the female rather than the male patient who is more concerned about the presence of forehead lines. These women are frequently quite determined to eliminate any vestige of the appearance of a forehead wrinkle. A cautious and empathetic cosmetic physician will remind such patients that the absolute absence of forehead wrinkles, especially at full contracture or while expressing an emotion, may not be particularly attractive or appropriate. It portrays an individual as too artificial and mask-like in appearance, and thus should not be one's ultimate goal. Because of the levator function of the frontalis, its antagonistic interaction with the depressor muscles of the glabella and periorbital area, and the potential risk of overtreatment causing brow ptosis, there are many who believe treating the frontalis with OnaBTX-A is not as easy as one might expect.[41]

Functional Anatomy of Horizontal Forehead Lines (See Appendix 2)

The horizontal forehead lines are produced by the contraction of the muscle fibers of the frontalis, the only levator muscle of the upper third of the face (Figure 13.54). The function of the frontalis is to elevate the eyebrows, the skin of the brow and forehead, and to oppose the depressor action of the muscles of the glabella and brow. Its superior aspect also retracts and lowers the scalp as a function of its participation in the occipitofrontalis galea aponeurotic complex.

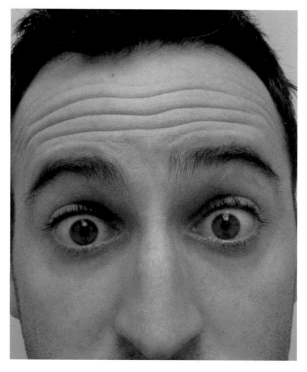

Figure 13.53 Abrupt contraction of the frontalis expresses surprise or even fear.

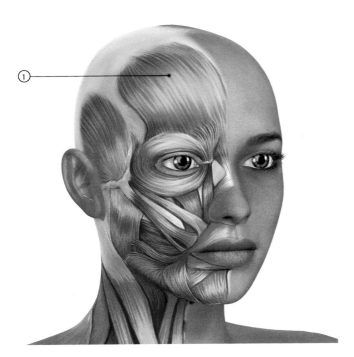

Figure 13.54 Frontalis, the only levator muscle of the forehead.

The frontalis is a pair of quadrilaterally shaped, distinct muscles whose fibers are oriented vertically, contracting in a vertical direction and producing the horizontal wrinkles of the forehead. The frontalis lies beneath a thick layer of sebaceous skin and subcutaneous tissue and has no attachment to bone. The frontalis is indirectly connected to the occipitalis by the epicranial, membranous galea aponeurotica, which attaches to both muscles on either side of the scalp vertex, the occipitalis posteriorly and the frontalis anteriorly. The frontalis originates from the membranous galea aponeurotica superiorly and inserts into the subcutaneous tissue and skin of the brow inferiorly at the level of the superciliary ridge (or arch) of the frontal bone. The fibers of the frontalis also interdigitate with muscle fibers of the brow depressors, that is, the procerus, corrugator supercilii, depressor supercilii, and orbicularis oculi. In some patients, there can be a downward extension of the membranous galea aponeurotica in the midline composed of little or no muscle fibers (Figure 13.54). Injections of OnaBTX-A into this area are ineffective and unnecessary when no muscle fibers are present.[77] However, in some men and even women, there are well-developed muscle fibers in the center of the forehead (Figures 13.52b and 13.55) which can be detected by light palpation over the area while the patient actively raises and lowers the eyebrows. A study of cadavers using punch biopsies to determine the location of frontalis muscle fibers at three different locations along the vertical axis in the forehead midline, revealed a diminishing presence of muscle fibers in the upper forehead.[30] Fibers of the paired frontalis intersected and overlapped in the midline at the level of the eyebrows in 100% of cases. At 2 cm above the eyebrows the two bellies of the frontalis interdigitated only in 40% of cases studied and at 4 cm above the eyebrow line no intersecting frontalis fibers were found in the midline. However, when functional muscle fibers of the frontalis can be detected in the center of the forehead, injections of OnaBTX-A in the midline of the forehead are needed to produce the desired effect (Figures 13.52b and 13.55e,f).

Dilution (See Appendix 3) When Treating Horizontal Forehead Lines

Controlled widespread diffusion can be a desired effect when injecting OnaBTX-A into the forehead. To avoid brow ptosis, the muscle fibers of the frontalis must remain fully functional 1.5–2.5 cm above the eyebrow, which is predicated on the resting position of the eyebrows (i.e., 3–4 cm above the actual bony orbital margin). Then higher dilutions and larger volumes of OnaBTX-A can be injected into the upper forehead. Consequently, injectors will use anywhere from 1 to 4 mL of non-preserved or preserved saline to reconstitute a 100 U vial of OnaBTX-A when treating the forehead.[39,78] The dilution recommended by the manufacturer and approved by the FDA and specified in the OnaBTX-A product's package insert is 2.5 mL of nonpreserved sterile saline or 4 U of OnaBTX-A per 0.1 mL of solution.

Dosing: How to Correct the Problem, (See Appendix 4), (What to Do and What Not to Do) Whenx Treating Horizontal Forehead Lines

Injections of OnaBTX-A into the frontalis for cosmetic purposes were approved by the FDA in October, 2017. The intricate and essential interaction of the frontalis with the brow depressors makes it virtually impossible not to treat the forehead when one is treating glabellar frown lines.

A typical dose for injecting the forehead in women is approximately 8–18 U of OnaBTX-A. However, the FDA approved dose for treating the forehead with Ona-BTX-A is 20 units. This can be injected either subcutaneously or intramuscularly at four to six sites across the forehead with 1–4 U of OnaBTX-A placed into each site at intervals of approximately 1.5–2.5 cm apart on either side of a deep crease (Figure 13.56).[78,79] For men, the typical dose is approximately 16–32 U of OnaBTX-A and occasionally higher.[80-82] These doses can be injected at 4–12 or even more sites either subcutaneously or intramuscularly depending on the height and width of the forehead, with up to 6–8 U of OnaBTX-A placed into each site, depending on the strength of the frontalis (Figures 13.56b and 13.57).[57,81] Some patients, either men or women, can have many rows of fine to moderate forehead wrinkles, whereas others can have one or two rows of deeply set folds and furrows. The number and dosage of the OnaBTX-A injections will depend on many factors, including the number and depth of the wrinkles, the size, shape, and strength of the muscle and the height, width, and shape of the forehead (Figure 13.57).[41,57,81,82] More often than expected, and unbeknownst to the individual, a patient will present with asymmetrical eyebrows prior to their first treatment with OnaBTX-A. Patients must be made aware of their idiosyncratic anatomical differences which must be documented both in the patient's clinical chart and in his or her photographic record. Sometimes the eyebrows can be made symmetrically level with each other with carefully placed injections of OnaBTX-A (Figure 13.58) and sometimes they cannot (Figure 13.59).

The patient usually is injected in an upright sitting or semireclined position. The pattern of injection across the forehead can vary depending on the anatomical dimensions of the forehead and the strength of the frontalis. To determine the overall muscular strength of the frontalis, lightly palpate the forehead at rest and during maximum eyebrow elevation. One can randomly inject 1–4 U of OnaBTX-A subcutaneously or intramuscularly at any point on the forehead that is at least 2–2.5 finger breadths (i.e., 2.5–4.0 cm) above the superior margin of the bony orbit (Figures 13.60 and 13.61).

Otherwise, one can use the on-label recommended technique and total dose of 20 units of OnaBTX-A for treating horizontal forehead lines for both men and women. To identify the recommended injection points one must first locate the superior extent of functionally active frontalis, which is usually approximately 1 cm above the highest horizontal forehead crease. Then locate the lowest row of treatable horizontal wrinkles, by identifying the midway point between the superior margin of active frontalis and the eyebrows. This midway

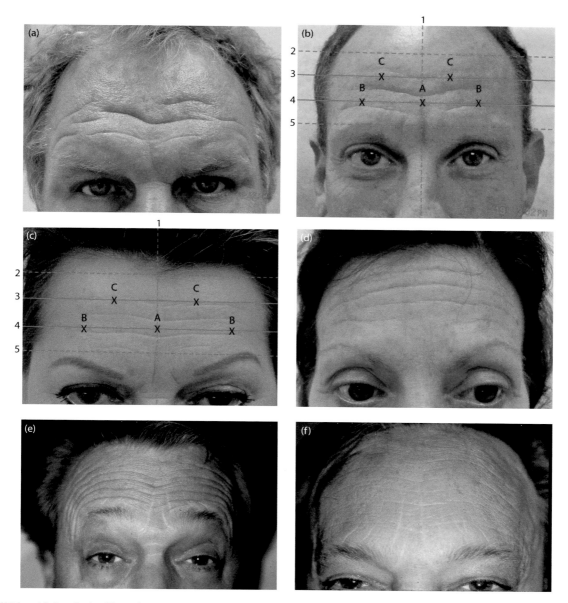

Figure 13.55 (a, b) Men with deep forehead lines; the 58-year-old patient in (b) works outdoors. (c, d) Some women can have a well-developed frontalis in the middle of their forehead. Neither of these women works outdoors. Note the on-label recommended injection points for treatment of the forehead on a patient (b) with a receding hairline and (c) with a fixed hairline: (1) midline; (2) superior margin; (3) upper treatable row; (4) lower treatable row; (5) inferior margin at upper level of eyebrows, and see text for location of injection points. (e, f) This 63-year-old man who spends a lot of time outdoors has a well-developed frontalis, seen here raising his eyebrows (e) before and (f) 2 weeks after an OnaBTX-A treatment. Note the non-tanned skin in the base of the forehead furrows (f) after treatment.

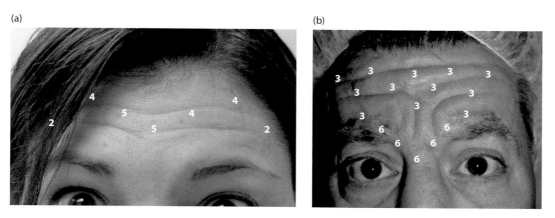

Figure 13.56 (a) Typical injection sites in a woman with an average sized forehead. (b) Typical injection sites in a man with an average sized forehead.

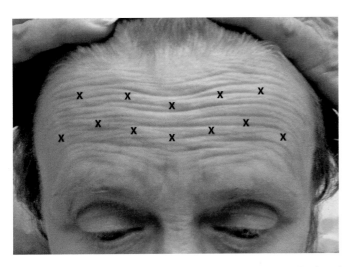

Figure 13.57 Random pattern injections into a forehead that is high and wide with multiple parallel wrinkles. This patient had 2 U of OnaBTX-A injected at each site.

point must be at least 2 cm above the eyebrows. Thirdly, the upper row of treatable horizontal wrinkles can be found midway between the superior margin of active frontalis and the lower row of treatable wrinkles. Five injections of 4 units of OnaBTX-A are approved for a total of 20 units placed at the intersection of the upper and lower rows

of treatable horizontal wrinkles with the following vertical landmarks (see Figure 13.55c):

1. On the lower row of treatable horizontal wrinkles first inject 4 units of OnaBTX-A at the midline of the face.
2. On the same lower row of treatable wrinkles, inject another 4 units of OnaBTX-A on the right and 4 units on the left side of the face, approximately 0.5–1.5 cm medial to the anterior temporal fusion line or temporal crest (see Figure 13.69).
3. On the upper row of horizontal wrinkles, midway between the central and lateral injection points of the lower row, inject another 4 units of OnaBTX-A on the right and 4 units on the left side of the face (see Figure 13.55c).

However, as one develops a more refined injection technique, improved and more natural appearing results can be realized when one injects BoNT starting just lateral to the midline, approximately 2–4 cm above the medial aspect of the eyebrows. From this starting point, injections are applied across the forehead at three or four points in an upward and downward pattern following the curvature of the arc of the eyebrows and maintaining the same distance of 2–3 cm above and parallel to the upper border of the eyebrows. The highest point of injection should be directly over the highest point of an arched eyebrow (Figures 13.60 and 13.61). This pattern will keep the OnaBTX-A high enough above the eyebrows and allow the lower muscle fibers along the transverse length of the frontalis to gently lift

(a)　　　　　　　　　　　　　　　　(b)

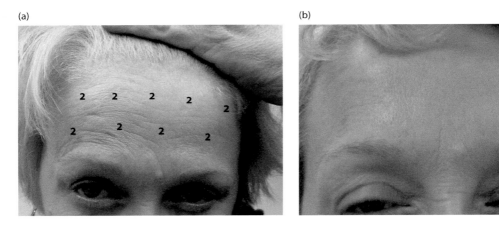

Figure 13.58 (a) This 68-year-old patient with an average sized forehead and low-set eyebrows was unaware that her right eyebrow was higher than her left. (b) After OnaBTX-A treatment they were symmetrical. Note the higher dosing on the right versus the left.

(a)　　　　　　　　　　　　　　　　(b)

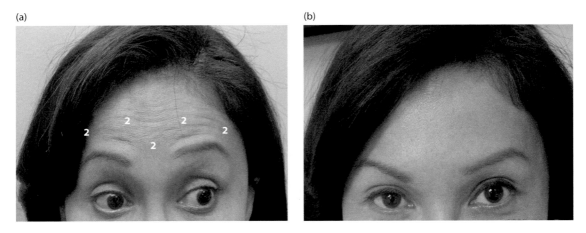

Figure 13.59 This 50-year-old patient has a high and narrow forehead and multiple rows of forehead wrinkles. Note the left eyebrow is higher than the right one (a) before and (b) after treatment with OnaBTX-A.

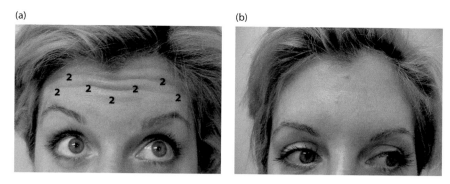

Figure 13.60 (a) A 40-year-old patient with a low and wide forehead with the right eyebrow higher than the left before treatment with OnaBTX-A. Note the position of the injection points: lower on the right lateral brow and higher over the left brow. (b) Note the position of the right eyebrow 1 week after treatment with OnaBTX-A.

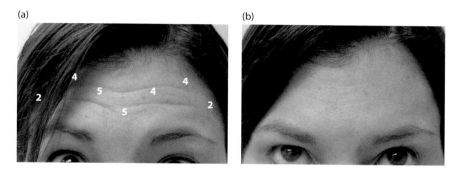

Figure 13.61 (a) This 36-year-old patient has an average low and narrow forehead with the right eyebrow higher than the left before a treatment of OnaBTX-A. (b) Two weeks after OnaBTX-A, the eyebrows are symmetrical.

and deliberately produce a naturally peaked and aesthetically pleasing arched eyebrow (Figures 13.2, 13.64, and 13.65). Injections that are too high above the lateral tail of the eyebrows may cause unaffected lower fibers of the lateral frontalis to excessively elevate the lateral aspect of the eyebrows, resulting in the so-called "Mephisto" or "Mr. Spock" look (Figures 13.62, 13.66, and 13.67). This occurred more frequently when a "V" pattern of injection was performed in the forehead (as discussed in the first edition of this text).

The simplest approach to treating the forehead in men is to inject as much as 25 U of OnaBTX-A or even more intramuscularly in a horizontal, linear fashion across the forehead, maintaining the same distance of approximately 3-4 cm above and parallel to the eyebrows and wrinkles (Figures 13.62 and 13.63). This pattern of injection minimizes the curvature of the eyebrows, resulting in a more masculine appearing eyebrow (Figure 13.63).

Another technique is to inject subcutaneously approximately 2–4 U of OnaBTX-A at sites approximately 2 cm apart and across the entire forehead horizontally at a point midway between the brow and the hairline also maintaining a constant distance above the eyebrows (Figures 13.58 and 13.63). This is advisable if the hairline is set low and if there are only one or two rows of horizontal wrinkles across the forehead (Figure 13.68).

In most patients, muscle fibers of the frontalis do not extend any more laterally than the anterior temporal fusion lines. If the width of the forehead is narrow, that is, less than 12 cm between the right and left anterior temporal fusion lines, or temporal crests, then four or five subcutaneous injections of 2–4 U of OnaBTX-A at each injection site across the forehead are sufficient (Figure 13.59). One can feel the anterior temporal fusion line by first identifying the zygomatic process of the frontal bone, which is the superior aspect of the upper lateral wall of the bony orbit (Figure 13.69). Its posterior edge continues upward, as a palpable protruding ridge along the lateral edge of the frontal bone, and arches upward and backward, delineating

the anterior and superior boundary of the temporal fossa. If an individual has a wider brow, that is, more than 12 cm between the right and left anterior temporal fusion lines, then five, six, or possibly more injection points across the forehead are probably necessary, with 2–4 U of OnaBTX-A injected at each site subcutaneously in women (Figures 13.57, 13.65 and 13.66). The stronger the frontalis, the more units of OnaBTX-A will be required to produce the desired effect (Figures 13.66 and 13.68).

Gentle massage upward and laterally at the injection sites for a few seconds helps relieve the acute and transient pain of a transcutaneous injection and can help disperse the toxin locally. Prolonged or heavy-handed massage, especially in a downward direction, can disperse the liquid OnaBTX-A beyond the intended area of injection, weakening adjacent lower muscle fibers and producing an unwanted brow ptosis.

OUTCOMES (RESULTS) WHEN TREATING HORIZONTAL
FOREHEAD LINES (SEE APPENDIX 5)

An adequate result when treating the frontalis is to completely eliminate the horizontal lines of the forehead when the patient is at rest, and to provide the ability for some movement and minimal wrinkling when the patient is animated or actively expressing an emotion. Ideally, weakening of the frontalis should last at least 3 full months when a sufficient dose of OnaBTX-A is injected. Frequently, after repeat treatments and occasionally even after the first treatment session in some patients, the effects of OnaBTX-A weakening can last as long as 4–6 months after it is injected.[41] Overgenerous intramuscular injections of the frontalis with high doses of OnaBTX-A will eliminate totally all movement of the muscle, even with forced contraction, creating a flat mask-like and motionless forehead and even some degree of brow ptosis especially in patients (young or old) with inelastic skin. There usually is never a good aesthetic reason for such total myorelaxation of the frontalis or any other muscle of facial expression even if the effect is only temporary. In addition, the overall duration of results usually

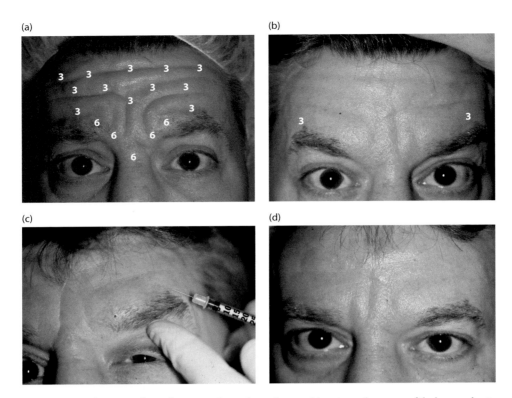

Figure 13.62 (a) Typical injection points and amount of units for a man who works outdoors and has strong depressors of the brow and a strong levator of the forehead causing very deep furrows. Before treatment with OnaBTX-A injections. (b) Same patient 2 weeks after the initial OnaBTX-A treatment and before an additional 6 U of OnaBTX-A. Note the elevated "Mephisto" or "Mr. Spock" lateral eyebrows and where an additional 3 U of OnaBTX-A were injected on each side to lower the lateral frontalis above the tail of the eyebrows, in this man who usually has straighter eybrows. (c) Same patient having a touch-up injection of 3 U of OnaBTX-A bilaterally 2 weeks after his initial OnaBTX-A treatment. (d) Same patient 5 weeks after the initial OnaBTX-A treatment and 3 weeks after a touch-up treatment. Note the less arched lateral brows and iatrogenic brow ptosis.

is not extended in any muscle when OnaBTX-A is injected at a higher dose than that which is recommended or normally sufficient for the individual's present problem.[79]

Occasionally and especially with the initial treatment of forehead wrinkles, the effect of OnaBTX-A weakening may not occur symmetrically, and there may be wrinkling on one side of the forehead and not on the other, even at rest. It is imperative that the physician warns the patient of this before treatment and requires the patient to return 2–3 weeks after a treatment session so that any minor asymmetries can be corrected. This is easily accomplished by injecting 1–2 U of OnaBTX-A in the vicinity of the persistent asymmetric wrinkling and muscle hyperactivity (Figures 13.62 and 13.67).[60] Remember, this should always be done at least 2–3 cm above the bony orbital rim, so as not to produce brow ptosis inadvertently. This is particularly important for those patients who have some degree of dermatochalasis and multiple rows of low-lying horizontal forehead lines (Figure 13.70a). By allowing the lower fibers of the frontalis to remain active, there typically may be a wrinkle or two directly above the eyebrow and a degree of asymmetric brow elevation that might persist. Total elimination of these particularly persistent wrinkles directly above the lateral aspect of the eyebrows usually cannot be reduced without causing some amount of brow ptosis (Figure 13.70b,c). Most of the time, these narrow horizontal lines immediately adjacent to, if not within, the upper lateral border of the eyebrows can be identified during pretreatment physical examination and management planning, and the patient should be made aware of them (Figures 13.63, 13.67, 13.70, and 13.71). The patient also should be given the option to eliminate these lines by other cosmetic procedures (e.g., fillers, energy-based therapy, or both), before initiating injections of OnaBTX-A. These minor horizontal forehead lines usually are the

manifestation of excessively lax skin and a hyperactive frontalis being recruited in a compensatory manner to elevate a weighty brow to prevent brow hooding and visual field obstruction. The patient is better off totally ignoring these lines. If they remain after the injections of OnaBTX-A have completely taken effect and still are extremely bothersome to the patient, they can be treated by injecting intradermally a minimal amount of highly diluted OnaBTX-A adjacent to the wrinkle. However, no matter how dilute and how little the amount of OnaBTX-A is injected, brow ptosis still may result. Otherwise, injections of a soft tissue filler, preferably a hyaluronic acid (e.g. a cohesive polydensified matrix hyaluronic acid to minimize the Tyndall effect) product 2–4 weeks later, can diminish these wrinkles while bolstering the lax, excessive brow skin and creating an overall additional aesthetic enhancement to the lateral brow and periorbital area.

Complications (Adverse Sequelae) When Treating Horizontal Forehead Lines (See Appendix 6)

When treating the frontalis with OnaBTX-A, appropriate injection patterns and meticulous injection techniques are extremely important in avoiding brow ptosis.[54,57,83] This is best accomplished by remaining at least 3–4 cm above the supraorbital bony margin or 2–3 cm above the eyebrow depending on the idiosyncratic anatomy of the individual patient being treated. This will enable the muscle fibers of the frontalis to remain functional with an adequate resting tone in the area directly above the brow so that the eyebrows will not drop and produce hooding over the upper eyelids (Figures 13.67 and 13.72).

In most patients, horizontal forehead lines are present in conjunction with glabellar frown lines. In these patients, the current preferred practice is to treat the upper third of the face during the

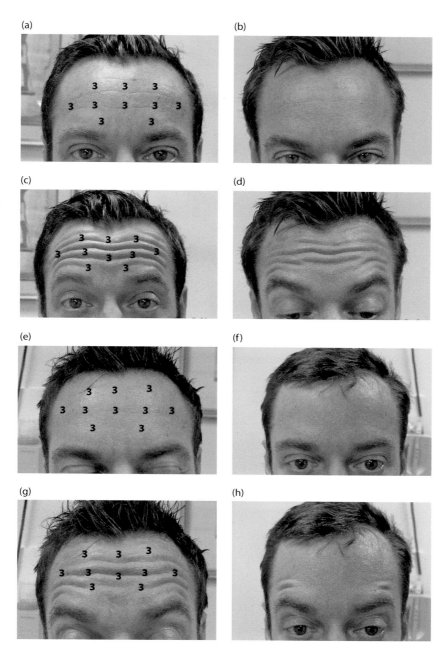

Figure 13.63 (a) A 40-year-old patient at rest before and (b) 3 weeks after an OnaBTX-A treatment of only the forehead. (c) Same patient raising his eyebrows before and (d) 3 weeks after an OnaBTX-A treatment of only his forehead. (e) Same patient at rest before and (f) 1 week after his fourth OnaBTX-A treatment of only his forehead. (g) Same patient raising his eyebrows before and (h) 1 week after his fourth OnaBTX-A treatment of only his forehead.

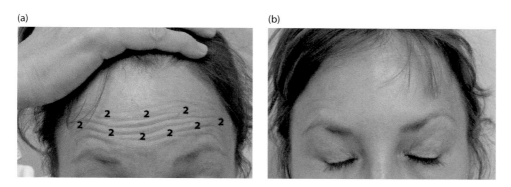

Figure 13.64 (a) Injection sites for a 38-year-old patient with a high and wide forehead and an asymmetrically lower right eyebrow. (b) After treatment.

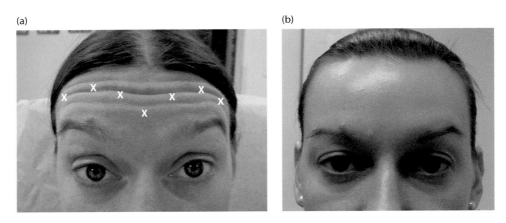

Figure 13.65 (a) Typical injection sites in a woman with an average sized forehead. (b) Same patient 2 weeks after an OnaBTX-A injection.

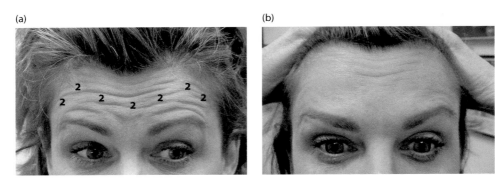

Figure 13.66 A 45-year-old patient raising her eyebrows (a) before and (b) 3 weeks after OnaBTX-A treatment of only the forehead.

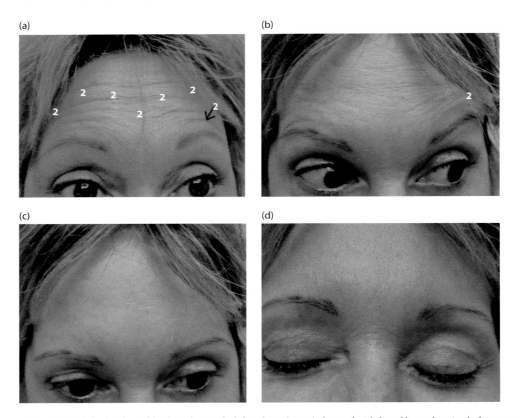

Figure 13.67 (a) A 54-year-old patient with forehead wrinkles directly over the left eyebrow (arrow) observed with forced brow elevation before treatment. (b) Same patient 2 weeks after initial treatment with OnaBTX-A. Note the left brow is now higher than the right brow with forced eyebrow elevation. An additional 2 U of OnaBTX-A was injected during this follow-up visit. (c) Same patient 5 weeks after the initial treatment with OnaBTX-A and 3 weeks after a touch-up of 2 U of OnaBTX-A. The left eyebrow remains slightly elevated laterally at rest with eyes wide open (d) but not with the eyes closed.

(a)

(b)

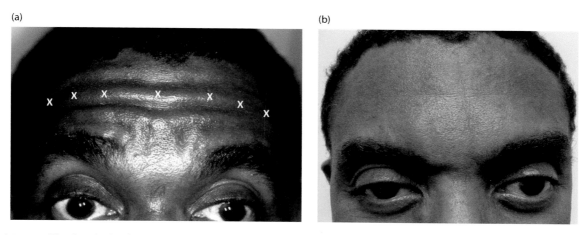

Figure 13.68 A 51-year-old male with a low forehead and 2 rows of horizontal wrinkles. Seen here (a) before and (b) 1 month after an onabotulinutoxinA treatment.

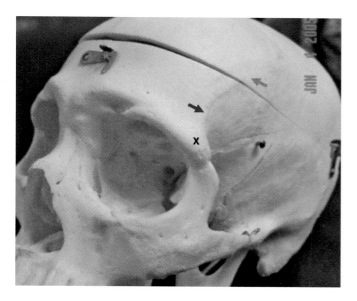

Figure 13.69 The location and extent of anterior and superior temporal fusion line on a skull: X, zygomatic process of the frontal bone; blue arrow: anterior temporal fusion line; red arrow: superior temporal fusion line.

same session.[42,43,47,48,55,71,80] The resting tone of the glabellar depressors (corrugator supercilii, depressor supercilii, procerus, orbicularis oculi) is usually slightly stronger than the resting tone of the brow elevator (frontalis). Therefore, if the brow depressors are not treated contemporaneously with the brow elevator, brow ptosis may be difficult to prevent because of the overriding downward pull of the depressors (Figure 13.73). Maintaining an adequate resting tone of the lower fibers of the frontalis just over the brow (approximately 2–4 cm) will help prevent brow ptosis (Figure 6.72).

If excessive doses of OnaBTX-A are injected into the center of the forehead, a drop of the mid forehead skin and soft tissue can occur, producing a bulge of skin to appear in the center of the glabella. This usually is accompanied by a weighing down of the medial aspect (heads) of the eyebrows and an unattractive downward sloping or a downward pointing of the heads of the eyebrows. This also may give some patients an unsettling sensation of a peculiar "heaviness" in the center of their forehead and brow. To avoid this all-too-common tell-tale evidence of being "over-Botoxed," injections should not be given too low directly in the center of the forehead, especially if there is a paucity of central forehead wrinkles, indicating an absence of frontalis muscle fibers. Before injecting this area, one should be

sure that there are strong and active frontalis muscle fibers in the center of the forehead, like those seen in Trindade's "omega" pattern of glabellar frown lines[27] (see Figure 13.22). To diminish an excessively downward sloping of the medial aspect of the eyebrows and glabellar soft tissue, injections of OnaBTX-A can be placed into the medial brow depressors: 3–5 U into each depressor supercilii, which also will diffuse into the medial fibers of the orbital orbicularis oculi, and 4–10 U into the procerus in the center of the glabella. This might relieve some of the forceful downward pull of the central glabellar soft tissue, especially in Trindade's "inverted omega" pattern of glabellar frowning (see Figure 13.23), and elevate the medial heads of the eyebrows. There is no antidote for brow ptosis, which can last as long as the OnaBTX-A injections are effective. Concomitant injections of low-dose, low-volume OnaBTX-A precisely placed into the superficial fibers of the lateral, upper orbital orbicularis oculi also is essential in reducing the extent of lateral brow ptosis.

Clinical experience has indicated that when a more concentrated dose of OnaBTX-A is used (i.e., dilutions of 1 mL per 100 U vial of OnaBTX-A) minimal volumes are injected and migration of the OnaBTX-A is negligible.[39] The results also seem to last longer. On the other hand, to prevent total paralysis of muscle movement, especially with forced contraction of the frontalis, a different approach can be utilized when attempting to aesthetically reduce horizontal forehead lines. Since there does not seem to be any agreement in the literature on which dilutions should be used when reconstituting a 100 U vial of OnaBTX-A, or which dosage regimens are most effective, one then can inject the forehead with the same total number of units of OnaBTX-A, but with a more dilute solution.[39,78,81] Namely, a 100 U vial of OnaBTX-A can be reconstituted with 2–4 mL of saline when used solely for injecting the frontalis. This dilution allows one to inject a greater volume of OnaBTX-A and disperse it over a wider area of the forehead, providing an effect that is less intensely paralyzing.[78] However, injecting large volumes of diluted OnaBTX-A possibly might limit the duration of its effectiveness. As long as nontargeted muscle fibers (i.e., those of the lower frontalis) are not directly in the wake of the intended toxin diffusion, higher dilutions may be a more forgiving alternative injection technique, especially for the neophyte injector. It is the total number of units that is important when treating patients with OnaBTX-A or any other BoNT and not the total volume used.

Other more common adverse sequelae that occur with an injection of OnaBTX-A are related more to the actual physical injection rather than to the material injected. All of these adverse events are transient and generally do not last longer than 24–36 hours. They include ecchymoses, local edema, erythema, and pain at the injection and

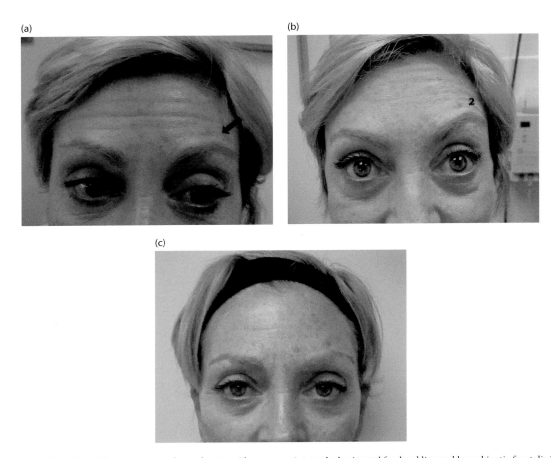

Figure 13.70 (a) A 62-year-old patient with compensatory brow elevation. The arrow points to the horizontal forehead line and hyperkinetic frontalis immediately above the left lateral brow. (b) Same patient after OnaBTX-A. Note the hyperkinetic lower lateral frontalis on the left. Two weeks after the initial treatment, 2 U of OnaBTX-A were injected 2–2.5 cm above the lateral left brow at a point of maximum contraction of the frontalis. (c) Same patient 5 weeks after initial treatment and 3 weeks after touch-up over the left eyebrow.

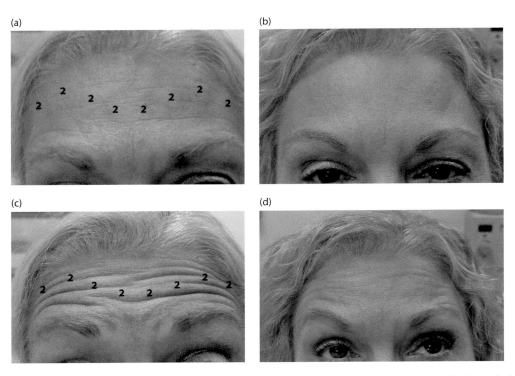

Figure 13.71 A 52-year-old patient with mild forehead wrinkling at rest (a) before and (b) 3 weeks after an OnaBTX-A treatment of only the forehead. The same patient raising her eyebrows (c) before and (d) 3 weeks after an OnaBTX-A treatment of only the forehead. Note the persistent wrinkles just above both lateral eyebrows.

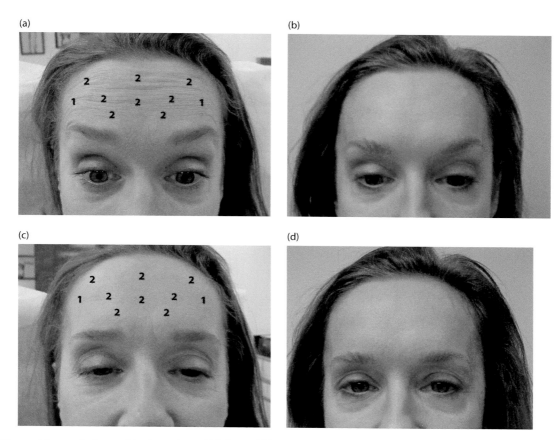

Figure 13.72 A 32-year-old woman is shown raising her eyebrows (a) before and (b) 1 month after treatment of only the forehead. The same patient is shown at rest (c) before and (d) 1 month after treatment of only the forehead. Note the gentle arching of the brows after treatment with OnaBTX-A.

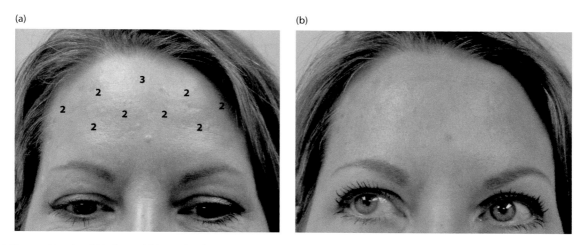

Figure 13.73 A 53-year-old patient (a) before and (b) 2 weeks after an OnaBTX-A treatment of only the forehead. Note the slight bilateral brow ptosis after treatment when the glabella is not adequately treated.

adjacent sites (Figure 13.40). For some patients, a dull and transient headache with or without general body malaise occurs after injections of OnaBTX-A that can last beyond 24–72 hours.[72] The occurrence of headache immediately after an OnaBTX-A injection seems paradoxical since OnaBTX-A injections are now FDA approved for treating tension and migraine headaches.[1,73] Serious reactions, particularly of the immediate hypersensitivity type such as anaphylaxis, urticaria, soft tissue edema, and dyspnea have been extremely rare.[76] When they occur, appropriate medical treatment must be instituted immediately.

Figures 13.74 through 13.81 are additional examples of different patients treated with OnaBTX-A for horizontal forehead lines. Many of them had their glabellas treated at the same time.

Treatment Implications When Injecting the Frontalis
1. Identify and document brow or forehead asymmetries prior to treatment with OnaBTX-A.
2. Injections of OnaBTX-A in the forehead can be placed subcutaneously or intramuscularly.

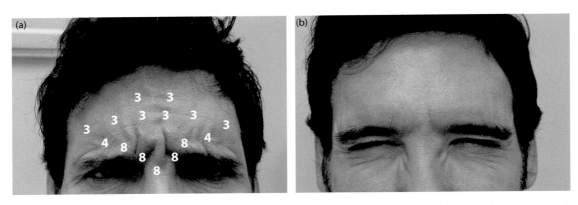

Figure 13.74 A 48-year-old patient frowning (a) before and (b) 3 weeks after an OnaBTX-A treatment of forehead and glabellar frown lines.

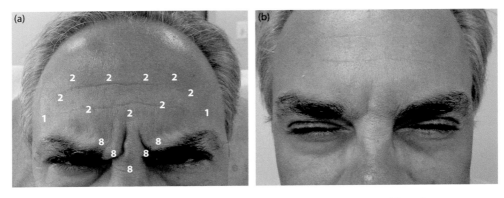

Figure 13.75 A 56-year-old patient frowning (a) before and (b) 2 weeks after an OnaBTX-A treatment for forehead and frown lines.

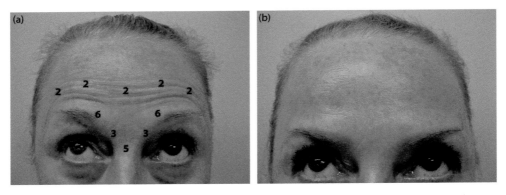

Figure 13.76 A 64-year-old patient raising her eyebrows (a) before and (b) 3 weeks after an OnaBTX-A treatment for forehead and frown lines. Note the "medial dip" of the glabella.

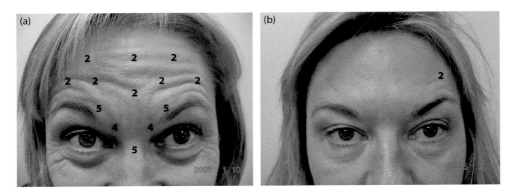

Figure 13.77 A 59-year-old patient raising her eyebrows (a) before and (b) 3 weeks after an OnaBTX-A treatment for forehead and frown lines. An additional 2 U were given over the left brow.

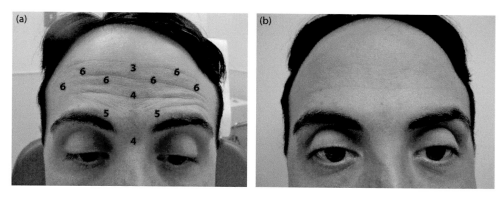

Figure 13.78 A 42-year-old patient raising his eyebrows (a) before and (b) 2 weeks after an OnaBTX-A treatment for forehead and frown lines.

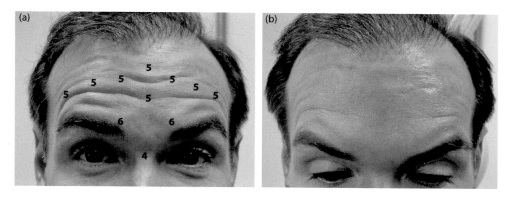

Figure 13.79 A 52-year-old patient raising his eyebrows (a) before and (b) 2 weeks after an OnaBTX-A treatment for forehead and frown lines. Note the "medial dip" of the glabella.

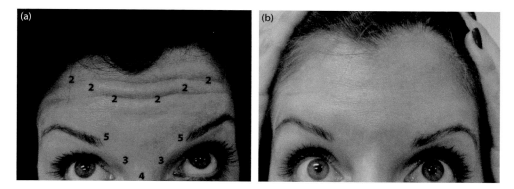

Figure 13.80 A 45-year-old patient raising her eyebrows (a) before and (b) 2 months after an OnaBTX-A treatment for forehead and frown lines.

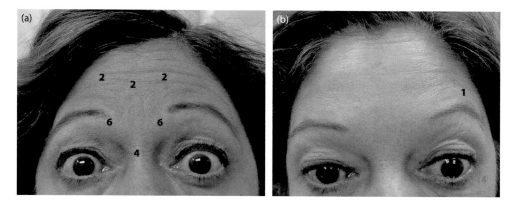

Figure 13.81 A 61-year-old patient raising her eyebrows (a) before and (b) 2 weeks after an OnaBTX-A treatment for forehead and frown lines. Note the higher left eyebrow before treatment and the additional 1 U at the follow-up visit.

3. Treating the frontalis with OnaBTX-A is best done in conjunction with treating the glabellar frown lines and lateral canthal crow's feet lines.

4. Weaken the frontalis; do not paralyze it.

5. The lower horizontal forehead lines may not be treatable if brow ptosis is to be avoided, especially in older patients.

6. Post-treatment forehead asymmetry can be corrected with 1 or 2 units of OnaBTX-A given into the hyperactive fibers of the frontalis, 2–4 weeks after a treatment session.

7. Avoid injecting the center of the forehead with OnaBTX-A to prevent a downward projection of the medial aspect of the eyebrows and central glabellar soft tissue, especially when this area is devoid of frontalis muscle fibers.

PERIORBITAL AREA: LATERAL CANTHAL LINES

Introduction: Problem Assessment and Patient Selection

One of the first signs of aging is the presence of wrinkles that radiate outwardly away from the lateral canthus, which are sometimes referred to as "crow's feet" (Figure 13.82). Depending on a person's skin type, history of sun exposure, and muscle strength, crow's feet can appear in someone as young as 20 years of age. The natural thinness and abundance of the skin in the lateral periorbital area make this site prone to wrinkling. These lateral canthal lines initially appear only during animation, then eventually accentuate while smiling, laughing, or squinting and become increasingly more noticeable with time. Their presence causes one to appear perpetually tired and fatigued and even older than one's current age. For a woman, crow's feet are the bane of her appearance, particularly when make-up accumulates in the depths of the creases. For men, crow's feet are a sign of hard work and fun in the sun.

When lateral canthal wrinkles are caused by the contraction of the lateral aspect of the orbital orbicularis oculi, they are referred to as *dynamic* wrinkles. They are the result of infolding and pleating of the overlying skin as the muscle contracts when a person animates. Lateral canthal wrinkles radiate in a horizontal direction away from the lateral canthus (Figure 13.82). These horizontal wrinkles are perpendicular to the direction of the contraction of the lateral muscle fibers of the orbital orbicularis oculi, which run mostly in a vertical direction around the lateral canthus (Figure 13.83). These dynamic lateral canthal wrinkles have been treated successfully

in an off-label manner with injections of BoNTs for many years (Figure 13.84). However, since 2013, the treatment of lateral canthal lines for cosmetic purposes was approved by the FDA, and now they can be treated with an on-label indication.[39,84–87]

In some patients, however, intrinsic chronologic aging combined with extrinsic photodamage are the major contributing factors that produce lateral canthal wrinkles. These types of wrinkles are always present whether a person is actively animating, and therefore are referred to as *static* wrinkles. When the bulk of crow's feet are the result of static wrinkles, injections of OnaBTX-A will be less effective. Only surgical suspension techniques, different resurfacing and energy-based rejuvenation procedures, or injections of soft tissue fillers can help efface static wrinkling of the lateral canthus. However, when the bulk of the crow's feet are produced by the hyperactivity of the lateral orbital orbicularis oculi, then injections of BoNT can play a significant role in diminishing the wrinkling and rejuvenating the face (Figure 13.84).

Functional Anatomy of Lateral Canthal Lines (See Appendix 2)

The orbicularis oculi is a broad, flat, subcutaneous layer of concentric muscle fibers, elliptical in overall shape. It encircles the globe, covering the eyelids and extending beyond the peripheral margins of the bony orbit: beyond the superior border of the eyebrows; approximately 3 cm lateral to the lateral canthus and as low as the mid cheek. It differs from the other facial muscles in that it has loose connective tissue superficial and deep to it. The other facial muscles are within and closely bound to the superficial fascia or the superficial musculoaponeurotic system (SMAS). Eyelid skin is the thinnest in the body and has underdeveloped dermal pilosebaceous and sweat glands. Eyelid skin is attached to the underlying orbicularis oculi by fine connective tissue that is devoid of fat but replete with a vascular network of arterial and venous anastomoses. The thinness of the skin and the fine underlying connective tissue readily permit eyelid skin to become distensible and collect interstitial fluid. The orbicularis oculi functions as the sphincter or protractor of the eyelids.[88]

The orbicularis oculi is divided into three component parts, the *orbital*, *palpebral*, and *lacrimal* parts (Figure 13.85).[28–30] These constituent parts of the orbicularis oculi are confluent and act in unison to form the eyelid protractors. The *orbital* part of the orbicularis oculi is the outermost and thickest portion of the muscle that forms

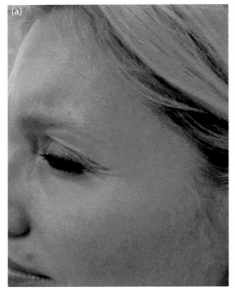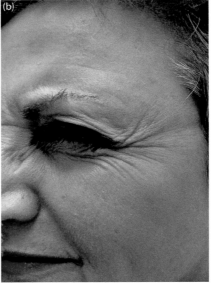

Figure 13.82 (a) Crow's feet accentuated by squinting in a 31-year-old patient. (b) Same condition in a 68-year-old patient.

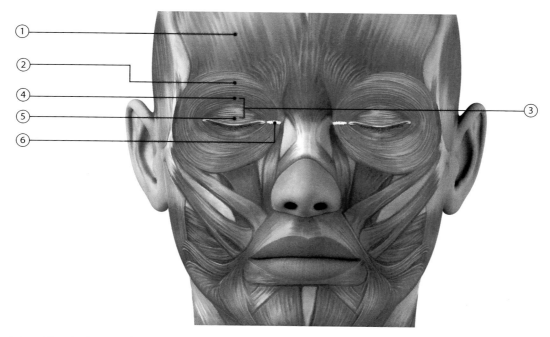

Figure 13.83 Frontal view of the *orbital* portion of the orbicularis oculi. Note the muscle fibers are oriented vertically around the lateral canthus, hence crow's feet (lateral canthal lines) radiate away from the lateral canthus in a horizontal direction, that is, perpendicular to the direction of muscle contraction. 1, frontalis; 2, orbicularis oculi *orbital* portion; 3, orbicularis oculi, *palpebral* portion; 4, preseptal; 5, tarsal; 6, lacrimal. (See Appendix 2—muscle attachments.)

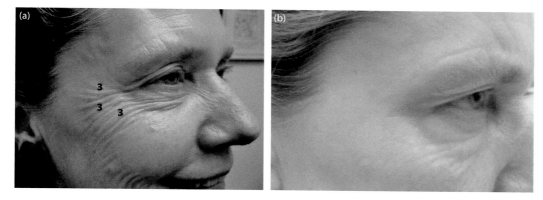

Figure 13.84 (a) Squinting produces a myriad of lateral orbital wrinkles in this 64-year-old patient before a treatment of OnaBTX-A into her crow's feet. (b) Same patient squinting 3 weeks after OnaBTX-A injections.

a complete ellipse around the bony orbit. The orbital orbicularis oculi originates on the anterior aspect of the inferior and superior bony orbital rim; that is, from the nasal component of the frontal bone, the frontal process of the maxilla, and the medial palpebral ligament. Its fibers form complete ellipses, without interruption even in its lateral aspect, where there is no bony attachment. In its superior aspect, the orbital orbicularis oculi interdigitates with the lower muscle fibers of the frontalis and lies over the corrugator supercilii. Medially, the orbital orbicularis oculi interdigitates with the central fibers of the frontalis, the depressor supercilii and the procerus. The orbital orbicularis oculi inserts into the soft tissue of the brow, anterior temple (superficial temporalis fascia), the cheeks (interdigitating with fibers of the levator labii superioris alaeque nasi, levator labii superioris, and zygomaticus major and minor) (see Chapter 14), and medial and lateral canthal tendons. Contraction of the orbital orbicularis oculi approximates the upper with the lower eyelids, as with forced, volitional eyelid closure (tight eye closure). Forced eyelid closure depresses the skin of the forehead, draws medially the skin of the temples and the medial

and lateral aspects of the eyebrows. The skin of the cheeks is pulled upward as well. Forced eyelid closure also compresses the globe and lacrimal sac, initiating the flow of tears into the nasolacrimal duct (see lacrimal pump below, Figure 13.132). With eyelid closure, the muscle fibers of the superior component of the orbital orbicularis act more as a depressor of the upper eyelid, while the muscle fibers of the inferior component of the orbital orbicularis act more as an elevator of the lower eyelid. Frequent squinting and incessant forced contraction of the orbital orbicularis oculi contribute to the formation of lateral canthal lines and lower eyelid wrinkles, as well as lower eyelid orbicularis hypertrophy and lateral brow and canthal attenuation.[64]

Certain medial fibers of the orbital orbicularis oculi have been referred to by some as the depressor supercilii. However, the depressor supercilii in recent anatomic studies has been identified as a distinct and separate pair of muscles, which insert into the undersurface of the skin at the medial aspect of the eyebrows (see above page 114). The depressor supercilii pulls the eyebrow downward when it contracts (see Figure 13.85).[28,29,31–36,77]

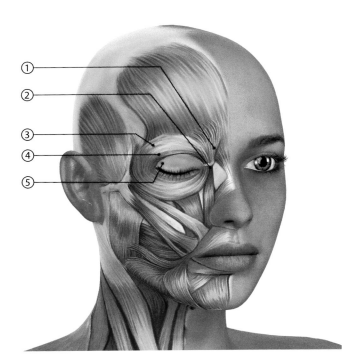

Figure 13.85 The depressor supercilii inserts into the undersurface of the skin just medial to the medial fibers of the *orbital* orbicularis oculi. They assist in depressing the medial eyebrows downward. The *palpebral* part of the orbicularis oculi is subdivided into the *preseptal* and *pretarsal* portions. The *lacrimal* part of the orbicularis oculi lies posterior to the medial canthal ligament. 1, depressor supercilii; 2, orbicularis oculi, lacrimal portion; 3, orbicularis oculi, *orbital* portion; 4, orbicularis oculi, *palpebral* portion, *preseptal*; 5, orbicularis oculi, *palpebral* portion, *pretarsal*. (See Appendix 2—muscle attachments)

The fibers of the *palpebral* part of the orbicularis oculi are half-ellipses which arise from the medial palpebral ligament, the bone on either side of the ligament, and the lateral canthal tendon. The palpebral orbicularis oculi is further subdivided into *pretarsal* and *preseptal* portions (Figure 13.85). The pretarsal orbicularis oculi sits directly above the tarsal plates of the eyelids. The preseptal orbicularis oculi surrounds the pretarsal fibers and courses superficially over and around the orbital septum at the junction between the bony orbit and eyelid. The preseptal fibers arise from the bifurcation of the medial palpebral ligament, while the upper and lower pretarsal fibers traverse laterally to join and form the lateral palpebral raphe or retinaculum.

Contraction of the palpebral orbicularis oculi provides the sphincteric action of the eyelids and gently closes them involuntarily, as with blinking or during sleep. The lower eyelids are drawn up medially and the upper eyelids are pulled down laterally, resulting in a counterclockwise sphincteric closure of the eyelids. Contraction of the pretarsal component of the palpebral orbicularis oculi is responsible for involuntary eyelid closure. It has a lesser effect on the development of lines or soft-tissue malposition than the orbital or preseptal divisions of the orbicularis oculi. Contractions of the preseptal muscle fibers are mainly responsible for blinking and gentle eyelid closure. Contractions of the superior palpebral orbicularis oculi lowers the upper eyelid. This action is opposed by the contractions of both the levator palpebrae superioris and Müller's muscle, which raise the upper eyelid. The palpebral orbicularis oculi should not be treated with OnaBTX-A for cosmetic purposes except in certain situations and only by the most experienced injector because it can cause loss of intentional and involuntary eyelid closure.

The *lacrimal* part of the orbicularis oculi is located posterior to the medial palpebral ligament and lacrimal sac (Figure 13.85; see also Figure 13.132). Its fibers arise from the upper part of the lacrimal crest and travel posteriorly to the lacrimal sac and insert onto the upper and lower tarsal plates medial to the lacrimal puncta. Contraction of the lacrimal orbicularis oculi draws the eyelids and lacrimal papillae posteriorly against the globe, thereby placing the lacrimal puncta in direct contact with the lacrimal lake. Compression on the lacrimal sac dilates it, facilitating the lacrimal pump by creating negative back pressure within the canalicular system, and allowing tears to flow into the nasolacrimal duct (see Figure 13.132).

Because crow's feet are enhanced during smiling and laughing, the contraction of the risorius and zygomaticus major and minor also contribute to the formation of these lateral canthal rhytides.

The zygomaticus major originates anterior to the zygomaticotemporal suture line deep to the orbital orbicularis oculi and travels diagonally toward the corner of the mouth (Figure 13.86). It decussates with the modiolus and inserts into the skin and mucosa of the corners of the mouth. The zygomaticus major pulls the angle of the mouth superiorly, laterally, and posteriorly when a person laughs and smiles.

The zygomaticus minor originates at the zygomatic bone posterior to the zygomaticomaxillary suture line, just anterior to the origin of the zygomaticus major, travels downward and forward and inserts into the mediolateral aspect of the upper lip (Figure 13.86). It helps draw the oral commissures posteriorly and superiorly, especially with laughing, smiling, and other similar facial expressions. The zygomaticus minor also helps to create and elevate the nasolabial fold and to elevate the upper lateral aspect of the upper lip, producing the expression of disdain. Forceful contraction of this muscle can deepen crow's feet and enhance soft-tissue redundancy at the lateral canthus.

The risorius is band like, usually poorly developed, and lies at the upper border of the facial platysma (Figure 13.86). It does not originate from bone, but from the connective tissue and fascia overlying the parotid gland, platysma mandibularis, masseter, and mastoid process. The risorius travels horizontally across the face, superficially to the platysma, intermingles with other muscles within the modiolus,

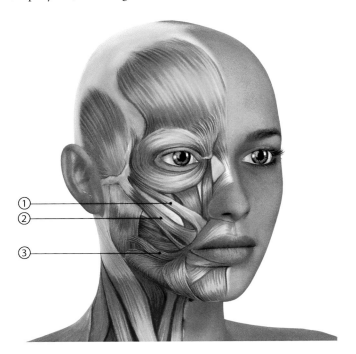

Figure 13.86 Zygomaticus major assists in lifting the lateral upper lip and oral commissure. Zygomatic minor elevates the upper lip more centrally. Risorius is the muscle of laughter and moves the commissure laterally and slightly upward. 1, zygomaticus minor; 2, zygomaticus major; 3, risorius. (See Appendix 2—muscle attachments)

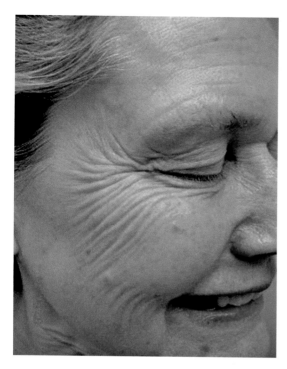

Figure 13.87 Crow's feet accentuated by squinting or smiling in a 64-year-old patient. Contraction of the risorius, zygomaticus major, and zygomaticus minor accentuates the lower aspect of her crow's feet and extends them radially down the cheeks.

and inserts into the skin of the oral commissure. The risorius at times can be indistinguishable from the platysma. The risorius can stretch the lower lip and displace the skin of the cheek posteriorly when laughing, grinning, or smiling, producing dimples in some individuals. Along with the platysma and zygomaticus major, the risorius moves the oral commissures during different facial expressions, downward, upward, and laterally. Consequently, when a person laughs, smiles, or grins they contract the risorius and zygomaticus major and minor, which also accentuate the lower aspect of their crow's feet that extend radially down the cheeks (Figure 13.87) (see Chapter 14).

Dilution for Treating LATERAL CANTHAL LINES (See Appendix 3)
When injecting OnaBTX-A in the periorbital area, it is imperative that minimal volumes be precisely placed. This will necessitate reconstituting a 100 U vial of OnaBTX-A with only 1 mL of normal saline. The recommended and approved method of reconstituting a 100 U vial of OnaBTX-A with 2.5 mL of normal saline may not be the best dilution for precise dosing when injecting precise amounts of OnaBTX-A in areas of the face other than the glabella.

Dosing: How to Correct the Problem (What to Do and What Not to Do) When Treating LATERAL CANTHAL LINES (See Appendix 4)
In September 2013, the FDA approved the use of OnaBTX-A injections for the cosmetic treatment of lateral canthal rhytides, also known as crow's feet.[1,56,87,89]

When one performs injections of OnaBTX-A or any other injectable in the periorbital area, both the patient and the physician should remain unencumbered, comfortable, and without distractions. The patient should be in a sitting or semireclined position, approachable from both the left and right sides. When injecting OnaBTX-A in the lateral canthal area, one should stand on the *opposite* side of the area to be treated with the patient facing toward the injector. This will allow the physician to approach the lateral canthus with the

tip of the needle pointed lateral to and away from the patient's eye. Stretching the skin over the target area with the nondominant hand under ample lighting enables the physician to visualize the plethora of blood vessels that lie just beneath the surface of the skin in this area (Figure 13.88a).

There are two injection patterns that were approved by the FDA for injecting OnaBTX-A in the lateral canthal area (Figure 13.88b–e). These recommended patterns are nearly the same injection patterns that have been used in earlier clinical trials when safety, efficacy, and dosing of OnaBTX-A for lateral canthal rhytides were being investigated. The one injection pattern is indicated when the lateral canthal wrinkles radiate outwardly in parallel lines away from the lateral canthus toward the temporal fossa. Injections of onaBTX-A should commence from a starting point in the center of the lateral canthus (Figure 13.88d: AX). This central injection starting point (point AX) should be at least 1.5–2.0 cm lateral to the lateral canthus and bony orbital rim, where 4 U OnaBTX-A can be injected (Figure 13.88b and d: AX). The second injection point (point BX) (Figure 13.88d: BX) is approximately 1.5–2.0 cm superior and at a 30° angle anteriorly from the first point (point AX) where 4 U of OnaBTX-A can be injected, while always remaining 1.5–2.0 cm lateral to the bony orbital rim. The third injection point (point CX) (Figure 13.88d: CX) is angled at the same 30° angle but in an inferior direction to the first injection point (Figure 13.88d: AX). With this third and inferiorly placed injection of 4 U of OnaBTX-A, it is imperative to remain superiorly positioned to the upper border of the zygomatic arch (i.e., above the Frankfurt plane) and no more medially than an imaginary vertical line passing through the lateral canthus. The Frankfurt plane is identified as an imaginary horizontal line that passes from the superior border of the external auditory meatus to the inferior margin of the bony orbit (Figure 13.88f).

The second recommended injection pattern is for those patients whose majority of lateral canthal rhytides appear below an imaginary horizontal line that bisects the lateral canthus (Figure 13.88c and e). The three injection points of 4 U of OnaBTX-A each should be placed approximately 1.5–2.0 cm lateral to the lateral canthus and reaching a point not more inferiorly to the superior border of the zygomatic arch (Frankfurt plane) and not more medially to an imaginary vertical line that passes through the lateral canthus (Figure 13.88e).

Since the skin of the periorbital area is thin, the tip of the needle should be inserted no more deeply than 2–3 mm below the skin surface, bevel pointing downward. Raising a wheal at each injection point will guarantee the injections are given at the proper depth (Figure 13.88b and c). This will allow the OnaBTX-A to diffuse slowly and evenly into the underlying lateral muscle fibers of the orbital orbicularis oculi. While injecting OnaBTX-A around the lateral canthus, it is important to remain at least 1.5–2.0 cm lateral to the lateral bony orbital rim.[1,87,88] The approved recommended dose for the cosmetic treatment of lateral canthal wrinkles is 4 U of OnaBTX-A injected into each of three sites subcutaneously at the lateral periorbital area 1.5–2.0 cm apart from each other for a total dose of 12 U of OnaBTX-A at each lateral canthus (Figure 13.89). Men may need slightly higher dosing, approximately 15–20 U per side for comparable results[1] (Figure 13.90). Because there can be variable patterns of the lateral canthal lines from one person to the other, OnaBTX-A treatments should be individualized for each patient. Generally, the lateral canthal lines can be identified as upper eyelid creases, lateral canthal creases, or lower eyelid or malar creases (Figure 13.91). Depending on a patient's age and amount of skin laxity, the lower malar creases can continue over the malar aspect of the cheeks as far down as the corners of the mouth. Characteristically, a patient can possess any one or multiple patterns of creases that can even be different in shape and severity from the right-to-left side of the face (Figure 13.92).[90] Even though

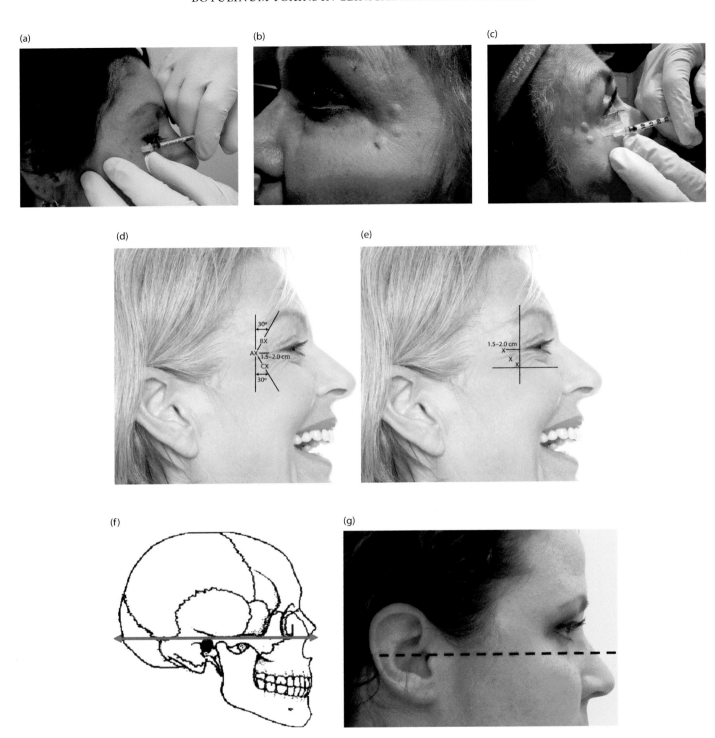

Figure 13.88 (a) Technique of injecting crow's feet or lateral orbital orbicularis oculi. Note the injector stands on the opposite side, pointing and inserting the needle away from the lateral canthus and globe. Stretching the skin with the non-dominant hand assists in visualizing superficial periocular vasculature. (b) Raising a wheal at each injection point will guarantee the injection is given at the proper depth in the crow's feet. (c) Note the wheals of injected OnaBTX-A. (d, e) Injection patterns approved by the FDA. (d) is the most common pattern; (e) is the less common pattern. Pattern (d) is recommended for lateral canthal wrinkles that radiate outwardly in parallel lines starting from a point in the center of the lateral canthus. The central starting point (AX) should be injected at least 1.5–2.0 cm lateral to the lateral canthus and bony orbital rim. The second injection point (BX) is approximately 1.5–2.0 cm superior to (AX) and placed at a 30° angle anteriorly, while always remaining 1.5–2.0 cm lateral to the bony orbital rim. The third injection point (CX) is angled in the same direction but inferior to injection point (AX), and must remain superiorly positioned to the upper border of the zygomatic arch (Frankfurt plane) and no more medially to an imaginary vertical line that passes through the lateral canthus. Pattern (e) is recommended for patients in whom the majority of lateral canthal rhytides appear below an imaginary horizontal line that bisects the lateral canthus. The 3 injection points should each be placed approximately 1.5–2.0 cm lateral to the lateral canthus, remaining superiorly positioned to the superior border of the zygomatic arch (Frankfurt plane) and no more medially than an imaginary vertical line that passes through the lateral canthus. (f, g) the Frankfurt plane: an imaginary horizontal line that passes from the superior border of the external auditory meatus to the inferior margin of the bony orbit.

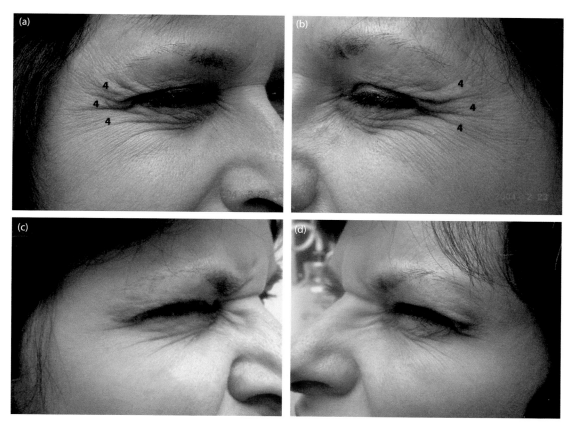

Figure 13.89 A 53-year old woman at rest (a, b) before and (c, d) 6 weeks after treatment with OnaBTX-A. Note the assymetric placement of the injections because of the asymmetric pattern of wrinkling.

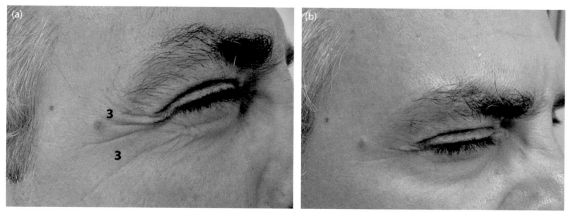

Figure 13.90 A 56-year-old man squinting (a) before and (b) 2 weeks after a treatment with OnaBTX-A.

Kane identified four different patterns of crow's feet, he concluded that the actual patterns manifested by patients were of no true anatomic significance. What mattered mostly was the recognition that there is a diversity in the motion of an individual's orbicularis oculi creating different crow's feet patterns and consequently they should be treated with varying doses of OnaBTX-A accordingly. In addition, a person may have a certain percentage of either static or dynamic wrinkles, but only the dynamic ones are reducible by injections of OnaBTX-A. With experience, a physician injector will come to realize that the number of injection sites and the dose of OnaBTX-A injected will depend on the pattern, depth, and severity of the lateral canthal wrinkling as well as the thickness of the skin and the presence or absence of blood vessels (Figures 13.93 and 13.94).[41–43,78,80,88,90] Men,

generally, will be satisfied with less of a reduction in wrinkling of the lateral canthi, especially during animation such as smiling and laughing (Figure 13.90).

Since lateral canthal wrinkles have been treated with OnaBTX-A for many years by early injectors before the current recommended dosing and injection techniques were approved, different injection techniques were already devised for diverse clinical presentations.[56,84–87] In order to avoid puncturing any one of the many superficial vessels found in and around the lateral canthus, the total dose of OnaBTX-A can be injected intradermally or subcutaneously as a single bolus at one or two sites, producing one or two wheals on the surface of the skin (Figure 13.95). The wheals of OnaBTX-A are then gently massaged toward the temple and away from the orbital fossa in an

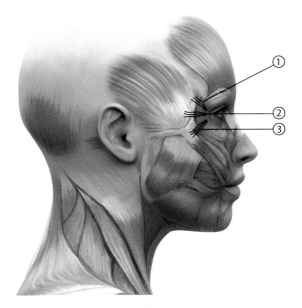

Figure 13.91 Different patterns of crow's feet: 1, upper eyelid; 2, lateral canthal; and 3, lower eyelid or malar eyelid creases.

upward and downward direction. By carefully kneading a bolus of OnaBTX-A around the lateral canthus, the injected OnaBTX-A is dispersed subcutaneously and over the muscle fibers of the lateral orbital orbicularis oculi. This maneuver can prevent post-injection ecchymoses only if none of the periorbital vessels are punctured. The

bolus of OnaBTX-A is always injected 1.5–2.0 cm lateral to the lateral bony orbital margin.

When treating crow's feet, especially at the level of the lower eyelid and lateral malar prominence, it is extremely important to inject OnaBTX-A in the intradermal or superficial subcutaneous plane, where the superficial muscle fibers of the orbital orbicularis oculi insert.

One must avoid deep injections placed inferiorly to the upper border of the zygoma because this will adversely affect and weaken the upper lip levators and result in asymmetry in the lower face and dysfunctional perioral movements.[91] The duration of effect of OnaBTX-A treatments of the lateral canthi usually is about the same as that seen in other areas of the face. At least 3 months and sometimes up to 4 or more months of diminished crow's feet can be obtained with proper dosing and accurate placement of the injections. For some patients, the duration of effect is extended with repeated treatments of OnaBTX-A.

Outcome (Results) When Treating Lateral Canthal Lines

When crow's feet are dynamic because they arise from the contractions of the orbital orbicularis oculi, injecting the proper amount of OnaBTX-A with the correct technique will significantly diminish wrinkling of the area with the least amount of adverse effects (Figure 13.96). However, if the crow's feet are mostly static and the result of photodamage and chronological aging, then the improvement from injections of BoNT will be disappointing, especially if the patient was not warned of this prior to treatment. It is important always to assess and discuss a particular problem and its solution in detail with the patient before initiating a course of treatment with OnaBTX-A. It is also in the best interest of both patient and physician to document the

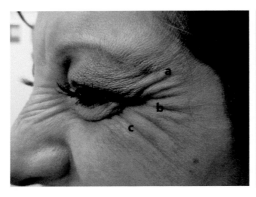
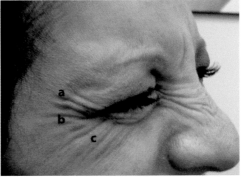

Figure 13.92 Different patterns of crow's feet: a, upper eyelid; b, lateral; and c, lower eyelid and malar creases of the left and right side of a 49-year-old patient squinting before a treatment of OnaBTX-A.

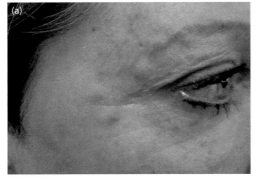
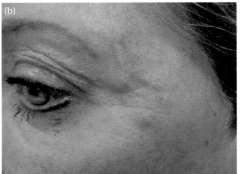

Figure 13.93 (a, b) Notice the shallow blood vessels that lie just beneath the surface of the skin, which are more obvious on the left in this 59-year-old female. Also, note the asymmetric application of superficial boluses of injected OnaBTX-A on the surface of the skin (a, four on the right; b, 2 on the left).

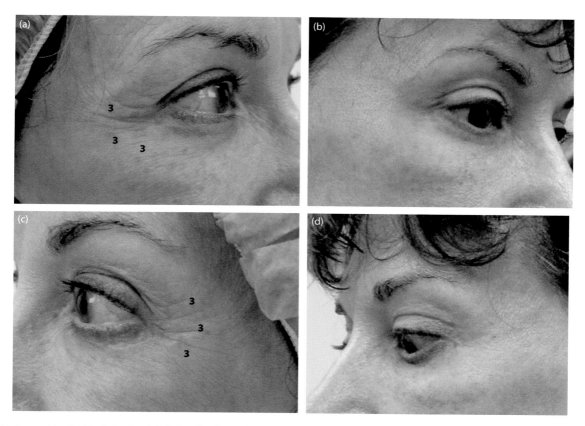

Figure 13.94 A 56-year-old patient (a,c) at rest and (b,d) 3 weeks after an OnaBTX-A treatment. Note the difference in pattern between the right and left crow's feet.

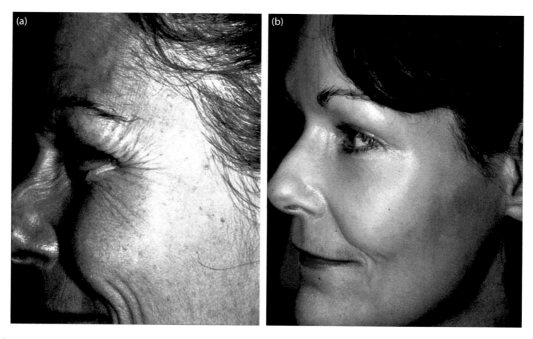

Figure 13.95 Patient's crow's feet (a) before and (b) 2.5 months after a treatment with OnaBTX-A as well as 2 months after full face CO_2 laser resurfacing.

pretreatment consultation both in writing and with photographs (see Appendix 4). The documentation should also include any remarks the patient may have voiced during the interview. All too often, a patient's memory of a physician's concerns and predictions expressed prior to treatment are quickly dismissed and easily forgotten by the patient after treatment.

Most of the time, the best way to diminish lateral canthal static wrinkling is by some form of ablative or non-ablative resurfacing, whether by fractionated laser or other energy-based treatments, dermabrasion, or chemical peeling and the addition of a soft tissue filler when appropriate (Figure 13.95) (see Chapter 7 by Alastair and Jean Carruthers). The different types of non-ablative facial rejuvenation techniques

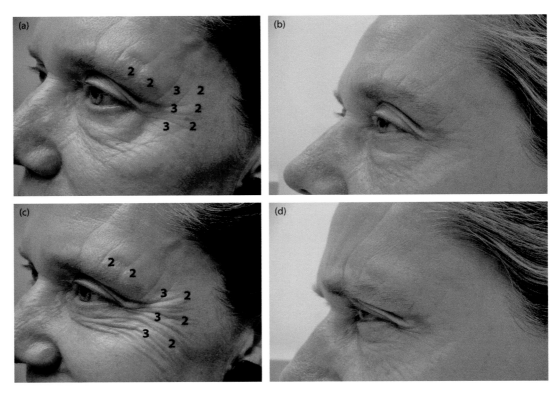

Figure 13.96 A 64-year-old patient at rest with deep, extensive, and recalcitrant crow's feet (a) before and (b) 1 month after OnaBTX-A. Same patient squinting (c) before and (d) 1 month after OnaBTX-A.

still cannot eliminate completely the deep and dense solar elastotic changes that create the pronounced crow's feet in the way many patients over 50 years of age would like. In such cases, oftentimes a treatment regimen of regularly scheduled OnaBTX-A injections after an ablative resurfacing procedure that is periodically augmented by injections of a soft tissue filler is the only way many patients will be able to realize the kind of facial improvement they are seeking (Figure 13.95). Prolongation of such improvements then can be accomplished on a regular basis, albeit infrequently throughout the year, with non-ablative laser, intense pulsed light, or other energy-based facial rejuvenation treatments and the daily application of topical retinoids, alpha hydroxy acids, or similar types of cosmeceuticals (see Chapter 17).

When the lateral orbital orbicularis oculi is exceptionally hyperkinetic, causing deep and elongated recalcitrant crow's feet that resist improvement with injections of OnaBTX-A placed in the recommended manner, additional injections placed posteriorly toward the lateral limits of the orbital orbicularis oculi in the temporal area may further efface those wrinkles (Figure 13.96).[92]

One should be cautious when treating the malar type of lower lateral canthal lines, because most of these lines may be produced by a hyperfunctional zygomaticus major. If the patient possesses redundant skin around the lateral canthus, then injecting OnaBTX-A into the lower crow's feet area can create additional skin folding over the lateral malar prominence and exacerbate the oblique wrinkling over the mid and lateral cheeks.[90] The potential for this may be identified prior to treating the patient with OnaBTX-A by having the patient smile forcibly and repeatedly. If their lower lateral canthal lines are continuous with oblique rhytides radiating down the mid and lateral cheeks, then caution must be taken when injecting the lower malar crow's feet (Figures 13.87 and 13.97). Soft tissue fillers or some form of energy-based resurfacing procedure may be the best way to rid the patient of these particularly difficult to treat types of rhytides. Treating the zygomaticus major with OnaBTX-A can easily

result in an asymmetric smile and a dysfunctional upper lip[91] (see Asymmetries below).

Complications (Adverse Sequelae) When Treating LATERAL CANTHAL LINES (See Appendix 6)

When injecting the lateral orbital orbicularis oculi, OnaBTX-A should be placed intradermally or subdermally, 1.5–2.0 cm lateral to an imaginary vertical line that passes through the lateral canthus. Also, the *intradermal* injections should *not* be placed below the level of the superior margin of the zygomatic arch. Otherwise, some of the muscle fibers of the levators of the lateral aspect of the upper lip and corners of the mouth (zygomaticus major and minor) will be affected and weakened by the spread of the OnaBTX-A.[90,91] This can occur because the zygomaticus major and minor originate at or near the lateral aspect of the superior margin of the zygomatic arch (Figure 13.86). If either the zygomaticus major or zygomaticus minor is inadvertently exposed to OnaBTX-A, the lateral one fourth of the ipsilateral upper lip will be weakened, causing a drooping of the upper oral commissure, an asymmetric smile, and possible drooling and dribbling from incontinence of food and liquid. If OnaBTX-A is injected or even spreads more medially and inferiorly to the superior margin of the zygomatic arch, then the central and deep upper lip levators (levator labii superioris, levator labii superioris alaeque nasi, and levator anguli oris) can be affected, causing a more profound interference with upper lip competence and basic sphincteric functions, resulting in dysarthria and dysphagia.[91]

Injecting subcutaneously small volumes of concentrated OnaBTX-A far enough (i.e., 1.5–2.0 cm) away from the lateral side wall of the bony orbit will prevent the unintended migration of OnaBTX-A medially and into the superior or inferior, or both, palpebral orbicularis oculi. If this occurs, weakening of the lateral canthal tendon occurs, producing lower eyelid retraction and possible ectropion, which manifests as rounding of the lateral canthus (Figure 13.98). Rounding can lead to secondary complications, initially manifesting as epiphora (tearing), then with

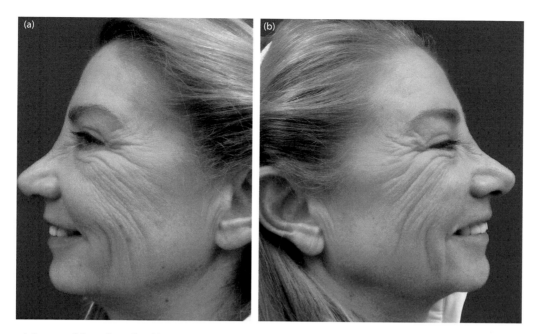

Figure 13.97 Lower crow's feet extend down the mid and lateral cheeks in this 62-year-old patient.

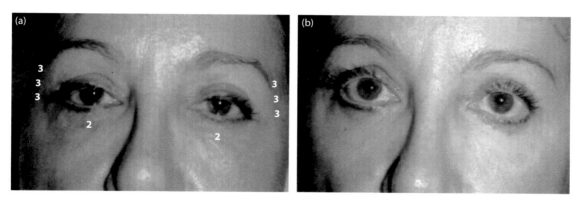

Figure 13.98 (a) Before 2 U of OnaBTX-A were injected into each lower eyelid along with 9 U of OnaBTX-A into the lateral canthus of a 55-year-old patient, 8 years postblepharoplasty. (b) Same patient 3 weeks later with asymptomatic lateral canthal rounding and lower eyelid ectropion. Note the scleral show and unnatural and unattractive rounding of the lateral canthi.

unabated eyelid weakness and prolonged corneal exposure, secondary xerophthalmia (dry eye) can easily develop, which eventually can result in debilitating corneal damage (superficial punctate keratitis).[64,70]

Because of their position within the orbit, the lateral and inferior rectus, or inferior oblique are especially disposed to accidental diffusion of injected OnaBTX-A through the orbital septum. This results when any BoNT is injected too close to the lateral canthus, which is closer than 1.5–2.0 cm from the bony rim of the orbit. If any of the extraocular muscles are inadvertently weakened by improper injection techniques of OnaBTX-A, diplopia and strabismus will result. If any of these serious complications does occur, immediate consultation with an ophthalmologist is imperative.

Overzealous treatments of OnaBTX-A in the lateral periorbital area given in high doses with high volume also can result in brow ptosis, ectropion, diplopia, lagophthalmos, xerophthalmia and keratitis sicca, and even superficial punctate keratitis because of corneal exposure. Direct injection of OnaBTX-A into the pretarsal orbicularis oculi has been reported as the cause of diminished tear secretion resulting in ocular irritation, xerophthalmia, and an abnormal Schirmer's test after treatment of lateral canthal rhytides.[93] This occurred because the pretarsal orbicularis oculi was inadvertently

weakened by a poor injection technique and the patient was unable to fully contract (blink) and activate the "lacrimal pump" (see Figure 13.132). The possibility of just simple diffusion of the OnaBTX-A into the muscle fibers of the orbicularis oculi or into the lacrimal gland as the cause for the reduction in tear secretion was excluded because the xerophthalmia remitted as the strength of the orbicularis returned.[93]

Brow ptosis is caused by the diffusion of OnaBTX-A into the lower fibers of the frontalis when OnaBTX-A is injected rapidly and forcefully, or when the area is massaged too vigorously after injection (Figure 13.99). Patients can cause brow ptosis if they manipulate the injected area excessively immediately after a treatment session, enough to disperse the OnaBTX-A beyond the targeted area. Injecting large volumes of low concentrations of OnaBTX-A also increases the risk of dispersion of product beyond the targeted muscle. Ectropion occurs when OnaBTX-A diffuses into the lower palpebral orbicularis oculi and the muscular sling of the lateral orbicularis is inadvertently weakened by the injections of OnaBTX-A, especially in someone who has had a previous interventional eyelid procedure such as a blepharoplasty, deep chemical peeling or laser resurfacing, and so on. This is generally seen as lower eyelid retraction manifesting as excessive rounding of the contour of the lateral canthus (Figure 13.98).[64]

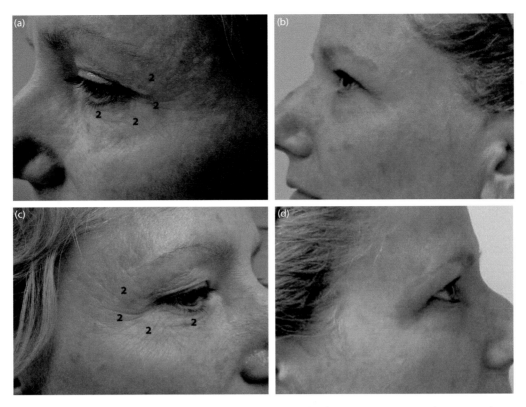

Figure 13.99 A 49-year-old woman (a, c) before and (b, d) after she developed brow ptosis 2 weeks after OnaBTX-A treatment for reasons unknown: patient manipulation or physician's technique or both.

Excess skin permits the eyelids and the periorbita to function normally. In the lateral canthal area, when the orbital orbicularis oculi contracts it elevates the redundant lateral eyelid skin and usually redistributes it locally. However, when the lateral orbital orbicularis oculi is completely denervated by a BoNT, this no longer occurs and the redundant lower eyelid skin forms a visible roll or folds of skin (Figure 13.100).[90] In severe cases, even at rest, there can be this extra roll of skin seen at the junction of the lower lateral eyelid and submalar cheek skin.[90] In rare instances, when the lateral orbital orbicularis oculi is repeatedly and consistently weakened with BoNT treatments and the crow's feet remain perpetually and completely effaced, subsequent muscle atrophy results in a flattening of the lateral periorbita. Consequently, when the lateral upper lip levators (zygomatic major and minor) are still functioning normally and the patient smiles emphatically, there may appear a peculiarly abrupt change in the contour of the upper lateral malar area with the lateral canthus.[90] As the lower lateral muscle fibers of the orbicularis oculi wrap around the lateral canthal angle they become horizontal in orientation. Normally when the patient smiles, these horizontal fibers of the inferior orbital orbicularis oculi contract and elevate the skin of the lateral submalar cheek in a vertical direction. When the zygomaticus complex along with this accessory elevator function of the inferior orbital orbicularis oculi move the skin and soft tissue of the lateral submalar cheek laterally and upward, they enhance the formation of a malar mound.[87] When the lateral canthal area is consistently and completely denervated with injections of a BoNT, there is a loss of upper cheek elevation by the orbital orbicularis oculi. This will cause any lax skin just inferior to the lower eyelid to become redundant and fold onto itself when a person laughs or intensely smiles. In younger patients who still have tight and elastic periorbital skin, an abrupt contour difference between the lower lateral periorbita and the upper zygoma may become annoyingly apparent (Figure 13.100). However, in older patients with loose,

inelastic skin, a full smile may create the unnatural appearance of a ledge separating flatter lower lateral canthal skin from fuller submalar cheek skin (Figure 13.100). There also can be some flattening of the normally occurring upper cheek malar mound. For these patients, a hyaluronic acid soft tissue filler in the lateral malar and canthal deficit is the best way to correct such a problem (Figure 13.100d).

The incidence of the usual transient adverse sequelae that accompany a transcutaneous injection, including pain, erythema, edema, and ecchymoses can be partially mitigated with the use of ice before and after injections, and the application of a local topical anesthetic. The anatomy of the periocular area, however, makes occluding the topical anesthetic to expedite its effect somewhat difficult and impractical. The patient also should be reminded to stop at least two weeks prior to treatment any alcoholic beverages, and non-essential, self-administered medications, such as aspirin, nonsteroidal anti-inflammatory drugs (NSAIDs), and other over-the counter medications, and food supplements that increase coagulation time.

There has not been a confirmed serious case of spread of toxin effect away from the injection site when OnaBTX-A has been used at the recommended dose to treat crow's feet lines.[1]

Figures 13.101 through 13.105 are some examples of different patients treated with OnaBTX-A to reduce their crow's feet (lateral canthal lines).

Treatment Implications When Injecting the Lateral Orbicularis Oculi (Crow's Feet)

1. All periocular injections of OnaBTX-A should be done under adequate lighting to visualize the abundant vasculature and placed in the lower dermis or superficial subcutaneous tissue to avoid bruising.
2. Inject OnaBTX-A slowly, placing the needle 1.5–2.0 cm lateral to the bony orbital rim and directing it away from the globe in

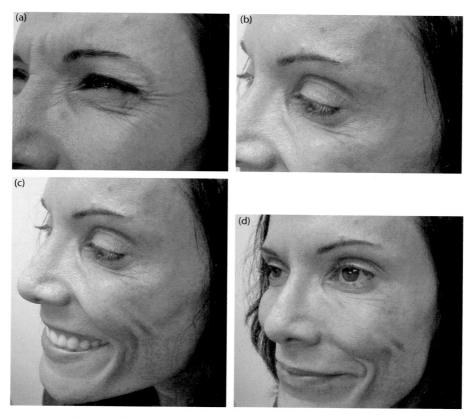

Figure 13.100 A 40-year-old patient is seen (a) before and (b) 2 weeks after OnaBTX-A treatment of the lateral canthal wrinkles. Note the flattening of the lateral canthal area due to weakening of the orbicularis oculi. Same patient seen with lateral malar deficit smiling (c) before and (d) immediately after a hyaluronic acid filler treatment.

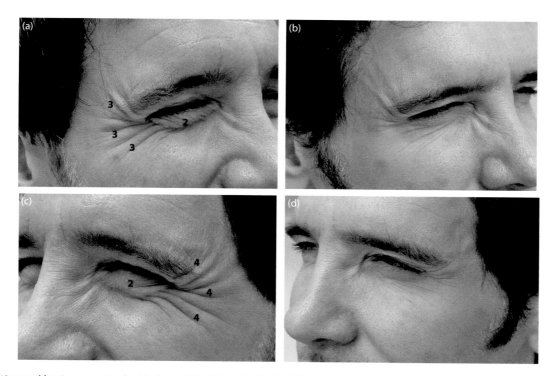

Figure 13.101 A 48-year-old patient squinting (a, c) before and (b, d) 3 weeks after OnaBTX-A treatment. Note the difference in wrinkle patterns between the right and left crow's feet.

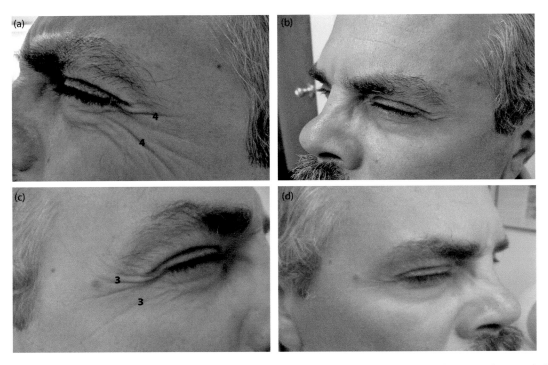

Figure 13.102 A 56-year-old squinting (a, c) before and (b, d) 2 weeks after an OnaBTX-A treatment. Note the difference in the patterns between the left- and right-side crow's feet.

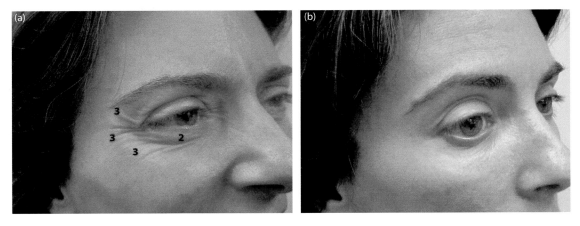

Figure 13.103 A 46-year-old patient squinting (a) before and (b) 2 weeks after an OnaBTX-A treatment.

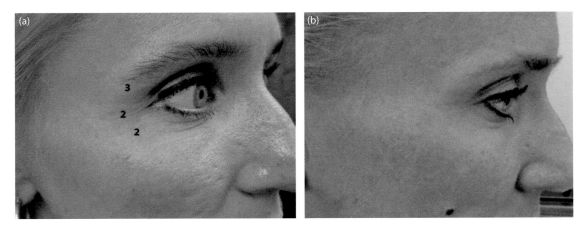

Figure 13.104 A 41-year-old patient at rest (a) before and (b) 4 weeks after an OnaBTX-A treatment.

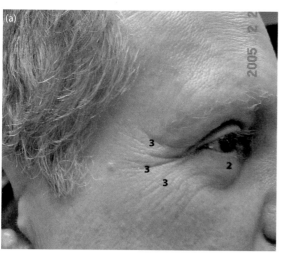 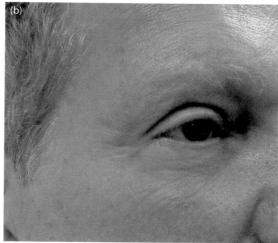

Figure 13.105 This 64-year-old patient at rest (a) before and (b) 6 weeks after an OnaBTX-A treatment.

the lateral canthal area to avoid injury to the eye, diplopia, and other adverse sequelae.

3. Older patients will have varying degrees of improvement after a treatment of OnaBTX-A, depending on the amount of photoaging, redundant skin, and static wrinkling present.

4. Post-treatment ecchymoses can last over one week, fallaciously suggesting incompetence and a substandard injection technique by the injector. Stop self-administered aspirin, non-steroidal anti-inflammatory drugs (NSAIDs), and other non-essential medications, and all home remedies that increase coagulation time at least two weeks before a treatment session. The application of ice before and moderate point pressure to the skin with ice after an injection of OnaBTX-A can reduce the extent of ecchymoses.

5. Different doses of OnaBTX-A can be injected into each lateral canthus in the same patient depending on the pattern and extent of their lateral canthal wrinkling.

6. Injecting the lower lateral canthus with large volumes of OnaBTX-A can produce upper lip asymmetry and cheek ptosis if the upper lip levators, zygomaticus major and minor are inadvertently affected. Therefore, inject OnaBTX-A lateral to an imaginary vertical line that passes through the lateral canthus, and place the needle above the superior margin of the zygoma (Frankfurt plane) while remaining 1.5–2.0 cm away from the bony orbital rim.

7. Precisely dosed and accurately placed low-volume OnaBTX-A injections are essential to avoid adverse sequelae in the periorbital area.

PERIORBITAL AREA: EYEBROW LIFT

Introduction: Problem Assessment and Patient Selection

With the progression of time and the accumulation of hours spent outdoors, the skin of the face as well as the rest of the body becomes more inelastic, causing the skin to sag and drape more loosely. This can result in the overhanging of skin of the lateral brow with the uniquely characteristic appearance of hooding or ptosis of the lateral eyebrows[92,94] (Figure 13.106). The thick skin of the lateral brow, when it becomes ptotic, gives the bearer a "heavy," down-trodden look. It makes one appear tired, overburdened with worries, and preoccupied with concerns. High, arched lateral eyebrows convey an expression of happiness, vigor, approval, confidence, and sensuality. However, depressed, low lying or flat lateral eyebrows convey an expression of sadness, fatigue, anxiety, disdain, and disapproval. Lateral brow hooding frequently intensifies with advancing age. The physical appearance of lateral brow hooding generally affects men at a later age than women, but men as well as women with this problem eventually will benefit from an upper eyelid blepharoplasty, brow lift, or both when the hooding progresses and peripheral vision is impeded. In the meantime, myorelaxation with BoNTs will forestall the inevitable by

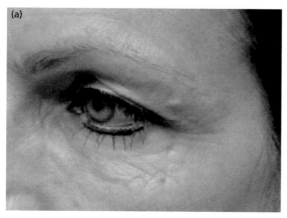 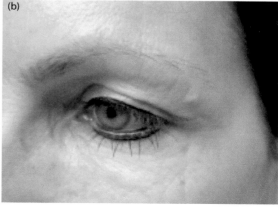

Figure 13.106 This 49-year-old patient is shown (a) before and (b) 3 weeks after OnaBTX-A was injected into the lateral aspect of the orbicularis oculi. Note the muscle fibers of the lower lateral frontalis raising the tail of the eyebrow and diminishing lateral hooding of the lateral aspect of the upper eyelid.

elevating the lateral brow and providing one with many more years of a more youthful, less tired appearance.

The overall appeal of the contour and shape of an individual's eyebrows depends on many factors, including age, sex, ethnicity, culture, and current fashion trends. The size, shape, and position of the eyebrows can vary widely, inherently dependent on the shape of the face (i.e., long, oval, heart, round, square, or diamond) (Figure 13.107).[99,96] Consequently, in clinical practice the "ideal eyebrow" cannot be universally applied to all faces. One should not force a particular shape of eyebrow on a given face because eyebrows that appear

(a)

SHAPE	DIAGRAM	PHOTO	EFFECT
Curved			Defaults to a thoughtful expression. Gives a more professional look.
Angled			Makes the face appear more youthful.
Soft angled			Similar to above, but its peak is softer, more subtle and feminine. This is often referred to as the ideal brow.
Round angled			Makes a face appear rounder. Softens faces and emphasizes the "heart" in a heart shaped face.
Flat			Makes the face appear shorter and more oval. Great for longer face. Natural look.

(b)

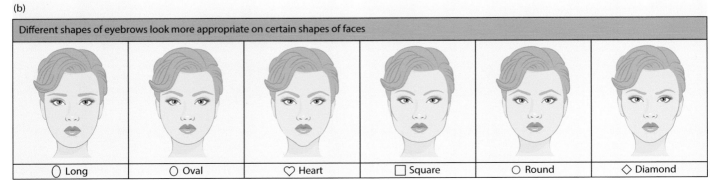

Different shapes of eyebrows look more appropriate on certain shapes of faces					
◯ Long	◯ Oval	♡ Heart	☐ Square	◯ Round	◇ Diamond

Figure 13.107 (a) Different shapes of eyebrows and how they affect the overall shape of the face. (b) Different shapes of eyebrows look more appropriate on certain shapes of faces:

aesthetically pleasing on one face may look abnormal and unattractive on another face. To produce acceptable results with injections of BoNT, each patient's face must be evaluated individually. It is incumbent on the physician injector to perform a detailed pretreatment assessment of how an individual's eyebrow shape and position conform to the contours of the "ideal brow" and to the aesthetic appearance of that particular individual's face.

The ideal contour and apex of the female eyebrow has been debated for decades. In May 1974, Westmore presented for the first time a paper on "Facial Cosmetics in Conjunction with Surgery" at the Aesthetic Plastic Surgery Society meeting in Vancouver, British Columbia, Canada, where he described specific morphologic characteristics of the "ideal" female eyebrow.[97] Westmore placed the apex of the female eyebrow arch over the lateral limbus. He indicated that the medial portion of the eyebrow should begin just above a vertical line drawn from the lateral edge of the ala nasi through the medial canthus. He further detailed how the lateral extent of the eyebrow should intersect a tangential line connecting the lateral canthus and the lateral aspect of the ala nasi. Lastly, the medial and lateral aspects of the eyebrow should fall within the same horizontal plane (Figure 13.108). The medial head of the eyebrow should have a "clubhead" configuration, and there should be a gradual tapering laterally toward the tail of the eyebrow into a point.

In 1985 Angres proposed a different paradigm for the "ideal female brow," which was predicated on the width of an individual's medial intercanthal space.[98] He believed that properly shaped and positioned eyebrows could create the illusion of a perfectly balanced face even if the eyes were too close together or too far apart. Normal or average intercanthal distances range from approximately 30–35 mm, roughly equal to the width of one eye (palpebral length = 28–30 mm). Angres felt that one therefore

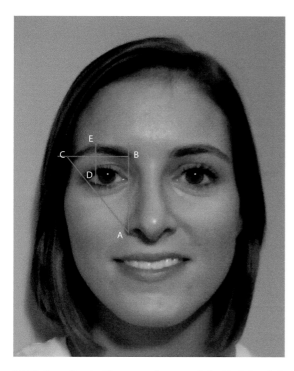

Figure 13.108 According to Westmore, the apex of the ideal female brow (E) should be positioned over the lateral limbus (D); the medial portion lying just above a vertical line drawn from the lateral ala through the medial canthus (AB); the lateral extent intersecting a tangential line connecting the lateral canthus and lateral ala (AC); and the medial and lateral aspects falling within the same horizontal plane (BC).

should consider the patient's intercanthal distance when assessing a patient's ideal eyebrow position (Figure 13.109).[98] If the medial intercanthal distance is normal, as it usually is in patients with oval-shaped faces, the medial aspect of the eyebrow should start at a vertical line that bisects the medial canthus (Figure 13.109a). The apex of the eyebrow, then, was more aesthetically appealing centered at the mid-pupillary line, or even slightly lateral as far as the edge of the lateral limbus, with the eyebrow ending slightly obliquely above the lateral canthus (Figure 13.109a). However, if the intercanthal distance is increased with wide-set eyes, as can be found with individuals of Asian or African ancestry, the eyebrow should begin medial to the medial canthus (Figure 13.109b). The apex of the arch should be above the *medial* edge of the limbus, or no farther lateral than the midpupillary line, and the tail of the eyebrows should end directly above the lateral canthus. These dimensions give the illusion of bringing the eyebrows closer together. On the other hand, a narrower intercanthal distance of close-set eyes seen in individuals with narrow faces, requires the eyebrow to start lateral to the vertical line that bisects the medial canthus (Figure 13.109c). The apex of the eyebrows should appear just above the *lateral* edge of the limbus, or slightly lateral to it, and the tail of the eyebrow should end at an acutely oblique angle from the lateral canthus (Figure 13.109c). This will draw one's attention temporally instead of nasally, making close-set eyes appear farther apart.[98]

Because Westmore's "ideal female eyebrow" was based on an oval face, there were many modifications to his standard measurements, depending on the facial shape of the subjects used in a particular clinical study. Cook and colleagues along with Gunter and Atrobus proposed that the apex of the eyebrow should appear more laterally, approximately halfway between the lateral limbus and the lateral canthus.[99,100] They also indicated that the medial brow should start as a continuation of the superciliary ridge and it should appear lower than the lateral brow. Roth and Metzinger compared the eyebrow apex of fashion models with a group of randomly selected volunteer women.[101] They found that the apex of the eyebrow should be more lateral than the lateral limbus, but just medial to the lateral canthus. In addition, the lateral brow should be higher than the medial brow on the horizontal plane, but never taking into account the shape of the face in their descriptions. Subsequently, Biller and Kim used independent Asian and Caucasian female evaluators to identify the preferred location of the eyebrow apex in Asian versus Caucasian women models. The fact that Asians tend to have a greater intercanthal distance compared to Caucasians played no significant role in the evaluators' preference to the location of the ideal eyebrow apex. In general, the evaluators, regardless of their ethnicity, favored a more lateral brow apex in younger faces, and a more medial brow apex in older ones, irrespective of the ethnicity of the models evaluated.[102]

In a similar study, Schreiber, et al. designed a study to define the dimensions of an aesthetically pleasing eyebrow from the perspective of the general public.[103] They surveyed 100 individuals in their local community and asked them to rank 27 photographs of models and of pre- and postblepharoplasty patients as either "attractive" or "unattractive." The result of their study revealed the general public prefers the eyebrow to be placed in a lower position than what was observed postoperatively and what is currently described in the literature. The study respondents felt many of the post-blepharoplasty eyebrows were placed too high, resulting in a look of constant surprise. They also preferred the arch of the eyebrow be positioned more laterally in relation to the lateral limbus than what was done postoperatively (Figure 13.108).[103]

In summary, current principles of eyebrow aesthetics dictate that the overall shape of the "ideal female eyebrow" in an *oval* face should appear as the continuation of the aesthetic dorsal line of the nose as

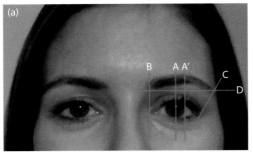
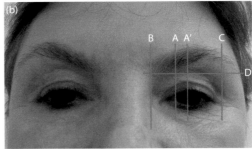
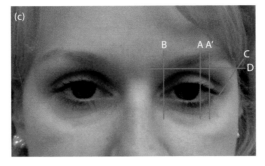

Figure 13.109 Brow position, as seen in oval, round, and narrow facial shapes. (a) Normally spaced eyes and brow position in an oval face. With a normal intercanthal distance, the apex of the brow should be centered above the mid-pupillary line (A) or at the lateral edge of the lateral limbus (A′). The medial aspect of the eyebrow should start at a vertical line that bisects the medial canthus (B). The eyebrow should end slightly obliquely above the lateral canthus (C), and lie approximately 1–2 cm above the horizontal line that joins the tail and the head of the eyebrow (D). (b) Wide-set eyes and brow position in a round face. The apex of the eyebrow should be positioned above the medial edge of the limbus (A) or close to the midpupillary line (A′). The eyebrow should begin medial to the medial canthus (B). The tail of the eyebrow should end directly above the lateral canthus (C), and lie on the same horizontal plane as the head of the eyebrow (D). (c) Close-set eyes and brow position in a narrow face. The apex of the eyebrow can appear just above the lateral edge of the limbus (A) or slightly lateral to it (A′). The eyebrow should start lateral to the vertical line that bisects the medial canthus (B). The tail should end at an acutely oblique angle from the lateral canthus (C) and lie approximately 2–4 cm below the horizontal line that joins the tail and the head of the eyebrow (D). (From Angres GG. *Annals of Ophthalmology* 1985; 17(10): 605–11.)

it curves laterally onto the superciliary ridge toward the medial brow (Figure 13.107). The ideal female eyebrow should begin at a point approximately 1 cm above the supraorbital rim where an imaginary vertical line drawn from the lateral border of the ala nasi transects the inner canthus. The eyebrow should end laterally where it meets an oblique line drawn from the most lateral point of the ala nasi through the lateral canthus. The medial and lateral ends of the eyebrow should lie on approximately the same horizontal plane with the tail of the eyebrow 1–2 mm higher than the head of the eyebrow. The apex of the arc of the eyebrow should lie on a vertical line directly above or slightly lateral to the lateral limbus of the iris of the eye (at the approximate junction of the medial two-thirds and the lateral one-third of the eyebrow). In some women whose overall facial shape is not exactly oval, the brow can peak at the lateral canthus instead of the lateral limbus.

Finally, when the face is not oval, make-up can assist one in subtly modifying Westmore's "ideal brow." Make-up artists, in particular, can change the position and shape of the eyebrows, thereby creating the illusion of the "ideal" oval face.[95,98,101,102] Certain face shapes may look more attractive with these compensatory modifications in brow position than strictly adhering to the traditional dimensions of the Westmore ideal brow.[104] For example, a square face favors soft curves of the eyebrows with the apex of the arch lateral to the lateral limbus and the tail of the eyebrow directed at the center of the ear. This makes the angles of the face seem less harsh and appears to decrease the distance between the upper and lower halves of the face. A long and thin face may look more attractive with a straighter, less-arched eyebrow, with the tail pointing closer to the top of the ear. This gives the illusion of reducing the length of the face. A round face is enhanced with a high arch that also points to the top of the ear to enhance the angularity of the face[95,104] (Figure 13.110). Last,

the overall silhouette of a female eyebrow should be that of the wings of a gull.

The position of the eyebrows and where they sit over the supraorbital arch is also very important. Cook et al. observed that in women the apex of the arch of the eyebrow usually is found well above the supraorbital bony rim, whereas in men it is located at the level of the orbital bony rim.[99] Not only does the male eyebrow differ in position from the female eyebrow, but it commonly also differs in shape. Usually, the ideal female eyebrow sits approximately 5 mm above the bony orbital margin, nicely arched and has a club-shaped medial portion[96,99] (Figure 13.108). Normally, however, the male eyebrow is flatter (less arched), thicker and

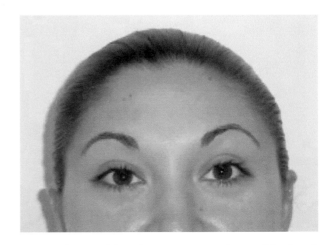

Figure 13.110 The apex of the eyebrow in someone with a round face is preferentially close to the lateral canthus.

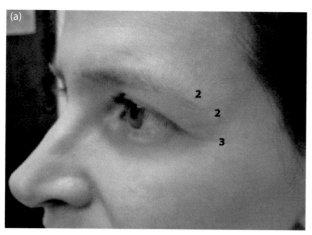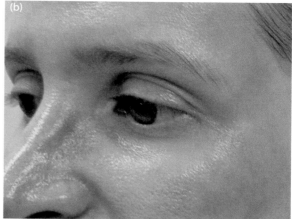

Figure 13.111 A 40-year-old at rest (a) before and (b) 3 weeks after OnaBTX-A treatment. Note the difference in the lateral brow height.

more prominent laterally and positioned lower, sitting on the superciliary arch just above the superior bony orbital margin[96,99,100] (Figure 13.4).

Functional Anatomy of the Eyebrow Lift (See Appendix 2)

The form and function of the eyebrows are essential in making the eyes and the whole face appear aesthetically pleasing. While the eyebrows play a significant role in preventing perspiration from running into the eyes, women in particular, are often dissatisfied with the natural shape of their eyebrows and incessantly thin and reshape them.[28] The reason for lateral brow ptosis is multifactorial. As the skin and supportive soft tissues of the periorbita become inelastic and redundant, the lower lateral fibers of the frontalis become less efficient in elevating the heavy mass of periorbital skin and soft tissue above the lateral bony orbital. In addition, the antagonistic muscle movements of repeated frowning and the strong contractions (i.e., depressor action) of the vertical fibers of the lateral orbital orbicularis oculi, in conjunction with the ineffective levator action of the lateral frontalis, progressively produce a downward drooping of the lateral eyebrow[96] (Figure 13.111). Anatomical studies of cadavers have shown that there is a fat pad beneath the eyebrow, which is secured to the supraorbital ridge by dense fibrous attachments. Because the supraorbital ridge extends to only over the medial one-half to two-thirds of the orbit, the lateral part of the eyebrow lacks deep tissue and structural support, causing it to droop more easily along with the frontal skin as the frontalis becomes more relaxed with age.[92] Since the lateral eyebrow has less support from deeper structures than what the medial eyebrow has, the balance of forces acting on the eyebrow selectively depresses the lateral aspect of the brow. In time, the subgalea fat pad glide plane facilitates increased brow mobility and the gravitational downward migration of the galea and preseptal fat pads. Therefore, brow ptosis is promoted by: (1) the relaxation of the lateral frontalis resting tone; (2) the forces of gravity pulling down on the lateral brow soft tissues; and (3) the corrugator supercilii in conjunction with the lateral muscle fibers of the orbital orbicularis oculi antagonistically pulling down on the frontalis and directly affecting the descent of the lateral brow.[94] (See above for a full description of the glabellar levator and depressor muscles.)

Dilution for Lifting the Eyebrow (See Appendix 3)

Treating the periorbital area should be done with low volume, highly concentrated OnaBTX-A. Therefore, reconstituting a 100 U vial of OnaBTX-A with 1 mL of normal saline is best for accurate injections with precise dosing and minimal trauma when a 3/10 mL

Becton-Dickenson U-100 insulin syringe with a 31-gauge needle is used.[37]

Dosing: How to Correct the Problem, (What to Do and What Not to Do) When Lifting the Eyebrow

To elevate and enhance the arching of the lateral eyebrow, especially in women, 2–4 U or even more of OnaBTX-A can be injected intradermally or subdermally into the lateral brow depressor, that is, the lateral orbital orbicularis oculi, in the vicinity of its maximal contraction. This often is seen clinically as corrugations in and around the tail of the eyebrow (Figure 13.112). They commonly are located where the lateral aspect of the superciliary arch meets the lower aspect of the anterior temporal fusion line at the zygomatic process of the frontal bone (Figures 13.69 and 13.113). Depending on the idiosyncratic anatomy of the patient being treated, intradermal injections can be placed just above, below or within the hairs of the lateral aspect and tail of the eyebrow (Figure 13.114). One or usually no more than three equally spaced injections of 2–4 U of OnaBTX-A can be given intradermally in this area of maximal muscle contraction, placed no more medially than the mid-pupillary line. Higher doses can be used with a lesser number of injection points. Injecting OnaBTX-A superficially in this area reduces the depressor action of the horizontal and vertical muscle fibers of the orbital orbicularis oculi at the lateral aspect of the brow, and allows the muscle fibers of the lower lateral frontalis to elevate the lateral eyebrow (Figure 13.115).

With the patient in the sitting or semireclined position, have the patient forcibly elevate and depress the eyebrows. This will allow one to assess the depressor strength of the lateral orbital orbicularis oculi and the levator strength of the lateral frontalis. After determining the dose of OnaBTX-A needed, have the patient once again forcibly elevate the eyebrows. Facilitate and maintain this upward movement by supporting the skin of the brow with the thumb and index finger of the nondominant hand (Figures 13.116 and 13.117). This maneuver allows the lower muscle fibers of the frontalis to rise, thereby uncovering and exposing the superficial muscle fibers of the upper orbital orbicularis oculi. With the needle pointing upward and away from the orbit and globe, inject *intradermally* approximately 2 U to no more than a total of 8 U of OnaBTX-A into one and usually no more than three injection sites along the lateral brow. In patients with very strong orbital orbicularis oculi who display a significant amount of lateral brow depression and hooding with or without corrugations, start the injections just lateral to the mid-pupillary line 2.5–3.0 cm above the supraorbital bony rim. Place the injections irrespective of where the eyebrow sits over the superciliary arch, because commonly

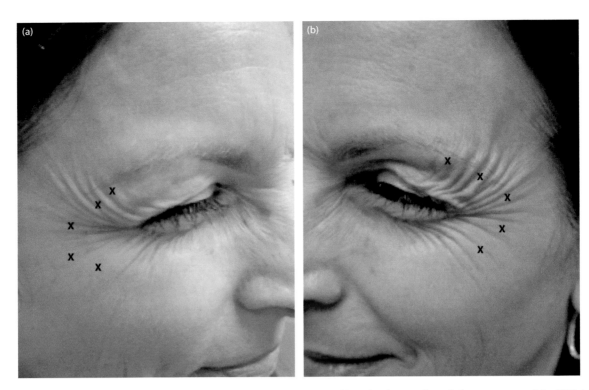

Figure 13.112 A 49-year-old patient with many wrinkles and corrugations of the upper lid and lateral eyebrow is shown before a treatment of OnaBTX-A. Note how the corrugations vary from right (a) to left (b). (X marks where 1–3 U of OnaBTX-A can be injected intradermally in the lateral aspect of the upper eyelid).

women's eyebrows are located higher than men's (Figure 13.114). Injecting OnaBTX-A subdermally or in the superficial subcutaneous tissue approximately 1 cm apart from each other and finish at a point where the superciliary arch meets the lower aspect of the anterior temporal fusion line (Figure 13.116). OnaBTX-A must be injected slowly and *superficially*. Raising a wheal at each injection point will guarantee the injections are given at the proper depth of the intradermal/subcutaneous interface (Figure 13.117). Ordinarily, in these patients with very strong orbital orbicularis oculi one to three

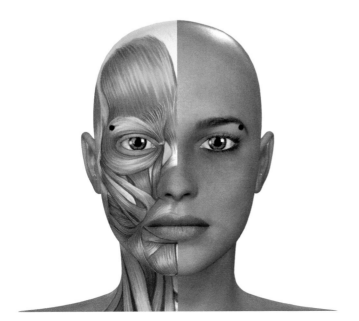

Figure 13.113 Location of the main injection point (•) when attempting to elevate the lateral aspect of the eyebrow.

intradermal injections of 2–3 U of OnaBTX-A placed into the lateral aspect of the brow also will suffice to produce an aesthetically pleasing lateral brow lift and a diminution of idiosyncratic lateral brow corrugations (Figures 13.118 and 13.119). This superficial injection technique will reduce the risk of the OnaBTX-A dispersing beyond the intended area and producing adverse sequelae, that is, brow and eyelid ptosis, ectropion, strabismus, diplopia, or xerophthalmia (see Complications below and Appendix 6).

Outcomes (Results) When Lifting the Eyebrow (See Appendix 5)

Lateral brow elevation is best appreciated as a decrease in hooding of the lateral aspect of the upper eyelid (Figure 13.120).[71,104] Elevating the eyebrows at their medial, central, or lateral aspects can be unpredictable when first attempted, but usually reproducible when the proper technique is used and specific clinical records and appropriate photographs are kept (see Appendix 4).[61] With the proper technique the complication rate is low and for some individuals the results might be subtle at best. Therefore, each patient's clinical record must include diagrammatic as well as sequential photographic documentation along with detailed progress notes if reproducible results are expected. The desirability of lifting the eyebrows for patients of different cultural backgrounds also will depend on current fashion trends and acceptable ethnic standards[102] (see Chapter 17 by Kyle Seo). The possibility of lifting the eyebrows will depend on the patient's overall physiognomy and idiosyncratic anatomy. The feasibility of doing so will depend on whether the physician is capable of injecting OnaBTX-A with a proper and reproducible technique. Typically, the effects of OnaBTX-A in the area of the lateral brow last as long as those of the glabella.

It is important to identify and remind each patient that attempting to eliminate the horizontal forehead lines that are positioned immediately above, adjacent to, or within the lateral eyebrows is virtually impossible without causing lateral brow ptosis (Figure 13.70). Those lines exist because they identify a person with compensatory brow lifting and

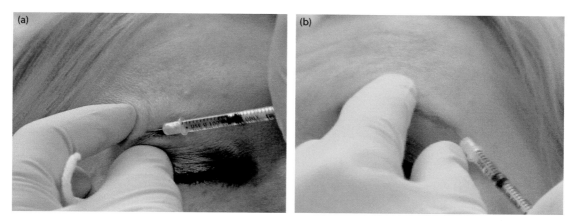

Figure 13.114 The exact location of injection points on the skin of an individual's lateral brow may vary according to the person's anatomy. Use the bony orbital rim and position of the superciliary ridge as the reference points for placing the injections and not the position of the eyebrows. Women's eyebrows usually are located higher than men's over the superciliary arch.

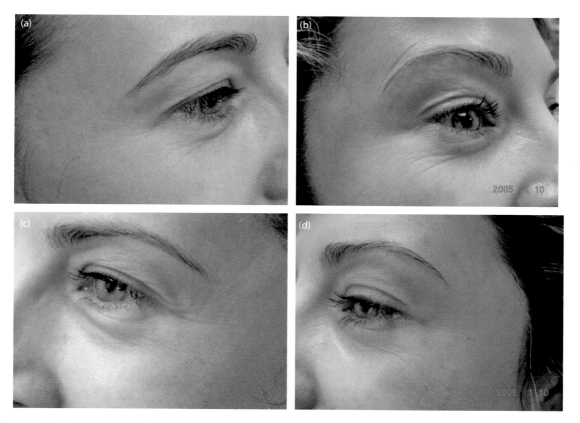

Figure 13.115 (a) Right lateral brow of a 45-year-old patient at rest and before a treatment of OnaBTX-A. (b) Note brow elevation 3 weeks after a treatment of OnaBTX-A of the lateral right brow. (c) Left lateral brow at rest and before a treatment of OnaBTX-A. (d) Note brow elevation 3 weeks after a treatment of OnaBTX-A of the lateral left brow.

their potential for secondary brow ptosis (Figure 13.36). Functioning lower fibers of the lateral frontalis are needed to raise the lateral brow. When there is excessive skin laxity and dermatochalasis in the area of the lower lateral forehead and lateral brow, the skin redundancy creating lateral orbital hooding and horizontal wrinkles immediately above the lateral brow may or may not be treatable by OnaBTX-A to the patient's satisfaction (Figure 13.121). For some patients, injections of a minimal amount of highly diluted OnaBTX-A can be attempted. Take 1/2 to 1 unit of OnaBTX-A and triple its volume with normal saline directly into the syringe. Then inject *intradermally* a minimal amount of this highly diluted OnaBTX-A directly into the wrinkles overlying the eyebrow. A fraction of a unit of OnaBTX-A is all that may be necessary to diminish those annoyingly persistent lines just adjacent to or within the eyebrow. Reduction of those lines with or without a minimal amount of brow ptosis may result. Otherwise, injections of a hyaluronic acid soft tissue filler in the affected brow might be a more suitable option to diminish the lines and avoid any amount of brow ptosis.

Complications (Adverse Sequelae) When Lifting the Eyebrow (See Appendix 6)

It is important to keep in mind when treating the forehead with OnaBTX-A, injections in the lateral aspect of the frontalis should not

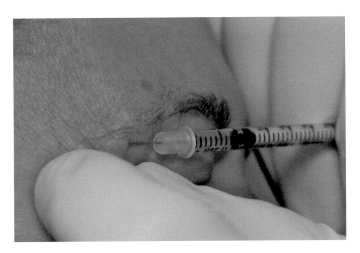

Figure 13.116 Most lateral injection point along the superciliary arch.

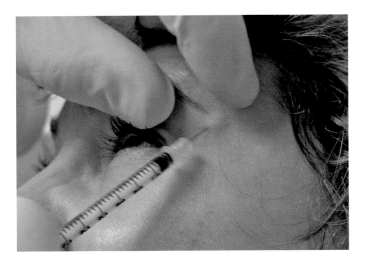

Figure 13.117 Raising a wheal at each injection point will guarantee the injection was given at the proper depth.

be done too high or too low. Injections that are *too high* can result in an excessively elevated lateral eyebrow, producing what is known as the Mephisto or "Mr. Spock" look. Injections that are *too low* will cause or accentuate brow ptosis and will negate any further attempt at lateral brow elevation until the strength of the lower lateral frontalis muscle fibers returns.

Xerophthalmia or dry eye can occur if OnaBTX-A is injected too deeply into the upper lateral aspect of the periorbital area and it diffuses either into pretarsal orbicularis oculi, diminishing the patient's ability to blink normally, or into the lacrimal gland, diminishing the patient's ability to secrete tears, or both.[93] When this occurs, regular instillation of commercially available artificial tears (i.e., ophthalmic normal saline) will be necessary until the lacrimal glands begin to function again and normal blinking returns. Consultation with an ophthalmologist also is recommended.

Forceful, deep, and rapid injections at the lateral canthus can cause the OnaBTX-A to spread into the bony orbit and weaken the lateral extraocular muscles, causing strabismus and diplopia. The best way to avoid these complications and other adverse sequelae is to inject OnaBTX-A *slowly* and *intradermally* with 2–3 U per injection point in women and 3–4 U per injection point in men. The dosage will depend on the strength of both the lateral brow depressors and the frontalis

and presence or absence of dermatochalasis, lateral orbital hooding and corrugations.

Figures 13.122 through 13.128 are some examples of different patients treated with OnaBTX-A to elevate their lateral brow.

Treatment Implications When Injecting the Lateral Eyebrows

1. Injecting 4–6 U of OnaBTX-A in the upper lateral eyebrow temporarily produces a lateral brow lift, widens the palpebral fissure, and corrects lateral canthal hooding when present.
2. Injections must be performed intradermally over the tail of the eyebrow, 2.5–3.0 cm above the supraorbital bony rim; otherwise the lacrimal gland will be affected and xerophthalmia may result. Raising a wheal confirms a superficial injection.
3. Before injecting OnaBTX-A intradermally, have patients raise their eyebrows elevating the lower fibers of the frontalis to uncover the upper fibers of the orbital orbicularis oculi in the vicinity of the lateral eyebrows.
4. Precise dosing, an accurate injection technique, and the superficial placement of OnaBTX-A into the upper lateral brow (orbicularis oculi) will avoid diffusion into the lower frontalis and the exacerbation of lateral orbital hooding.
5. Upper lateral orbicularis oculi injections placed intradermally 1.5–2.5 cm above and horizontally along the superciliary arch but lateral to the mid-pupillary line will diminish the skin corrugations of the lateral brow seen in some patients.
6. Maintain the strength of the lower lateral fibers of the frontalis and prevent worsening of lateral orbital hooding by injecting OnaBTX-A intradermally approximately 2.5–3.0 cm above the bony orbital rim along the superciliary arch. Prevent a Mephisto or "Mr. Spock" look by injecting OnaBTX-A *intramuscularly* into the lower fibers of the frontalis, 3–4 cm above the lateral bony orbit.
7. In patients with excessive skin laxity and dermatochalasis in the lateral brow and lower lateral forehead, injections of OnaBTX-A may not satisfactorily lift the lateral brow and relieve brow hooding. Injections of a soft tissue filler can be a corrective option.

PERIORBITAL AREA: LOWER EYELID LINES

Introduction: Problem Assessment and Patient Selection

Along with crow's feet and lateral brow ptosis, many people have additional folds and creases of the lower eyelids, which give them the appearance of being tired, sleep deprived, or even older than their current age. These lower eyelid "festoons" or "jelly rolls" are produced by hypertrophy of the palpebral (preseptal or pretarsal or both) orbicularis oculi along with some degree of skin laxity (blepharochalasis), retroseptal fat prolapse, and lymphedema (Figure 13.129).[28,77,102] These lower eyelid folds also contribute to the appearance of "dark circles" and baggy eyes that women and even men would prefer not to have. Likewise, a tired, disinterested, downtrodden, and unambitious demeanor is projected when the palpebral fissure is narrowed because of a hyperfunctional pretarsal orbicularis oculi. Various facial movements, primarily smiling or laughing, also will narrow momentarily the palpebral fissure. Injections of OnaBTX-A in the inferior preseptal orbicularis oculi will reduce excess lower eyelid wrinkling, and injections into the pretarsal orbicularis oculi will widen the vertical ocular aperture, and produce a more youthful, happier, and overall more pleasant and inviting appearance.

Functional Anatomy when treating LOWER EYELID LINES (See Appendix 2)

The orbicularis oculi helps protect the eyes from bright light, gusts of air, and fast flying projectiles. Those working outdoors or in a brightly

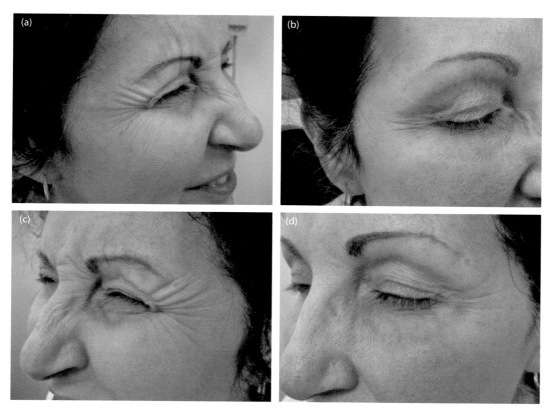

Figure 13.118 A 62-year-old patient (a) before and (b) 2 weeks after treatment with OnaBTX-A injection in the lateral aspect of her right brow. Note the lateral brow lift and diminution of the lateral brow corrugations. (c) before and (d) 2 weeks after treatment with OnaBTX-A injection in the lateral aspect of the left brow. Note the lateral brow lift and diminution of the lateral brow corrugations.

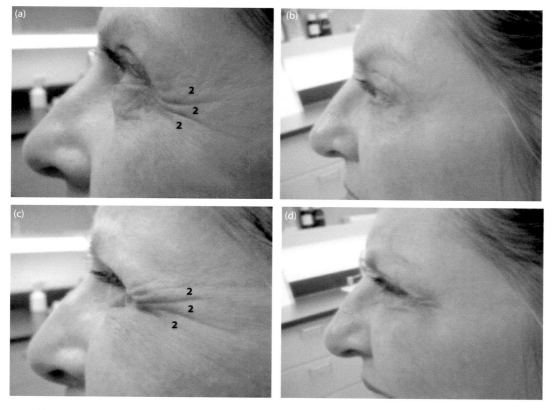

Figure 13.119 A 58-year-old patient is shown at rest (a) before and (b) 3 weeks after her OnaBTX-A treatment; and also squinting (c) before and (d) 3 weeks after her OnaBTX-A treatment.

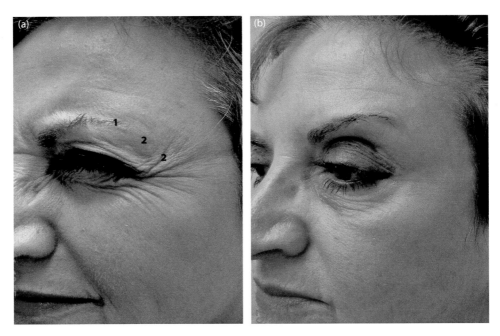

Figure 13.120 A 68-year-old patient (a) before and (b) 3 weeks after OnaBTX-A was injected into the lateral aspect of the orbicularis oculi. Note the elevation of the hooding of the lateral aspect of the upper eyelid.

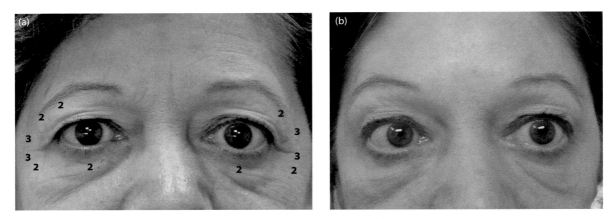

Figure 13.121 (a) A 61-year-old woman with dermatochalasis causing skin redundancy and orbital hooding bilaterally, with the injection pattern and number of units used for OnaBTX-A treatment. (b) Same patient 3 weeks after OnaBTX-A.

lit environment automatically maintain their orbicularis oculi in a constant hyperkinetic state of partial closure, as they continuously squint. This can cause the muscle fibers of the inferior orbicularis oculi to hypertrophy. In younger patients, hypertrophic palpebral orbicularis oculi can be observed as producing additional periorbital folds, and are sometimes referred to as "jelly rolls," especially in the vicinity of the lower eyelid (Figure 13.129). These lower eyelid folds can be diminished by OnaBTX-A (Figure 13.130). In older patients, however, the skin of the eyelids gradually becomes thin, redundant, and inelastic. The orbital septum attenuates, and becomes less effective. Because of a resultant weakening of the preseptal orbicularis oculi, the inferior periorbital fat bulges from behind the bulwark of the preseptal orbicularis oculi and creates characteristic suborbital "festoons" (Figure 13.131). OnaBTX-A injections of the already weakened and incompetent preseptal orbicularis oculi will enhance its inability to contain the periorbital fat and invariably will enlarge this type of suborbital festooning, and therefore should not be performed.[105]

Blinking is an essential, involuntary, semi-autonomic rapid closing of the eyelids. It helps remove irritants from the surface of the cornea and maintain its lubrication by spreading tears across the surface of the globe. A blink is initiated by both the simultaneous inactivation of accessory muscles of the upper and lower eyelids: the levator palpebrae superioris and the superior and inferior tarsal muscles, and the activation of the palpebral orbicularis oculi. A major function of the preseptal orbicularis oculi is its spontaneous and reflex sphincteric blinking action. Each blink of the eye distributes over the anterior surface of the globe the drops of tears that are secreted from the main and accessory lacrimal glands (Figure 13.132). Opening and shutting the eyes activates the so-called "lacrimal pump," shunting the secreted tears through the canalicular system, into the lacrimal sac, down the nasolacrimal duct, and into the nasal cavity out of the inferior meatus from under the inferior nasal turbinate.

As the secreted tears flow from the lacrimal glands into the upper lateral aspect of the orbit, they collect in the lower medial corner of the orbit to form the lacrimal lake. With the eyelids open, the lacrimal orbicularis oculi compresses the lacrimal sac and positions the patulous punctum in direct contact with the globe and the lacrimal lake. This allows the tears to flow into and through the patent

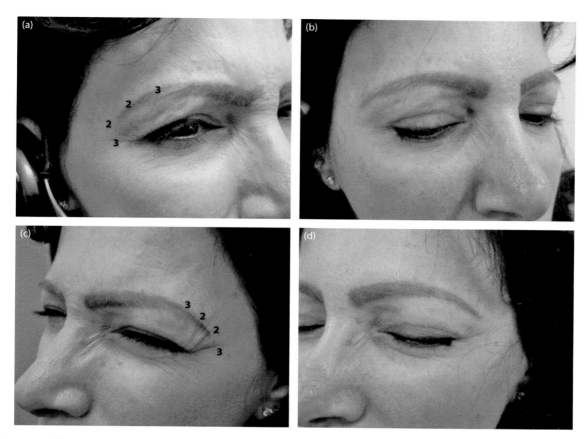

Figure 13.122 A 57-year-old patient squinting (a) before and (b) 3 weeks after OnaBTX-A treatment on the right and squinting (c) before and (d) 3 weeks after OnaBTX-A treatment on the left. Note the difference in lateral brow height and hooding.

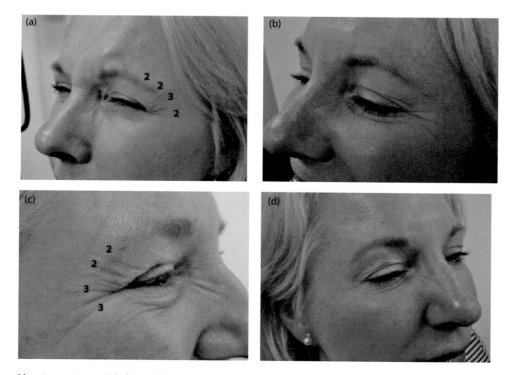

Figure 13.123 A 52-year-old patient squinting (a) before and (b) 3 weeks after OnaBTX-A treatment on the left and squinting (c) before and (d) 3 weeks after OnaBTX-A treatment on the right. Note the difference in lateral brow height and lateral brow hooding.

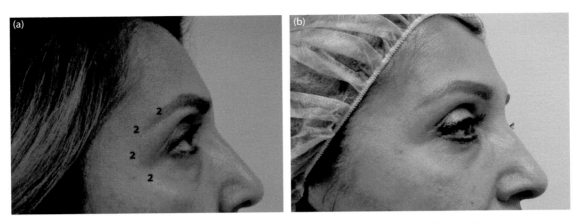

Figure 13.124 A 57-year-old patient at rest (a) before and (b) 2 weeks after OnaBTX-A treatment. Note the difference in the lateral brow hooding.

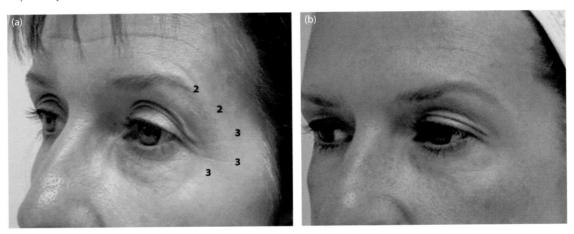

Figure 13.125 A 45-year-old patient is shown (a) before and (b) 2 weeks after OnaBTX-A was injected into the lateral aspect of the *orbital* orbicularis oculi. Note the reduction in the lateral brow hooding.

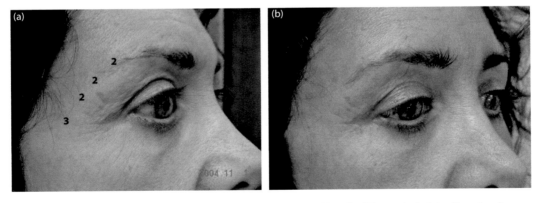

Figure 13.126 A 53-year-old patient at rest (a) before and (b) 3 weeks after OnaBTX-A treatment. Note the difference in the lateral brow hooding.

canaliculus. Contracting the superficial fibers of the pretarsal orbicularis oculi on blinking shuts the eyelids and distributes the tears over the anterior surface of the globe in a superior lateral to an inferior medial direction. Opening the eyes again causes the deep fibers of the pretarsal orbicularis oculi to contract again, shutting down the upper and lower canalicular system. Contemporaneously, the deep fibers of the preseptal orbicularis oculi pull on the lateral walls of the lacrimal sac, enlarging its lumen and contributing to the negative pressure gradient within the nasolacrimal canalicular system, which causes the tears to be aspirated into the lacrimal sac (Figure 13.132). On reopening the eyelids, the positive pressure within the canalicular system is recreated and the lacrimal sac collapses,

propelling the tears into the nasolacrimal duct, then through the inferior meatus under the inferior nasal turbinate and into the nasal cavity. Simultaneously, the puncta and canaliculi reopen to collect more tears from the lacrimal lake and the process recycles with each opening and shutting of the eyelids.[28,30]

Dilution: When treating LOWER EYELID LINES (See Appendix 3)

When treating the periorbital area with OnaBTX-A it is imperative to be precise with dosing and accurate with injecting minimal volumes of OnaBTX-A. Therefore, a 100 U vial of OnaBTX-A should be reconstituted with only 1 mL of normal saline (see Appendix 2).

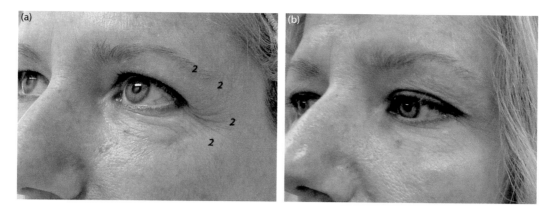

Figure 13.127 A 49-year-old patient at rest (a) before and (b) 3 weeks after OnaBTX-A treatment. Note the difference in the lateral brow height and hooding.

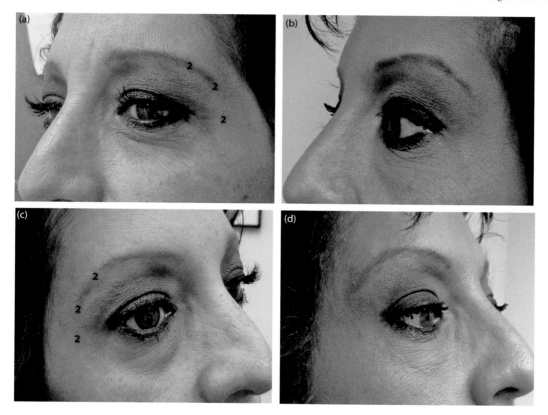

Figure 13.128 A 48-year-old patient at rest (a) before and (b) 2 weeks after OnaBTX-A treatment on the left and at rest (c) before and (d) 2 weeks after OnaBTX-A treatment on the right. Note the difference in the lateral brow height and hooding.

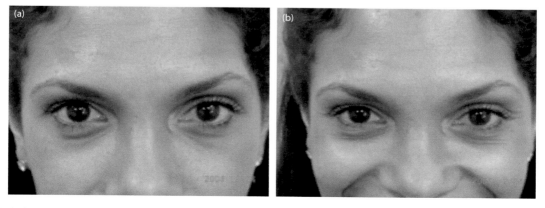

Figure 13.129 (a) Early festoons and wrinkles of the lower eyelid are seen in this 42-year-old patient at rest. (b) Same patient with periocular wrinkles exaggerated when she smiles. She also complained of dark circles under her eyes.

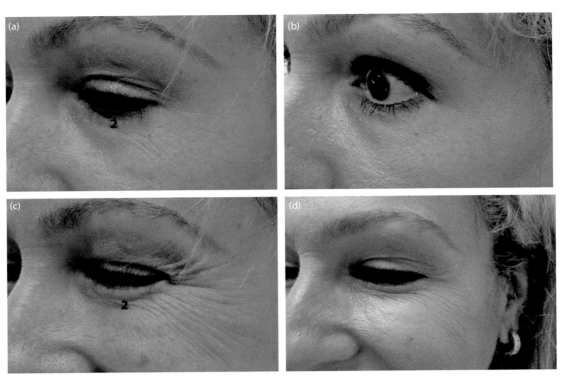

Figure 13.130 (a) Left lower eyelid of a 42-year-old woman at rest and before 2 U of OnaBTX-A were injected in the middle of the left lower eyelid. (b) Same patient at rest 3 weeks after OnaBTX-A. (c) Same patient smiling before 2 U of OnaBTX-A were injected in the middle of the left lower eyelid. (d) Same patient smiling 3 weeks after OnaBTX-A.

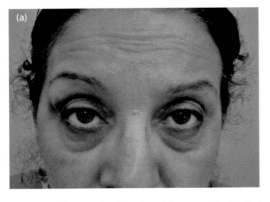
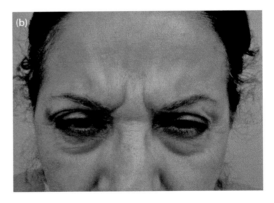

Figure 13.131 (a) This 64-year-old woman has thinning of the *preseptal* orbicularis oculi, which is seen as festoons of the lower eyelids. (b) Same patient squinting causes the *orbital* and *palpebral* portions of the orbicularis oculi to contract. Injections of OnaBTX-A in the lower eyelid will make the orbicularis oculi incompetent at rest and intensify her festooning and wrinkles with squinting. Therefore, OnaBTX-A injections in this patient in the lower eyelids should not be performed.

Dosing: How to Correct the Problem, (See Appendix 4), (What to Do and What Not to Do) When treating LOWER EYELID LINES

Appropriate candidates for OnaBTX-A treatment of the lower eyelids are those who have normal eyelid elasticity, determined by a normal snap-back test and a normal pinch (distraction) test. Most individuals under the age of 60 years who have not had any previous lower eyelid surgery, including blepharoplasty or some form of resurfacing, either by laser or chemical peeling, usually display normal snap-back and pinch tests and can be treated with injections of BoNT in the lower eyelids.

To perform a lower eyelid snap-back test, pull down on the lower lid with an index finger for 5 seconds. The patient is asked not to blink as the eyelid is released. A normal result is when the lower eyelid skin recoils spontaneously and immediately snaps back against the globe within 1 second. Minimal laxity is present if it takes 2 seconds for the eyelid to return to its neutral position against the globe. Laxity is moderate if it takes 3 or more seconds to return, while pronounced laxity is present if the patient must blink to return the eyelid against the globe. With severe laxity, the eyelid remains everted even after the patient blinks.[28]

To perform a pinch or distraction test, grasp the skin of the lower eyelid between the thumb and index finger. Gently pull the eyelid skin away from the globe. If the forward projection is less than 8 mm, then the eyelid's elasticity is ostensibly normal, and it can be treated with injections of OnaBTX-A.[28] When the snap-back and pinch tests indicate insufficient elasticity of lower eyelid skin, then they should not be injected with OnaBTX-A because the probability of postinjection lower eyelid retraction and even full-blown ectropion is high.

Another way to test the competency of the lower palpebral orbicularis oculi is to have the patient look forward in a relaxed manner and then gaze upward. If the lower eyelid flattens and pushes the periorbital fat inward, the preseptal orbicularis oculi is competent, tight, and can be

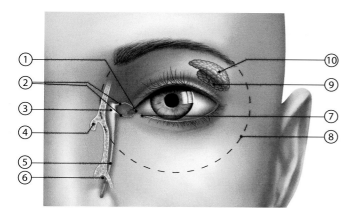

Figure 13.132 Tears are produced by the main (orbital) and accessory (palpebral) lacrimal glands. The distribution of these tears over the surface of the eye is achieved with each blink of the eyelids performing a wiping action of the marginal tear bed. The passage of tears into the nose occurs via the lacrimal drainage system, propelled by contraction of the palpebral orbicularis oculi. 1, plica semilunaris and lacrimal lake; 2, lacrimal canaliculi; 3, lacrimal sac; 4, middle nasal turbinate; 5, nasolacrimal duct; 6, inferior nasal meatus; 7, inferior lacrimal papilla and punctum; 8, outer limit of orbicularis oculi (orbital); 9, palpebral (accessory) lacrimal gland; 10, orbital lacrimal gland.

OnaBTX-A will only exacerbate the fat prolapse and festooning of the lower eyelids and should not be done. Lymphedema, on the other hand, is not altered by this maneuver.[28] In preparation for a treatment the patient should be looking directly forward in a sitting or a semireclined position. To prevent frightening the patient with the sight of the needle, the physician should approach the patient from the side while standing on the same side of the patient directly adjacent to the lower eyelid to be treated. As the injector approaches the patient with the needle, the patient should be asked to gaze directly upward and to take a deep breath without moving. Contemporaneously, the physician pulls the lower eyelid skin inferiorly with the index finger of the nondominant hand. The syringe barrel rests on the index finger while the needle tip is inserted at about a 45° angle into the pretarsal skin at a point 2–3 mm below the lower lid margin and 2–4 mm lateral to the mid-pupillary line. The needle tip then is advanced approximately 2–3 mm into the skin. It should remain at the depth of the lower dermis and not be advanced any deeper than the dermal/subcutaneous interface (Figure 13.133a). Even as the needle tip is advanced 2–3 mm within the skin, it should remain in its superficial position just lateral to the mid-pupillary line. When the tip of the needle is sufficiently through the skin and has reached its proper depth and location lateral to the mid-pupillary line, an injection of 2 U (i.e., 0.02 mL) of OnaBTX-A can be given. The liquid OnaBTX-A should remain within the thin eyelid tissue and not leak through or track out along the path of the needle puncture. The injector should observe the rise of a wheal of fluid, which should reassure the physician that an adequate dose of OnaBTX-A has been delivered at the proper superficial depth (Figure 13.133b and c). No additional drops of OnaBTX-A should escape from the needle as it is withdrawn out of the skin, provided there is no air within

treated with OnaBTX-A. If the lower eyelid bulge of fat becomes more pronounced and projects even farther anteriorly, especially when external digital pressure on the globe at the level of the upper eyelid is performed, then the lower preseptal orbicularis oculi is probably weak and incompetent allowing for the retroseptal fat pad prolapse. Injections of

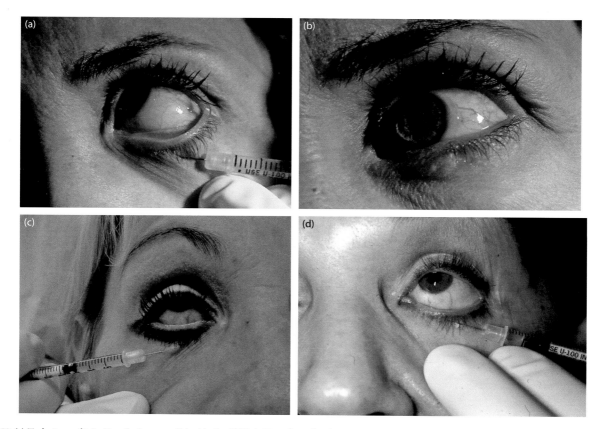

Figure 13.133 (a) Technique of injecting the lower eyelid with OnaBTX-A. Note the index finger of the non-dominant hand pulling down on the skin of the lower eyelid making it taut. The needle tip is inserted at a 45° angle and 2–3 mm down from the lid margin and approximately 2–3 mm deep within the deep dermal to subcutaneous layer. (b) Note the appearance of the wheal of OnaBTX-A. (c) The appearance of a wheal indicates that the bolus of OnaBTX-A has been delivered successfully and at the correct depth. (d) A microdroplet of air within the syringe wastes a drop of OnaBTX-A as it escapes out of the tip of the needle and onto the surface of the skin upon withdrawing the needle out of the skin.

the barrel of the syringe. Air within the syringe causes a positive pressure gradient inside the barrel, forcing some BoNT fluid out of the needle as it exits the skin, even without any digital pressure on the plunger of the syringe (Figure 13.133d). Delicate massage of the injected area directed laterally will distract the patient and help disperse the OnaBTX-A safely along the superficial fibers of the palpebral orbicularis oculi. When this technique is executed in a calm and expeditious manner, the patient will not cower away from the needle pointed directly at her or his eye, and he or she may even compliment the physician on the painless fashion and ease with which the treatment was administered. An additional 1–2 U of OnaBTX-A can be injected intradermally or at the dermal/subcutaneous interface and approximately 2–3 mm below the lid margin, at a point halfway between the lateral canthus and the mid-pupillary line (Figure 13.134).[1,106,107] For most patients this second injection in the lower eyelid is superfluous. It may even lead to lateral lower eyelid retraction and other annoying adverse sequelae (Figure 6.98).

Outcomes (Results) When Treating LOWER EYELID LINES (See Appendix 5)

It was discovered serendipitously that an injection of 2–4 U of OnaBTX-A placed subcutaneously in the pretarsal orbicularis oculi of the lower eyelid at the mid-pupillary line, approximately 2–3 mm below the lid margin, can improve the rolls of festooning redundant skin that occur on and just inferior to the lower eyelid (Figures 13.129 and 13.130).[106] Pretarsal injections of OnaBTX-A in the lower eyelid also were found to produce a desirable relaxation of the pretarsal orbicularis oculi, which consequently increased the palpebral fissure both

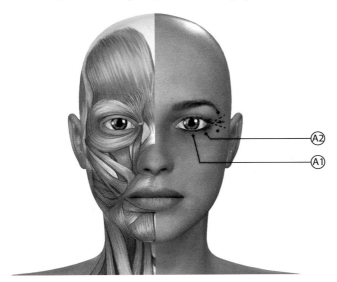

Figure 13.134 When treating the lower eyelid fold and festoons, one (A1) injection at the mid-pupillary line or a second (A2) injection halfway between the mid-pupillary line and the lateral canthus can be performed depending on the strength of the *palpebral* orbicularis oculi and the depth of the folds. Additional injections (•) of OnaBTX-A may be needed to treat crow's feet, the dosage of which will depend on the strength of the lateral *orbital* orbicularis oculi.

at rest and during smiling, laughing, and various other facial movements. The extent of the increase in vertical palpebral aperture was dependent on the amount of units injected into the pretarsal orbicularis oculi and whether crow's feet were treated at the same time. For those patients who were treated with only 2 U of OnaBTX-A injected in only one site in the lower eyelid at the pretarsal midpupillary line, the average increase in palpebral aperture (IPA) was approximately 0.5 mm at rest and 1.3 mm at full smile (Figure 13.134). When combined with a fixed dose of 12 U of OnaBTX-A given in three separate doses 1.5 mm apart at the lateral canthus to treat concomitant crow's feet, the average IPA was approximately 1.75 mm at rest and 2.9 mm at full smile (Table 13.1). Increasing the number of units of OnaBTX-A injected in the lower eyelid with or without concomitant treatment of the lateral canthi increased the IPA commensurately (Table 13.1).[107] There appeared to be a synergistic effect to the response of the lower pretarsal orbicularis oculi when the lateral orbital orbicularis oculi was contemporaneously treated during the same session. This technique of injecting the pretarsal orbicularis oculi produces an "openeyed look" that gives the patient the appearance of one who is vibrantly active and cheerfully youthful (Figure 13.135). In most cases, the second intermediary injection of OnaBTX-A between the lateral canthus and mid-pupillary line is not always necessary (A2 in Figure 13.134). It may even increase the chance for lateral canthal rounding and lower eyelid retraction (Figure 13.98). This technique of injecting the lower eyelids with OnaBTX-A in this study was especially popular among Asian patients who desire a more rounded, Western eyelid fissure.[106,107]

Complications (Adverse Sequelae) (See Appendix 6)

For first-time recipients of an infra-orbital treatment of OnaBTX-A, the presence of periorbital edema lasting a few hours to days may occur. This can be attributed to lymph stasis, possibly produced by a nondetectable attenuation of the sphincteric pumping action of the inferior preseptal orbicularis oculi, reducing the efficiency of lymph fluid clearance from the surrounding soft tissue.[64] Moreover, when there is a blatant reduction in lower eyelid tone, reduced blinking can compromise the action and efficacy of the "lacrimal pump," resulting in transient epiphora, until the lower eyelid tone returns (see Figure 13.132).

Rounding or retraction of the lateral canthus occurs when there is excessive weakening of the lateral upper or lower, or both, palpebral orbicularis oculi. However, injecting crow's feet at least 1.5–2.0 cm lateral to the lateral canthus can help avoid such an unwanted outcome. The second intermediate injection of the lower pretarsal orbicularis oculi (A2 in Figure 13.134) also has been found to cause rounding of the lateral canthus and retraction of the adjacent lateral aspect of the lower lid margin, especially when a full treatment of OnaBTX-A is injected into the adjacent upper and lower crow's feet area (Figure 13.98). Therefore, unless the patient has recalcitrant lower eyelid festoons that wrap around the lateral canthus and are continuous with deep and resistant lateral canthal lines, this second (A2 in Figure 13.134), intermediate, lateral pretarsal injection of OnaBTX-A should be withheld, and only the central pretarsal injection of the lower eyelid at the mid-pupillary line should be given (A1 in Figure 13.134).

Table 13.1 IPA—Increase in Palpebral Aperture at Rest and at Full Smile

	Pretarsal area treated alone			Pretarsal area treated together with crow's feet (12 U of OnaBTX-A)		
OnaBTX-A units	2 U	4 U	8 U	2 U	4 U	8 U
IPA at rest (mm)	0.5	1.75	1.95	1.75	2.2	1.5
IPA at full smile (mm)	1.3	2.5	4.5	2.9	2.9	4.0

Source: Adapted from Flynn TC et al. *Dermatol Surg* 2001; 27: 703–8.

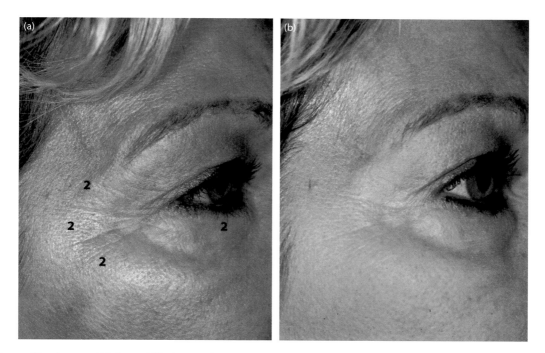

Figure 13.135 A 56-year-old patient seen (a) before and (b) after 2 U of OnaBTX-A was injected into the lower eyelid at the mid-pupillary line 2–3 mm from the lid margin. Note the wide-eyed look.

Lower eyelid orbicular hypertrophy manifests as bulging in the lower lateral aspect of the eyelid (pretarsal bulging). Fagien reported treating this bulging of the muscle with 0.5–1.5 U OnaBTX-A in each of two locations. One injection was given in the farthest point in the corner of the lower lateral canthus (pretarsal orbicularis oculi) just below the lid margin and the other in the middle of the lower eyelid pretarsal orbicularis oculi at the midpupillary line.[64] It is imperative that the pretarsal injections be placed 2–3 mm inferior to the lid margin into the deep dermis, barely reaching the subcutaneous tissue, and nowhere near the bony malar prominence, since most of the upper lip levators originate along the margin of the zygomatic arch (Figure 13.136). Otherwise, upper lip ptosis, asymmetry, and even sphincter incompetence of the upper lip can result. These adverse sequelae can occur when OnaBTX-A is injected too deeply and inferiorly along the zygomatic arch, because the levators of the lateral aspect of the upper lip (zygomaticus major and levator anguli oris) and even the levators of the central aspect of the upper lip (levator labii superioris, zygomaticus minor, and levator labii superioris alaeque nasi) can be weakened by the spread of the injected OnaBTX-A.

Injecting OnaBTX-A medial to the midpupillary line of the lower eyelid and in the center of the malar bone runs the risk of weakening the voluntary and involuntary sphincteric and levator function of the lower palpebral orbicularis oculi. This can compromise forced eyelid closure and the blink reflex. This in turn could both diminish the pumping action of the naso-lacrimal outflow and cause temporary epiphora or even an ectropion if overdosed. Xerophthalmia resulting from a supervening lagophthalmos can lead to corneal overexposure, desiccation (keratitis sicca), and punctate keratitis (corneal ulcers).[108] This can occur more readily in older patients who have attenuated muscular strength and a thinned orbital septum.

Postinjection ecchymoses are practically inevitable whenever the thin and vascular skin of the lower eyelid is injected (Figure 13.137). The use of a small insulin syringe with a super-fine needle (Becton-Dickinson U-100 Insulin 3/10 syringe with a 31-gauge needle) and a slow, *intradermal* injection technique may prevent or at least limit the extent of postinjection ecchymoses. Other maneuvers at preventing

postinjection bruising include pre- and post-treatment icing and ample overhead bright lighting that reveals the surface vasculature. Gentle stretching of the eyelid skin over the area to be treated prior to the injection also helps locate the numerous superficial vasculature present in the area and avoid ecchymoses (Figure 13.10c). After the injections, light massage and point pressure with ice can help reduce the incidence of bruising. Patients with fragile vasculature, as is commonly seen in middle-aged and older individuals, contribute to the

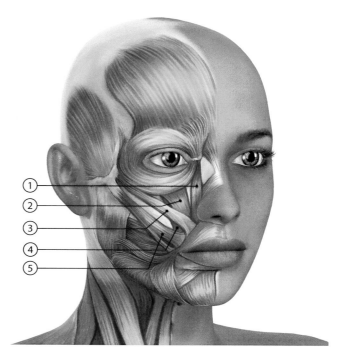

Figure 13.136 Upper lip levators: 1, levator labii superioris alaeque nasi; 2, levator labii superioris; 3, zygomaticus minor; 4, levator anguli oris; 5, zygomaticus major. (See Appendix 2—muscle attachments)

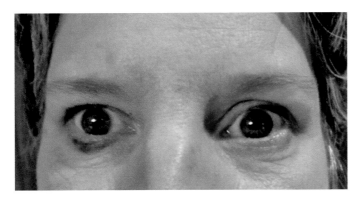

Figure 13.137 Two days after 2 U of OnaBTX-A were injected in both lower eyelids for the first time in a 53-year-old woman. The ecchymosis in the right eyelid lasted for about 10 days.

inevitability of frequently occurring lower eyelid ecchymoses, which should resolve in a few (approximately 10–12) days.

Pseudoherniation of the infraorbital fat pad can be unwittingly enhanced when OnaBTX-A is injected into the inferior palpebral (preseptal) orbicularis oculi in patients who have festooning caused by protruding periorbital fat in inelastic, incompetent lower eyelids. A worsening of pseudoherniation by OnaBTX-A is particularly easy to produce either in older patients who have a reduction and downward displacement of their suborbicularis oculi fat (SOOF) and a weakening of their orbital septum, or in patients who in the past have had a blepharoplasty or other type of lower eyelid surgery. In these patients, the tarsoligamentous sling support of their lower preseptal orbicularis oculi is compromised and ineffective (Figure 13.131).[105]

Injections of OnaBTX-A in the inferior preseptal, inferolateral canthal, and superior malar areas of patients with lax lower eyelid skin can compromise further the integral strength of the orbicularis oculi, accentuating the infraorbital festoons, instead of reducing them, and therefore should not be performed.[90]

In their dose-defining studies, Flynn et al. found no substantial adverse events in the patients treated with only 2 U of OnaBTX-A injected at one site pretarsally in the lower eyelid (Figure 13.134).[107] In those patients who had 4 U of OnaBTX-A injected pretarsally in two divided doses of 2 U each (Figure 13.134 A1, A2), less than half of them suffered from "dry eyes" and one patient could not wear her contact lenses.[106,107] There were additional, temporary adverse events that were more of an annoyance than a serious complication and they occurred after 8 U of OnaBTX-A were injected pretarsally in two divided doses of 4 U each into the lower eyelid (A1 and A2 in Figure 13.134). These untoward side effects included transient lower eyelid edema, which gave the patient an increased sense of lower eyelid fullness, persistently "dropped bags," and a sensation of puffy lower eyelids, which became worse toward the end of the day.[106,107] Also, there were patients who developed photophobia, and who were unable to go outdoors in bright light because they had difficulty with squinting and could not protect their eyes from sunlight. Still others were bothered by incomplete sphincteric eyelid closure, which caused stinging of their eyes when they washed their faces with or without soap. All of these annoyances remitted within 3 months from the time the 8 U of OnaBTX-A were injected into the two sites in the mid and lateral aspects of the pretarsal orbicularis oculi of their lower eyelids.

Figures 13.138 through 13.143 are some examples of different patients treated with OnaBTX-A to reduce folds and creases of the lower eyelids.

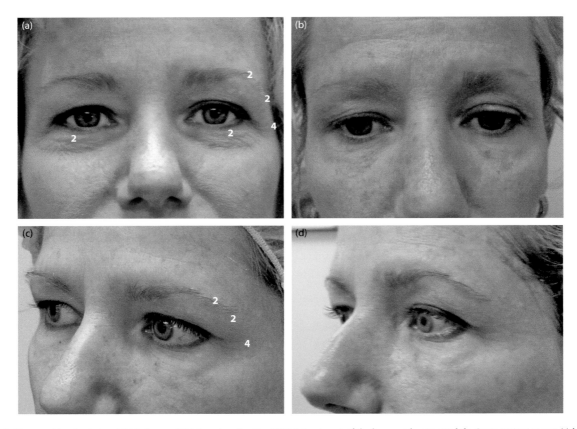

Figure 13.138 A 49-year-old patient at rest (a) before and (b) 3 weeks after OnaBTX-A treatment of the lower and upper eyelids. Same patient at rest (c) before and (d) 3 weeks after OnaBTX-A treatment of the lower and upper eyelids seen from the left side. Note the lifting of the brow and upper lid shown. Note the wide-eyed appearance with upward gaze.

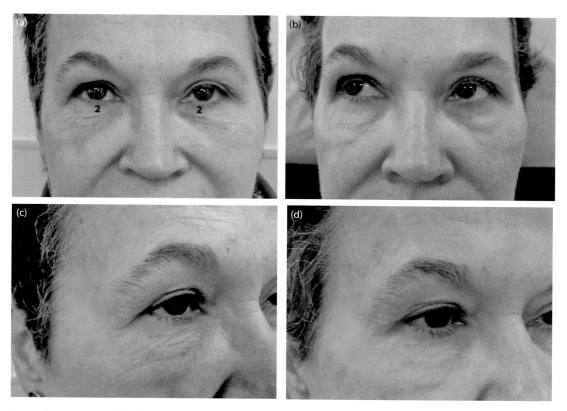

Figure 13.139 A 68-year-old patient at rest (a) before and (b) 5 weeks after OnaBTX-A treatment of the lower eyelids and 1 month after superficial CO_2 fractional laser ablation. Same patient at rest (c) before and (d) 5 weeks after OnaBTX-A treatment of the lower eyelids and 1 month after superficial CO_2 fractional laser ablation seen from the right side.

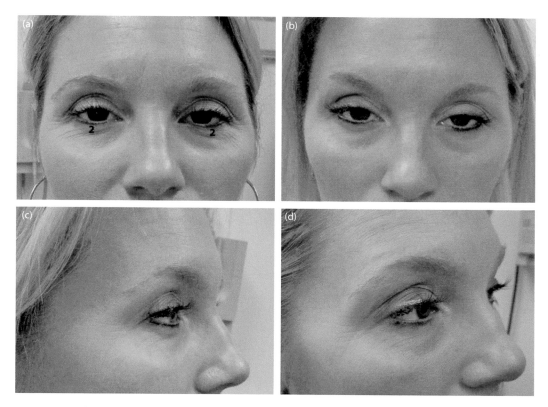

Figure 13.140 A 38-year-old patient at rest (a) before and (b) 1 month after OnaBTX-A treatment of the upper, and lower eyelids and lateral canthal crow's feet; at rest (c) before and (d) 1 month after OnaBTX-A treatment of the lower eyelids seen from the right side (note the concomitant brow lift).

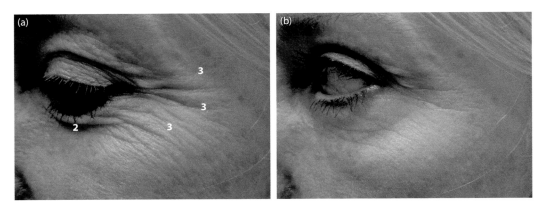

Figure 13.141 A 47-year-old patient at rest (a) before and (b) 2 weeks after OnaBTX-A treatment of the lower eyelids and crow's feet.

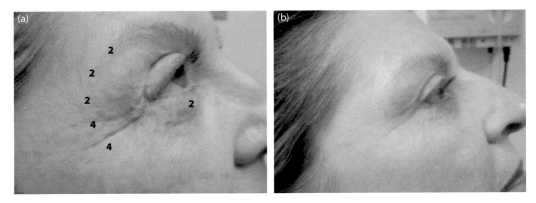

Figure 13.142 A 58-year-old patient is shown at rest and forward gazing (a) before and (b) 3 weeks after OnaBTX-A injection of the upper and lower lid and crow's feet. Note the reduction of the lower lid festoons and crow's feet.

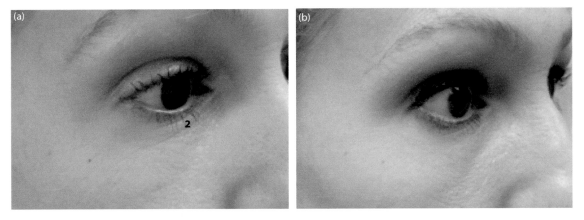

Figure 13.143 A 42-year-old patient is shown at rest and forward gazing (a) before and (b) 3 weeks after an OnaBTX-A injection of the right lower lid. Note the wide-eyed open look.

Treatment Implications When Injecting the Lower Eyelids

1. Lower eyelid injections of OnaBTX-A produce a "wide-eyed," youthful appearance.
2. Inject only 1–3 U and no more than 4 U of OnaBTX-A intra-dermally or into the dermal/subcutaneous interface 2–3 mm inferior to the lower eyelid margin into the pretarsal orbicularis oculi 2–4 mm lateral to the mid-pupillary line.
3. Overtreatment with pretarsal injections of OnaBTX-A and at the intermediate point between the lower eyelid lateral canthus and the mid-pupillary line increases the risk for lower eyelid ectropion, a rounded lateral canthus, inability to firmly shut the eyes, photophobia, epiphora, corneal desiccation, and various other adverse sequelae.
4. Pretarsal injections of OnaBTX-A in the lower eyelid *medial* to the mid-pupillary line may lead to excessive weakening of the lower eyelid, which may cause epiphora by weakening the blink reflex, or dry eyes by creating persistent lagophthalmos and unavoidable corneal exposure.

5. Deep injections of OnaBTX-A lower than 3–4 mm from the lower eyelid margin can result in lip asymmetry and cheek ptosis because of upper lip levator weakening.

6. Low-volume, highly concentrated injections of low doses of OnaBTX-A are recommended when injecting the superficial fibers of the lower pretarsal or preseptal orbicularis oculi.

7. Anyone who has had other periorbital cosmetic procedures and consequently has a sluggish snap-back test and an abnormal distraction test should not be treated with OnaBTX-A injections in the lower pretarsal or preseptal orbicularis oculi.

REFERENCES

1. Package insert on BOTOX®/BOTOX®. *Cosmetic*. Irvine, CA: Allergan, Inc; revised October 2017.
2. Package insert on Dysport®, Galderma Laboratories, L.P., Fort Worth, TX,–revised March 2012.
3. Package insert on Xeomin®, Merz Pharma, GmbH&Co KGaA, Am Pharmapark, D-06861, Dessal-RossLau, Germany—revised April 2014.
4. Brin MF, Boodhoo TI, Pogoda JM et al. Safety and tolerability of OnaBTX-A in the treatment of facial lines: A meta-analysis of individual patient data from global clinical registration studies in 1678 participants. *J Am Acad Dermatol* 2009; 61(6): 961–70, e1–e11.
5. Schlessinger J, Dover JS, Joseph J et al. Long-term safety of abobotulinumtoxinA for the treatment of glabellar lines: Results from a 36-month, multicenter, open-label extension study. *Dermatol Surg* 2014; 40: 176–83.
6. Rzany B, Flynn TC, Schlöbe Am Heinz M et al. Long-term results for incobotulinumtoxinA in the treatment of glabellar frown lines. *Dermatol Surg* 2013; 39: 95–103.
7. Scott AB. Botulinum toxin injection into extraocular muscles as an alternative to strabismus surgery. *Ophthalmology* 1980; 87(10): 1044–49.
8. Carruthers JA, Lowe NJ, Menter MA, Gibson J et al. A multicenter, double-blind, randomized, placebo-controlled study of the efficacy and safety of botulinum toxin type A in the treatment of glabellar lines. *J Am Acad Dermatol* 2002; 46: 840–9.
9. Monheit G, Carruthers A, Brandt F et al. A randomized, double-blind, placebo-controlled study of botulinum toxin type A for the treatment of glabellar lines: Determination of optimal dose. *Dermatol Surg* 2007; 33: s51–9.
10. Kane MA, Brandt F, Rohrich RJ et al. Evaluation of variable-dose treatment with a new U.S. botulinum toxin type A (Dysport) for correction of moderate to severe glabellar lines: Results from a phase III, randomized, double-blind, placebo-controlled study. *Plast Reconstr Surg* 2009; 124: 1619–29.
11. Brandt F, Swanson N, Baumann L et al. Randomized, placebo-controlled study of new botulinum toxin type A for treatment of glabellar lines: Efficacy and safety. *Dermatol Surg* 2009; 35: 1893–901.
12. Sattler G, Callender M, Grablowitz D, Walker T et al. Noninferiority of incobotulinumtoxinA, free from complexing proteins, compared with another botulinum toxin type A in the treatment of glabellar frown lines. *Dermatol Surg* 2010; 36: 2146–54.
13. Imhof M, Kühne U. A phase III study of incobotulinumtoxinA in the treatment of glabellar frown lines. *J Clin Aesthet Dermatol* 2011; 4: 28–34.
14. Prager W, Huber-Vorlander J, TauFigure AZ et al. Botulinum toxin type A treatment to the upper face: Retrospective analysis of daily practice. *Clin Cosmet Investig Dermatol* 2012; 5: 53–8.
15. Karsai S, Raulin C. Current evidence on the unit equivalence of the different botulinum neurotoxin A formulations and recommendations for clinical practice in dermatology. *Dermatol Surg* 2009; 35: 1–8.
16. Lorenc ZP, Kenkel JM, Fagien S et al. Consensus panel's assessment and recommendations of the use of 3 botulinum toxin type A products in facial aesthetics. *Aesthet Surg J* 2013; 33: 35s–40s.
17. Kane M, Donofrio L, Ascher B et al. Expanding the use of neurotoxins in facial aesthetics: A consensus panel's assessment and recommendations. *J Drugs Dermatol* 2010; 9(suppl): s7–s22.
18. Carruthers A, Kane MAC, Flynn TC et al. The convergence of medicine and neurotoxins: A focus on botulinum toxin type A and its application in aesthetic medicine—A global, evidence-based botulinum toxin consensus education initiative part I: Botulinum toxin in clinical and cosmetic practice. *Dermatol Surg* 2013; 39(3): 493–509.
19. Carruthers J, Fournier N, Kerscher M et al. The convergence of medicine and neurotoxins: A focus on botulinum toxin type A and its application in aesthetic medicine—A global, evidence-based botulinum toxin consensus education initiative part II: Incorporating botulinum toxin into aesthetic clinical practice. *Dermatol Surg* 2013; 39(3): 510–25.
20. Carruthers JDA, Carruthers JA. Treatment of glabellar frown lines with C. Botulinum-A exotoxin. *Dermatol Surg Oncol* 1992; 18: 17–21.
21. Blitzer A, Brin MF, Keen MS, Aviv JE. Botulinum toxin for the treatment of hyperfunctional lines of the face. *Arch Otolaryngol Head Neck Surg* 1993; 119: 1018–22.
22. Fulton JE. Botulinum toxin: The Newport Beach experience. *Dermatol Surg* 1998; 24(11): 1219–24.
23. Hankins CL, Strimling R, Rogers GS. Botulinum A toxin for glabellar wrinkles: Dose and response. *Dermatol Surg* 1998; 24: 1181–3.
24. Carruthers JD, Lowe NJ, Menter MA et al. Double-blind, placebo-controlled study of the safety and efficacy of botulinum toxin type A for patients with glabellar lines. *Plast Reconstr Surg* 2003; 112: 1089–98.
25. Wu Y, Zhao G, Li H et al. Botulinum toxin type A for the treatment of glabellar lines in Chinese: A double-blind, randomized, placebo-controlled study. *Dermatol Surg* 2010; 36(1): 102–8.
26. Rzany B, Ascher B, Monheit GD. Treatment of glabellar lines with botulinum toxin type A (Speywood Unit): A clinical overview. *JEADV* 2010; 24(Suppl 1), 1–14.
27. Trindade de Almeida AR, da Costa Marques ER, Banegas R et al. Glabellar contraction patterns: A tool to optimize botulinum toxin treatment. *Dermatol Surg* 2012; 38(9): 1506–15.
28. Fratila A, Attrasch C, Zubcov-Iwantscheff A. Structural and functional anatomy of the orbital region, Chapter 1. In: Fratila A, Zubcov-Iwantscheff A, Coleman WP. (ed). *Illustrated Guide to Eyelid and Perioral Surgery: Applied Anatomy, Examination, Blepharoplasty*. UK: Quintessence Publishing Co, Ltd; 2015, pp. 1–25.
29. Lamilla GC, Ingallina FM, Poulain B, Trévidic P. *Anatomy and Botulinum Toxin Injections*. Master Collection Volume 1. Paris, France: Expert 2 Expert SARL; 2015.
30. Standring S (ed). *Gray's Anatomy: The Anatomical Basis of Clinical Practice*. Chapter 30 and 33, 41st ed. Philadelphia: Elsevier; 2016.
31. Benedetto AV, Lahti JG. Measurements of the anatomical position of the corrugator supercilii. *Dermatol Surg* 2005; 31: 923–7.
32. Janis JE, Ghavanni A, Lemmon JA et al. Anatomy of the corrugator supercilii muscle: Part 1. Corrugator topography. *Plast Reconstr Surg* 2007; 120: 1647–53.
33. Knize DM. Muscles that act on glabellar skin: A closer look. *Plast Reconstr Surg* 2000; 105(1): 350–61.

34. Macdonald MR, Spiegel J, Raven RB et al. An anatomical approach to glabellar rhytides. *Arch Otolaryngol Head Neck Surg* 1998; 124: 1315–20.

35. Park JI, Hoagland TM, Park MS. Anatomy of the corrugator supercilii muscle. *Arch Facial Plast Surg* 2003; 5: 412–5.

36. Cook Jr. BE, Lucarelli MJ, Lemke BN. Depressor supercilii muscle: Anatomy, histology, and cosmetic implications. *Ophthalmic Plast Reconstr Surg* 2001; 17: 404–11.

37. Flynn TC, Carruthers A, Carruthers J. Surgical pearl: The use of the Ultra-Fine II short needle 0.3-cc insulin syringe for botulinum toxin injections. *J Am Acad Dermatol* 2002; 46: 931–3.

38. Alam M, Dover JS, Arndt KA. Pain associated with injection of botulinum A exotoxin reconstituted using isotonic sodium chloride with and without preservative: A double-blind, randomized controlled trial. *Arch Dermatol* 2002; 138: 510–14.

39. Trindade de Almeida AR, Secco LC, Carruthers A. Handling botulinum toxins: An updated literature review. *Dermatol Surg* 2011; 37: 1553–65.

40. Alam M, Bolotin D, Carruthers J et al. Consensus statement regarding storage and reuse of previously reconstituted neuromodulators. *Dermatol Surg* 2015; 41: 321–6.

41. Carruthers J, Fagien S, Matarasso SV et al. Consensus recommendations on the use of botulinum toxin type A in facial aesthetics. *Plast Reconstr Surg* 2004; 114(Suppl): 1s–18s.

42. Carruthers JDA, Glogau RG, Blitzer A et al. Advances in facial rejuvenation: Botulinum toxin type A, hyaluronic acid dermal fillers, and combination therapies: Consensus recommendations. *Plast Reconstr Surg* 2008; 121(Suppl): 5s–30s.

43. Raspaldo H, Baspeyras M, Bellity P et al. Upper- and mid-face anti-aging treatment and prevention using onabotulinumtoxin A: The 2010 multidisciplinary French consensus—part 1. *J. Cosmet Dermatol* 2011; 10: 36–50.

44. Jankivic J. Needle EMG guidance for injection of botulinum toxin: Needle EMG guidance is rarely required. *Muscle Nerve* 2001; 24: 1568.

45. Pribitkin EA, Greco TM, Goode RL, Keane WM. Patient selection in the treatment of glabellar wrinkles with botulinum toxin type A injection. *Arch Otolaryngol Head Neck Surg* 1997; 123: 321–6.

46. Carruthers A, Carruthers J, Samireh S. Dose-ranging study of botulinum toxin in the treatment of glabellar rhytides in females. *Dermatol Surg* 2005; 31: 414–22.

47. Carruthers A, Carruthers J. A single-center, dose-comparison, pilot study of botulinum neurotoxin type A in female patients with upper facial rhytids: Safety and efficacy. *J Am Acad Dermatol* 2009; 60(6): 972–79.

48. Carruthers A, Carruthers J. A single-center dose-comparison study of botulinum neurotoxin type A in females with upper facial rhytids: Assessing patients' perception of treatment outcomes. *J Drugs Dermatol* 2009; 8(10): 942–29.

49. Carruthers J, Carruthers A. Prospective, double-blind, randomized, parallel-group, dose-ranging study of botulinum toxin type A in men with glabellar rhytides. *Dermatol Surg* 2005; 31: 1297–303.

50. Flynn TC. Botox in men. *Dermatol Ther* 2007; 20: 407–13.

51. Monheit G, Lin X, Nelson D, Kane M. Consideration of muscle mass in glabellar line treatment with botulinum toxin type A. *J Drugs Dermatol* 2012; 11(9): 1041–45.

52. Keaney TC, Alster TS. Botulinum toxin in men: Review of relevant anatomy and clinical trial data. *Dermatol Surg* 2013; 39: 1434–43.

53. Bowe WP, Chekuri B, Eidelman ME. Neurotoxin techniques for men. *Cosmet Dermatol—A Supplement to Cutis* 2013: 22–8.

54. Alam M, Dover JS, Klein AW, Arndt KA. Botulinum A exotoxin for hyperfunctional facial lines: Where not to inject. *Arch Dermatol* 2002; 138: 1180–85.

55. Carruthers J, Carruthers A. Botulinum toxin type A treatment of multiple upper facial sites: Patient-reported outcomes. *Dermatol Surg* 2007; 33: s10–7.

56. Moers-Carpi M, Carruthers J, Fagien S et al. Efficacy and safety of OnaBTX-A for treating crow's feet lines alone or in combination with glabellar lines: A multicenter, randomized, controlled trial. *Dermatol Surg* 2015; 41: 102–12.

57. Benedetto AV. The cosmetic uses of botulinum toxin type A. *Int J Dermatol* 1999; 38: 641–55.

58. Lehrer MS, Benedetto AV. Boutlinum toxin—an update on its use in facial rejuvenation. *Cosmet Dermatol* 2005; 4: 285–97.

59. Binder WJ, Blitzer A, Brin MF. Treatment of hyperfunctional lines of the face with botulinum toxin A. *Dermatol Surg* 1998; 24: 1198–205.

60. Frankel AS, Kamer FM. Chemical browlift. *Arch Otolaryngol Head Neck Surg* 1998; 124: 321–23.

61. Huang W, Rogachefsky AS, Foster JA. Browlift with botulinum toxin. *Dermatol Surg* 2000; 26: 55–60.

62. Ahn MS, Cotton M, Maas CS. Temporal browlift using botulinum toxin A. *Plast Reconstr Surg* 2000; 105: 1129–35.

63. Carruthers A, Carruthers J. Eyebrow height after botulinum toxin type A to the glabella. *Dermatol Surg* 2007; 33: s26–31.

64. Fagien S. Temporary management of upper lid ptosis, lid malposition and eyelid fissure asymmetry with botulinum toxin type A. *Plast Reconstr Surg* 2004; 114: 1892–902.

65. Ramey NA, Woodward JA. Mechanisms of blepharoptosis following cosmetic glabellar chemodenervation. *Plast Reconstr Surg* 2010; 126(5): 248e–9e.

66. Steinsapir KD, Groth MJ, Boxrud CA. Persistence of upper blepharoptosis after cosmetic botulinum toxin type A. *Dermatol Surg* 2015; 41: 833–40.

67. McKinney P, Camirand A, Carraway JH et al. Secondary upper eyelid blepharoplasty. *Aesthet Surg J* 2004; 24(1): 51–9.

68. Zoumalan CI, Lisman RD. Evaluation and management of unilateral ptosis and avoiding contralateral ptosis. *Aesthet Surg J* 2010; 30(3): 320–8.

69. Malik KJ, Lee MS, Park DJJ. Lash ptosis in congenital and acquired blepharoptosis. *Arch Ophthalmol* 2007; 125(12): 1613–15.

70. Northington ME, Huang CC. Dry eyes and superficial punctate keratitis: A complication of treatment of glabellar dynamic rhytides with botulinum exotoxin A. *Dermatol Surg* 2004; 30: 1515–17.

71. Fagien S. Botulinum toxin type A for facial aesthetic enhancement: Role in facial shaping. *Plast Reconstr Surg* 2003; 112 (Suppl 5): 6s–18s.

72. Alam M, Arndt KA, Dover JS. Severe, intractable headache following injection with botulinum A exotoxin. *J Am Acad Dermatol* 2002; 46: 62–5.

73. Ashkenazi A, Silberstein S. Is botulinum toxin useful in treating headache? Yes. *Curr Treat Options Neurol* 2009; 11(1): 18–23.

74. Carruthers A, Carruthers J, and Cohen J. Dilution volume of botulinum toxin type A for the treatment of glabellar rhytides: Does it matter? *Dermatol Surg* 2007; 33: S97–104.

75. Sclafani AP, Jung M. Desired position, shape, and dynamic range of the normal adult eyebrow. *Arch Facial Plast Surg* 2010; 12(2): 123–7.

76. Cote TR, Mohan AK, Polder JA et al. Botulinum toxin type A injections: Adverse events reported to the US Food and Drug Administration in therapeutic and cosmetic cases. *J Am Acad Dermatol* 2005; 53: 407–15.

77. Wieder JM, Moy RL. Understanding botulinum toxin. Surgical anatomy of the frown, forehead, and periocular region. *Dermatol Surg* 1998; 24: 1172–4.

78. Hsu TS, Dover JS, Arndt KA. Effect of volume and concentration on the diffusion of botulinum exotoxin A. *Arch Dermatol* 2004; 140: 1351–4.

79. Carruthers A, Carruthers J, Cohen J. A prospective, double-blind, randomized, parallel-group, dose-ranging study of botulinum toxin type A in female subjects with horizontal forehead rhytides. *Dermatol Surg* 2003; 29: 461–7.

80. Rohrich RJ, Janis JE, Faigen S, Stuzin JM. The cosmetic use of botulinum toxin. *Plast Reconstr Surg* 2003; 112: 117s–87s.

81. Ozsoy Z, Genc B, Gozu A. A new technique applying botulinum toxin in narrow and wide foreheads. *Aesth Plast Surg* 2005; 39: 368–72.

82. Oliveira de Morais O, Reis-Filho EM, Pereira LV et al. Comparison of four botulinum neurotoxin type A preparations in the treatment of hyperdynamic forehead lines in men: A pilot study. *J Drugs Dermatol* 2012; 11(2): 216–19.

83. Matarasso SL. Complications of botulinum A exotoxin for hyperfunctional lines. *Dermatol Surg* 1998; 24: 1249–54.

84. Keen M, Kopelman JE, Aviv JE et al. Botulinum toxin A: A novel method to remove periorbital wrinkles. *Facial Plast Surg* 1994; 10(2): 141–6.

85. Matarasso SL. Comparison of botulinum toxin types A and B: A bilateral and double-blind randomized evaluation in the treatment of canthal rhytides. *Dermatol Surg* 2003; 29: 7–13.

86. Lowe NJ, Lask G, Yamauchi P. Bilateral, double-blind, randomized comparison of 3 doses of botulinum toxin type A and placebo in patients with crow's feet. *JAAD* 2002; 47: 834–40.

87. Carruthers A, Bruce S, de Coninck A et al. Efficacy and safety of OnaBTX-A for the treatment of crow's feet lines: A multi-center, randomized, controlled trial. *Dermatol Surg* 2014; 40: 1181–90.

88. Patrinely JR, Anderson RL. Anatomy of the orbicularis oculi and other facial muscles. In: Jankovic J, Tolosa E (eds). *Adv Neurol. Vol. 49; Facial Dyskinesias*. New York, NY: Raven Press; 1988.

89. Lowe NJ, Ascher B, Heckmann M. Double-blind, randomized, placebo-controlled, dose-response study of the safety and efficacy of botulinum toxin type A in subjects with crow's feet. *Dermatol Surg* 2005; 31: 257–62.

90. Kane MAC. Classification of crow's feet patterns among Caucasian women: The key to individualizing treatment. *Plast Reconstr Surg* 2003; 112(5): 33s–9s.

91. Matarasso SL, Matarasso A. Treatment guidelines for botulinum toxin type A for the periocular region and a report on partial upper lip ptosis following injections to the lateral canthal rhytids. *Plast Reconstr Surg* 2001; 108(1): 208–14.

92. Lemke BN, Stasior OG. The anatomy of eyebrow ptosis. *Arch Ophthalmol* 1982; 100: 981–6.

93. Matarasso SL. Decreased tear expression with an abnormal Schirmer's test following botulinum toxin type A for the treatment of lateral canthal rhytides. *Dermatol Surg* 2002; 28: 149–52.

94. Knize DM. An anatomically based study of the mechanism of eyebrow ptosis. *Plast Reconstr Surg* 1996; 97: 1321.

95. Alex JC. Aesthetic considerations in the elevation of the eyebrow. *Facial Plast Surg* 2004; 20: 193–98.

96. Yalcınkaya E, Cingi C, Söken H, Ulusoy S, Muluk NB. Aesthetic analysis of the ideal eyebrow shape and position. *Eur Arch Otorhinolaryngol* 2016; 273: 305–10.

97. Westmore MG. Facial cosmetics in conjunction with surgery. Paper Presented At: *Aesthetic Plastic Surgical Society Meeting*; May 7, 1974; British Columbia, Canada: Vancouver.

98. Angres GG. Blepharopigmentation and eyebrow enhancement techniques for maximum cosmetic results. *Ann Ophthalmol* 1985; 17(10): 605–11.

99. Cook TA, Brownrigg PJ, Wang TD et al. The versatile midforehead browlift. *Arch Otolaryngol Head Neck Surg* 1989; 115(2): 163–8.

100. Gunter JP, Antrobus SD. Aesthetic analysis of the eyebrows. *Plast Reconstr Surg* 1997; 99(7): 1808–16.

101. Roth JM, Metzinger SE. Quantifying the arch position of the female eyebrow. *Arch Facial Plast Surg* 2003; 5(3): 235–9.

102. Biller JA, Kim DW. A contemporary assessment of facial aesthetic preferences. *Arch Facial Plast Surg* 2009; 11(2): 91–7.

103. Schreiber JE, Singh NK, Klatsky SA. Beauty lies in the "Eyebrow" of the beholder: A public survey of eyebrow aesthetics. *Aesthetic Surg J* 2005; 25: 348–52.

104. Baker SB, Dayan JH, Crane A, Kim S. The influence of brow shape on the perception of facial form and brow aesthetics. *Plast Reconstr Surg* 2007; 119(7): 2240–7.

105. Goldman M. Festoon formation after intraorbital botulinum A toxin: A case report. *Dermatol Surg* 2003; 29: 560–1.

106. Flynn TC, Carruthers J, Carruthers A. Botulinum A toxin treatment of the lower eyelids improves infraorbital rhytides and widens the eye. *Dermatol Surg* 2001; 27: 703–8.

107. Flynn TC, Carruthers JA, Clark RE. Botulinum A toxin (BOTOX) in the lower eyelid: Dose-finding study. *Dermatol Surg* 2003; 29: 943–50.

108. Balikian RV, Zimbler MS. Primary and adjunctive uses of botulinum toxin type A in the periorbital region. *Otolaryngol Clin N Am* 2007; 40: 291–303.

14 Cosmetic uses of botulinum toxin A in the mid face
Anthony V. Benedetto

MID FACE
Introduction
With the increased demand for facial rejuvenation done by noninvasive techniques, many experienced injectors of botulinum neurotoxins (BoNTs) are now venturing below the upper face with treatments.[1] At this time, however, all these treatments in the United States (US) are not Food and Drug Administration (FDA) approved and are performed in an off-label manner. As with any other part of the face, it is imperative for the treating physician to be completely knowledgeable of the dynamic balance of the levator and depressor action of the mid face mimetic musculature if successful treatments with BoNTs are to be realized. The reciprocating action of opposing mimetic muscles can prove to be a bit more complicated in anatomical morphology and function in the mid and lower face and therefore more challenging to treat than in the upper face. Specifically, the muscles of the upper face are easily distinguishable from one another because of various topographic landmarks, making it easy to inject them with any BoNT. However, in the mid and lower face there is an interdependence of movement of superficial and deep mimetic muscles which also are adjacent to, and form part of, some of the muscles surrounding the mouth that function in the articulation of sounds, expression of emotions, and, or in mastication and deglutition. All adjacent mid face mimetic muscles interdigitate with each other and are invested by the superficial muscular aponeurotic system (SMAS). Many of them perform complementary and, at times, unrelated dynamic functions. The mimetic muscles of the mid and lower face have very specific functions, which are mostly centered around the mouth. These muscles can sometimes act as agonists, sometimes as antagonists, but always in a complex, synergisticly dynamic manner. They allow a person to smile, laugh, grimace, pucker the lips, or to make any other overt or subtle gesture with the mouth. These complex functions permit one to hold solids, liquid, or air within the mouth without loss of contents. They also allow one to release contents at will from the mouth either slowly or forcibly. These muscles allow for the fine motor movements necessary to produce either subtle whispering sounds or thunderous clamor. They also facilitate the actions of chewing, swallowing, and a myriad of other simple and complex movements that either explicitly or implicitly function in deliberate and involuntary motor movements that are so particular of an individual's mannerisms and personality. In addition, many of these superficial and deep muscles overlie a thicker mass of soft tissue as well as each other, creating an anatomy that is quite different from the forehead and brow. Consequently, if OnaBTX-A (OnaBTX-A) migrates beyond the targeted muscles when it is injected in the mid and lower face, unintended effects and adverse sequelae can easily occur. Therefore, when treating anyone with OnaBTX-A in the lower two-thirds of the face, low doses usually are effective and higher doses are not necessarily better but instead can be rather detrimental to the dynamic balance of normal facial mimetic function.

There are additional factors that contribute to the differences in the anatomy of the upper face as compared to that of the mid and lower face, which will determine how one injects OnaBTX-A when rejuvenating the face.[2] In the upper face, the skin can be thicker and more tightly adherent to the underlying musculature. Adverse outcomes in the upper face, if and when they occur, often are related to a variable uptake and diffusion of the injected OnaBTX-A. They usually present as asymmetries or cosmetic inconveniences which can be easily rectified in most cases with a few additional units of strategically placed OnaBTX-A. Generally, much higher doses of OnaBTX-A are needed in the upper facial musculature to produce a desired effect, and these treatments rarely cause any functional imbalance, except when severe ptosis occurs.

On the other hand, because of its compact spatial arrangement and indistinct borders, the diminutive mid and lower facial musculature should be treated with lower doses of OnaBTX-A that gently weaken targeted muscular movement while avoiding spread of the injected neurotoxin to adjoining muscles. Wrinkles in the mid and lower face tend to be more static in nature as compared to those in the upper face, which are more dynamic in origin.[3,4] Particularly in the mid face, wrinkles develop and are enhanced because of photodamage, volume loss, and soft tissue shifting.[5] These are some of the reasons why deep longstanding wrinkles and furrows in the mid and lower face generally cannot be totally effaced, no matter how much OnaBTX-A is injected. Persistent treatments with escalating doses of any BoNT can result in anatomic aberrations and functional imbalance without satisfactorily diminishing the unwanted wrinkles. This must be made perfectly clear to the patient prior to treatment so as not to disappoint the patient and frustrate the injector. To maintain anatomic symmetry while preserving normal muscular activity in the mid and lower face when treating a patient with injections of OnaBTX-A, it is absolutely necessary, more so than in the upper face, that accurately measured, minimal volumes of low doses of OnaBTX-A be precisely injected into specifically targeted muscles. Particularly during treatments of the mid face, the upper lip levators are easily affected by the slightest amount of OnaBTX-A diffusing from an injection of an adjacent muscle. This can readily cause a disruption in one or many of the complex motor functions of the lips (e.g., eating, drinking, speaking, and expressing emotion). Also, because of the intermingling of the muscle fibers of the orbicularis oris with those of the upper lip levators, which are invested with a thicker mass of subcutaneous soft tissue, OnaBTX-A injections of the mid face should be performed only by an expert injector.[6]

In most areas of the mid and lower face, however, better overall cosmetic results can be achieved with different soft tissue fillers, or with resurfacing techniques and many other types of interventional procedures (i.e., rhytidectomy, prosthetic implantation, and different soft tissue suspension techniques), while supplementary treatments with OnaBTX-A injections can be performed to enhance and prolong the final aesthetic outcomes[5–7] (see Chapter 7, by Alastair and Jean Carruthers).

NASOGLABELLAR LINES (SEE APPENDIX 2)
Introduction: Problem Assessment and Patient Selection
There are many individuals who form diagonal wrinkles and lines over the lateral walls of the nasal bridge near the root of the nose that radiate downward, toward the nasal alae. These diagonal lines accentuate and deepen when those individuals speak, smile, laugh, or frown. These lines are identified as nasoglabellar lines and politely referred to as "bunny" lines. They are particularly prevalent in those individuals who are constantly squinting, either because they have poor vision and refuse to wear corrective eyeware, or spend extended periods of time in front of computer screens at work or enjoy extended periods of time outdoors in bright light without protective, shaded eyeware. These nasoglabellar wrinkles are produced primarily by

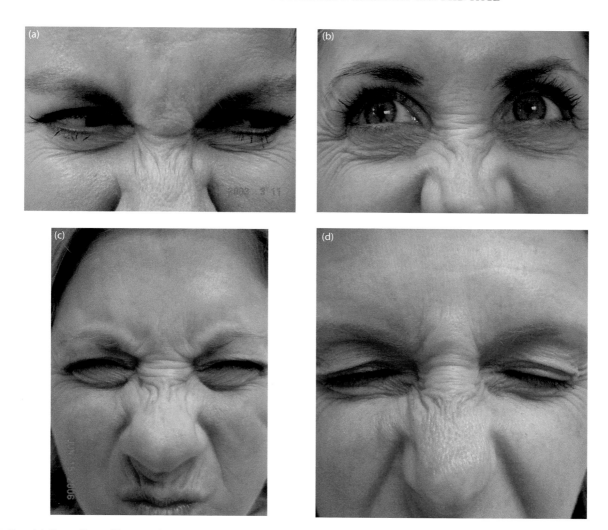

Figure 14.1 Nasoglabellar or "bunny" lines, produced by the transverse nasalis, are those vertical lines emanating from the lateral sides of the root of the nose before a treatment with OnaBTX-A. The transverse or horizontal lines across the root of the nose are produced by the procerus. Different patients have different wrinkle patterns possibly contributed by contractions of the medial aspect of the LLSAN, *orbital* orbicularis oculi, and anomalus nasi. Note the commonly seen nasoglabellar lines caused by the contraction of the transverse nasalis, which are accompanied by (a) nasociliary rhytides, (b) naso-orbicular and naso-alar rhytides, (c) nasociliary and naso-alar rhytides, and (d) naso-orbicular and naso-alar rhytides.

the contraction of the transverse portion of the nasalis. The pattern and depth of these wrinkles and lines can be different on either side of the midline (Figure 14.1). They are anatomically distinct both in location and source from the horizontal lines that span transversely across the nasal radix, which are produced by the downward pull of the procerus. When this radial fanning of longitudinal wrinkles of the upper lateral aspect of the nasal bridge occurs as a secondary, compensatory contraction of the transverse nasalis after treatment of glabellar frown lines with OnaBTX-A, the nasoglabellar lines have been demonstratively identified as the "BOTOX® sign" (Figure 14.2).[7] On the other hand, when these nasoglabellar lines occur naturally and before any treatment with a BoNT, they are referred to as "bunny lines" or a "nasal scrunch" (Figure 14.3).[7,8] Women who idiosyncratically produce nasoglabellar wrinkles find them to be annoying and unsightly because they can unintentionally project an attitude of disdain, dislike, or disapproval. These lines should be treated along with glabellar frown lines with injections of OnaBTX-A during the same treatment session. On the other hand, there are some individuals with inelastic, lax, redundant skin who elevate skin and soft tissue of the midface when they forcibly squint and produce deeply corrugated nasoglabellar rhytides. For these patients, whose nasoglabellar lines are not produced by the contraction of the transverse nasalis, but by

the elevation and pleating of submalar and lateral nasal skin, injections of OnaBTX-A are not helpful and futile (Figure 14.4).

Functional Anatomy of Nasoglabellar Lines (see Appendix 2)

Nasoglabellar lines are the result of the contraction of the upper or transverse portion of the nasalis, also known as the compressor naris. The nasalis is a thin, flat, paired, triangular-shaped muscle that can be divided into two parts: a *transverse* and an *alar* part.[9,10] The transverse nasalis originates from the maxilla, superior and lateral to the incisive fossa overlying the root of the canine tooth (Figure 14.5). Its fibers course medially and superiorly and expand into a thin aponeurosis over the bridge of the nose, which cross the midline and interdigitate with its contralateral paired transverse nasalis muscle fibers. Superiorly, the transverse nasalis inserts into the aponeurosis of the procerus, and inferiorly interdigitates with medial fibers of the *orbital* orbicularis oculi and the levator labii superioris alaeque nasi (LLSAN). Some fibers of the transverse nasalis also may attach to the skin of the nasolabial and alar folds along with the alar nasalis, also called the *posterior* dilator naris (Figure 14.6). (See the next section on "Nasal Flare" for a description of the alar part of the nasalis.) The transverse nasalis or "compressor naris" depresses the cartilaginous part of the nose, pushing the alae inwardly toward the nasal septum,

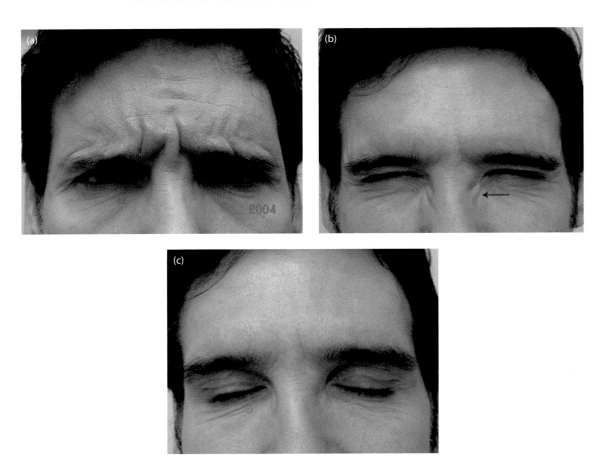

Figure 14.2 "BOTOX® Sign." (a) Patient frowning and without nasoglabellar lines prior to a treatment with OnaBTX-A. (b) Same patient frowning 3 weeks after an OnaBTX-A treatment of his glabellar frown lines. Note the compensatory nasoglabellar lines, that is, "BOTOX® Sign" (*arrow*). (c) Two weeks after a touch-up injection of OnaBTX-A in the transverse nasalis and 5 weeks after the original OnaBTX-A treatment. Note the compensatory nasoglabellar lines are gone.

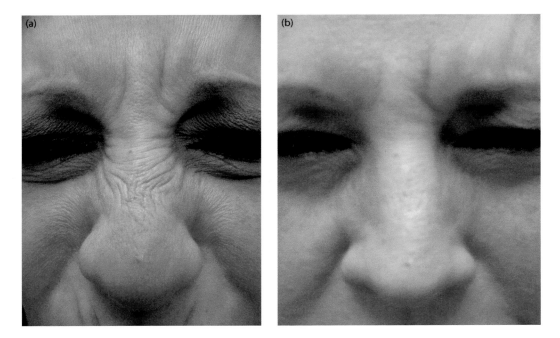

Figure 14.3 A 49-year-old patient frowning (a) before and (b) 3 weeks after a treatment with OnaBTX-A of both the glabella and nasoglabellar lines. Note the diminished nasoglabellar "bunny lines."

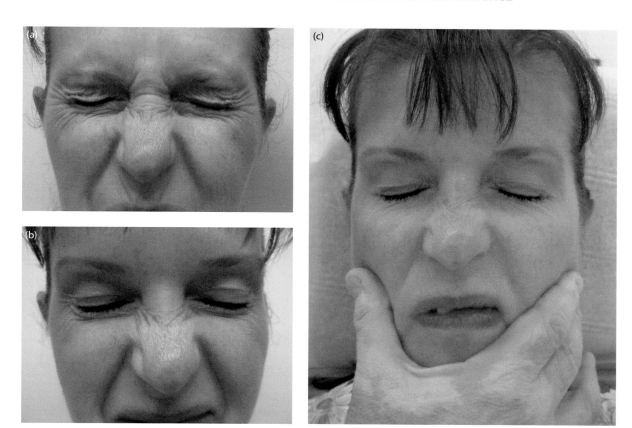

Figure 14.4 (a) In this 49-year-old patient, not all the nasoglabellar lines are produced by the contraction of the transverse nasalis, but rather (b) by the pleating of the submalar and lateral nasal skin as seen here two weeks after OnaBTX-A injections which were not entirely helpful in this patient and (c). Note the absence of the dorsolateral nasal lines created by forced upward movement of lax skin when the mid face skin is prevented from elevating.

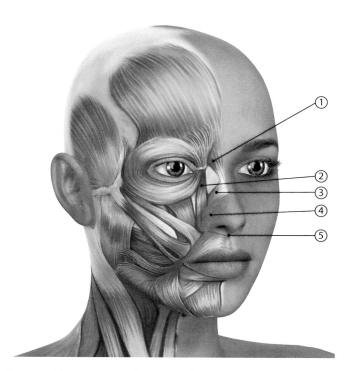

Figure 14.5 The transverse nasalis originates from the maxilla and inserts into the nasal bridge aponeurosis. 1, procerus; 2, levator labii superioris alaeque naris; 3, transverse nasalis (compressor naris); 4, alar nasalis (posterior dilator naris); 5, depressor septi nasi.

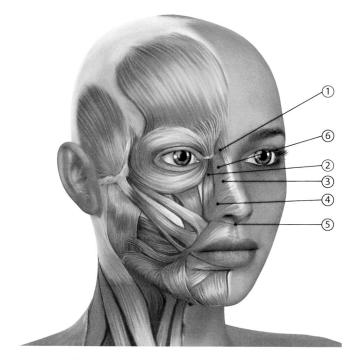

Figure 14.6 When present the anomalus nasi covers an area normally devoid of musculature between the orbital orbicularis oculi, LLSAN, and the procerus on the lateral side of the nasal bone. 1, procerus; 2, levator labii superioris alaeque naris; 3, transverse nasalis (compressor naris); 4, alar nasalis (posterior dilator naris); 5, depressor septi nasi; 6, anomalus nasi.

thereby compressing the nasal aperture at the junction of the vestibule and nasal cavity, and activating the internal nasal valve.[9,10] A recent study found that in the 36 of 40 (81%) cadavers examined, muscle fibers of the transverse nasalis interdigitated with superficial fibers of the LLSAN at the lateral side of the nose.[11] This might explain why some individuals can easily produce bunny lines and others cannnot. It is those individuals who have an ample amount of transverse nasalis fibers interdigitating with a substantial number of adjacent LLSAN fibers who will possess enough strength to move and wrinkle the mid to upper nasal bridge. While others, whose transverse nasalis does not form extensive interconnections with the LLSAN might just form weak bunny lines or might not be able to produce any at all. In fact, Trevidic and his plastic surgeon and anatomist colleagues believe that nasoglabellar lines are not formed by the transverse nasalis at all but only by the contraction of the LLSAN.[10] An alternative consideration for why some individuals can form bunny lines naturally and why others cannot is possibly because they might be the few individuals in the population (50% or 60%) that might have an additional muscle along the bridge and lateral aspect of the nose called the *anomalus nasi*. Letourneau and Daniel found an anomalus nasi present in 50% of their fresh cadaver dissections.[12] The anomalus nasi originated from the frontal process of the maxilla and it inserted into the nasal bone, the upper lateral cartilage, the procerus, and the transverse nasalis.[9,12–14] When present the anomalus nasi was found to cover an area normally devoid of musculature between the orbital orbicularis oculi, LLSAN, and the procerus on the lateral side of the nasal bone.[15] By its position and the direction of its muscle fibers the anomalus nasi appears to function by compressing and possibly elongating the nose (see also Tamura's bunny line patterns below) (Figure 14.6).

Nasoglabellar lines are produced by asking the patient to squint forcibly, as if intense light is shining in the eyes. If these lines become prominent without any upward movement of cheek skin, then the patient will most likely readily produce bunny lines after his or her glabellar lines are treated with OnaBTX-A (Figure 14.3). Therefore, such naturally occurring nasoglabellar lines should be elicited, identified, and demonstrated to the patient before any treatment with a BoNT. In this way, the patient will understand why the transverse nasalis should be treated in conjunction with glabellar frown lines. If the nasoglabellar lines are not treated at the same time as the glabellar lines, the patient will be more inclined to blame the physician and OnaBTX-A for the presence of these lines if and when they appear after treatment, whether the patient was aware of them before treatment. Therefore, it behooves the physician injector to disclose their presence to the patient prior to any treatment with OnaBTX-A, underscoring the necessity to include nasoglabellar frown lines as an integral part of their treatment (Figure 14.3).

However, when the transverse nasalis does not overtly contract and produce nasoglabellar wrinkling naturally, it is not necessary to treat the transverse nasalis in conjunction with the glabellar frown lines. On the other hand, if the nasoglabellar lines do become prominent, displaying the "BOTOX sign," after a patient's glabellar frown lines are treated with OnaBTX-A, then the nasoglabellar lines should be identified and treated during the obligatory follow-up visit, 2–3 weeks after an OnaBTX-A treatment session (Figure 14.2).

Dilution When Treating Nasoglabellar Lines (see Appendix 3)

To prevent the unintended widespread diffusion of OnaBTX-A beyond the point of injection, it is necessary that a minimum amount of OnaBTX-A be injected when treating nasoglabellar lines. Therefore, 1 mL of normal saline should be used to reconstitute the 100 U vial of OnaBTX-A when injecting nasoglabellar lines.

Dosing: How to Correct the Problem (see Appendix 4) (What to Do and What Not to Do) When Treating Nasoglabellar Lines

Myorelaxation of nasoglabellar lines can be accomplished by injecting 2–5 U of OnaBTX-A subcutaneously or intramuscularly into the lateral walls of the nasal bridge, just inferior to the nasal radix and anterior and superior to the nasofacial angle (Figure 14.7). This technique should position the needle well above the angular vessels and upper lip levators.[16–18] The skin and soft tissue are extremely thin and vascular in this area and advancing the needle tip a few millimeters here, goes a long way.

With the patient in the upright sitting or semireclined position, it is most important to perform the injections in such a way as to avoid injecting too low along the nasal sidewalls and into the nasofacial sulcus (Figure 14.8). Otherwise, either the LLSAN or the levator labii superioris (LLS), or both, may be weakened by the injected OnaBTX-A, since they both originate along the medial aspect of the malar prominence. If either of these levators is affected, then upper lip ptosis, asymmetry, and resultant functional changes of the mouth can occur. It appears men are not treated for this problem as frequently as women are. The dose of OnaBTX-A depends on the overall depth and location of the lines and strength of the transverse nasalis. A dose of 3–5 U of OnaBTX-A injected on each side of the nasal bridge may be necessary to diminish these lines. An additional 2–4 U may be required before the least amount of nasoglabellar wrinkling is totally eliminated, especially in those men and women who spend the better part of their day outdoors and whose nasalis

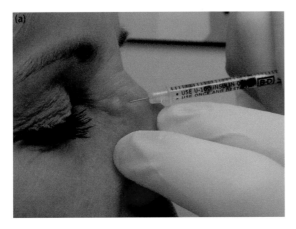
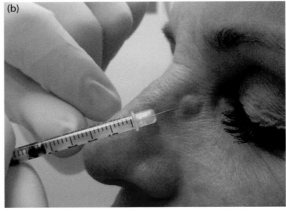

Figure 14.7 (a, b) Injecting the transverse nasalis anterior and superior to the nasofacial angle. Note the wheal of injected OnaBTX-A.

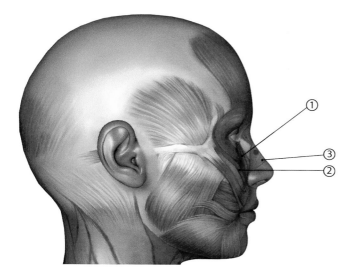

Figure 14.8 The blue dot (•) marks the point at which injections should be placed when treating the compressor naris (transverse nasalis) to avoid inadvertently weakening the levators of the central upper lip and injuring the angular neurovascular structures. 1, LLSAN; 2, LLS; 3, transverse nasalis. See Chapter 12, Figures 12.1 and 12.2.

is hypertrophic and hyperkinetic from constant squinting (see also Tamura's bunny line patterns).

Outcomes (Results) When Treating Nasoglabellar Lines (see Appendix 5)

Eliminating nasoglabellar lines along with glabellar frown lines gives an individual a relaxed, youthful appearance. When the nasoglabellar lines are not treated and the glabellar frown lines are, nasoglabellar lines in the presence of a smooth glabella produce an exceptionally unsightly effect (Figures 14.2 and 14.9).

Tamura et al.[19] found that they could successfully treat approximately 40% of their patients with nasoglabellar lines by injecting them with 3 U of OnaBTX-A on either side of the nasal side wall into the belly of the transverse nasalis (Figure 14.10). The other 60% of the patients in their study had persistent bunny lines that exhibited different linear patterns along the proximal and distal nasal bridge. They found that to further diminish these persistent bunny lines an additional 2 U of OnaBTX-A needed to be injected at different locations along either side of the nasal bridge according to the three different patterns they identified. They named the recalcitrant bunny lines according to their anatomic location as the *nasoalar* rhytides, *nasoorbicular* rhytides, and *nasociliary* rhytides (Figures 14.1 and 14.11). The additional OnaBTX-A treatments were given during the first follow-up visit, 4 weeks after the initial treatment

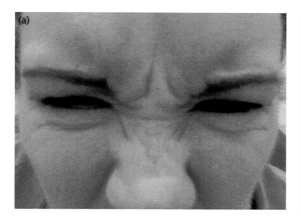
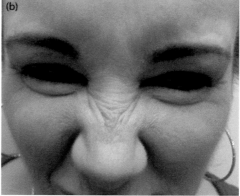

Figure 14.9 Note the presence of glabellar and nasoglabellar "bunny lines" before (a) and the compensatory contractions of the transverse nasalis 3 weeks after (b) an OnaBTX-A treatment of only glabellar frown lines. Patient insisted on not having her bunny lines treated.

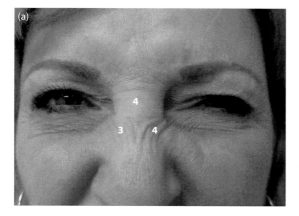
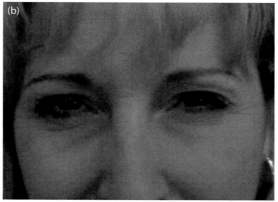

Figure 14.10 A 52-year-old patient frowning (a) before and (b) 2 weeks after a treatment with OnaBTX-A of both the glabellar (4 units into the procerus) and nasoglabellar (total of 7 units) lines. Note the stronger and deeper lines on the left which required an extra unit of OnaBTX-A and the diminished "bunny lines."

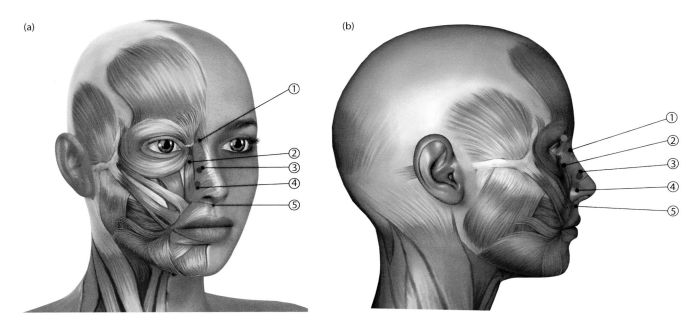

Figure 14.11 (a, b) Standard injection point for transverse nasalis: blue dot (•). Note the additional injections sites to diminish persistent nasoglabellar lines: red dot (•) for nasociliary rhytides; green dot (•) for nasoorbicular rhytides; purple dot (•) for nasoalar rhytides.

with OnaBTX-A. There were approximately 30% of the patients who had persistent wrinkling at the root of the nose, which extended superiorly toward the medial margin of the eyebrow and glabella caused by the contraction of the *orbital* orbicularis oculi adjacent to the ciliary arch, so they were identified as having *nasociliary* rhytides (Figures 14.1a, c and 14.11). Another 30% of the patients had persistent wrinkling of the root of the nose owing to contraction of the nasal portion of the orbital orbicularis oculi, so these patients were identified as having *nasoorbicular* rhytides (Figures 14.1b, and d and 14.11). The third pattern, identified as persistent naso-alar

wrinkles, occurred in both of the above subgroups and were felt to be the result of the contraction of the alar portion of the LLSAN (Figures 14.1b–d and 14.11). Each area of persistent wrinkling was produced by unaffected fibers of the underlying muscles after a standard treatment with OnaBTX-A, which required the additional 2 U of OnaBTX-A on either side of the nasal bridge to completely eliminate any residual nasoglabellar "bunny lines" (Figures 14.12 and 14.13).[19]

However, patients who recruit cheek and submalar skin and elevate it toward the nasal radix forming corrugations of skin along the lateral

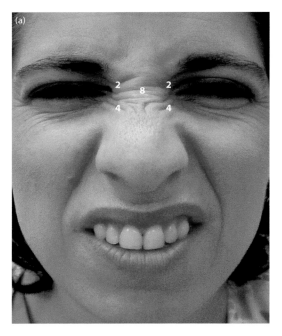

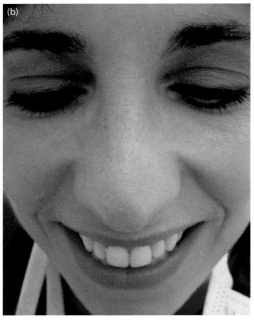

Figure 14.12 A 45-year-old patient frowning (a) before and (b) 3 weeks after a treatment with OnaBTX-A of both the horizontal glabellar and oblique nasoglabellar lines. The horizontal line across the root of the nose produced by the procerus were treated with 8 units of OnaBTX-A; the nasociliary lines were treated with 2 units of OnaBTX-A on either side of the nasal root and the nasoorbicular lines were treated with 4 units of OnaBTX-A on either side of the nasal bridge. Note the complete elimination of the "bunny lines."

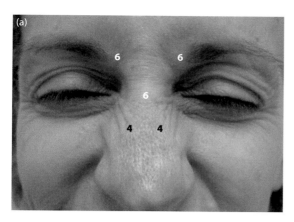
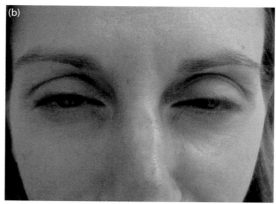

Figure 14.13 This 49-year-old patient is shown (a) before and (b) 3 weeks after an OnaBTX-A treatment. Note: Glabellar treatment units are shown in white, and the naso-glabellar units in black.

aspect of the proximal nose will not be helped by OnaBTX-A injections (Figure 14.4). Injections of OnaBTX-A will diminish only those rhytides that are formed by the contraction of the transverse nasalis and contributing ancillary muscle fibers, such as the medial portion of the *orbital* orbicularis oculi, alar portion of the LLSAN, and possibly an anomalus nasi when present (Figures 14.3, 14.6, 14.12, and 14.13). Usually, one can expect the effect of an OnaBTX-A treatment of naso-glabellar lines to last at least 3–4 months, or however long the glabellar frown lines remain effaced. In patients who previously had undergone a rhinoplasty, the results may be somewhat less than expected.[17–18,20,21]

Complications (Adverse Sequelae) When Treating Nasoglabellar Lines (See Appendix 6)

Injecting OnaBTX-A too deeply and low along the nasal sidewalls and into the nasofacial sulcus will allow it to diffuse into the upper lip levators (i.e., levator labii superioris alaeque nasi and levator labii superioris), since they both originate along the medial aspect of the malar prominence. If either of these levators is affected, the outcome can be an asymmetric smile and even ptosis of the upper lip, resulting in sphincter incompetence and functional difficulties with speaking, eating, and drinking.

Also, if the medial *palpebral* orbicularis oculi is weakened as the result of the unintended diffusion of OnaBTX-A, a diminution in the action of the lacrimal pump can occur, causing epiphora (excessive tearing) (see Chapter 13).[21] Diplopia also can result if the medial rectus is weakened by the inadvertent spread of OnaBTX-A caused by

overzealous dosing or incorrect placement of the injection. Vigorous massage to the area after the injection of OnaBTX-A can cause it to spread beyond the targeted area and produce the same untoward adverse results, even if dosing is appropriate and the injection technique is flawless. There is no antidote for any of these untoward post-treatment sequelae, and the patient is obligated to endure them until the effects of the OnaBTX-A remit. In the meantime, consultation with an ophthalmologist to help the patient cope with these alarming ocular problems is advisable.

It is important also to keep in mind that the angular artery and vein sit in the nasofacial angle and injections placed too low along the nasal sidewall and too deeply into the skin can result in an intra-vascular injection of the OnaBTX-A or injury to one of the vessels causing either ecchymoses (vein) or hematoma (artery). Therefore, intradermal or superficial subcutaneous placement of the needle tip is all that is necessary when injecting this area with a BoNT (Figure 14.7). There have been no reports of any adverse events from an intra-vascular injection of OnaBTX-A when less than 10 U is injected. Figures 14.14 through 14.19 are additional examples of different patients treated with OnaBTX-A for nasoglabellar lines.

Treatment Implications When Injecting Nasoglabellar Lines

1. Squinting will reveal the presence or absence of naturally occurring nasoglabellar lines in some individuals and are identified as "bunny lines." They should be elicited and recognized before treating glabellar frown lines with OnaBTX-A.

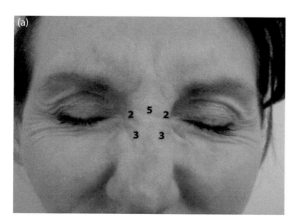
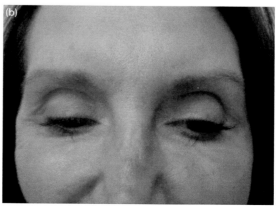

Figure 14.14 A 59-year-old patient frowning (a) before and (b) 3 weeks after a treatment with OnaBTX-A of both the glabellar and nasoglabellar lines. Note the diminished "bunny lines."

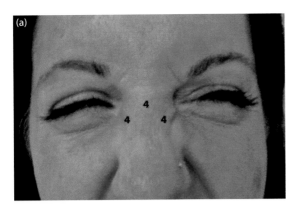
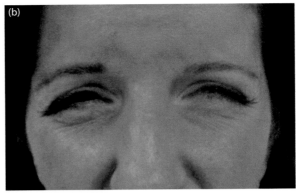

Figure 14.15 A 55-year-old patient frowning (a) before and (b) 4 weeks after a treatment with OnaBTX-A of both the glabellar and nasoglabellar lines (nasoalar). Note the diminished "bunny lines."

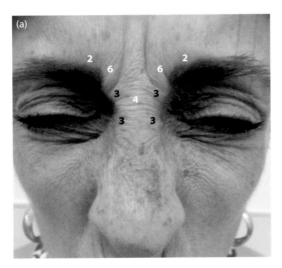
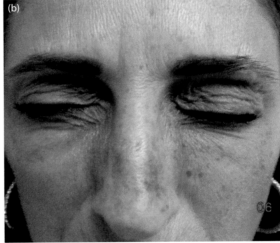

Figure 14.16 This 52-year-old patient has nasociliary, naso-orbicular, and naso-alar nasoglabellar lines. She is shown here (a) before and (b) 8 days after an OnaBTX-A treatment. *Note:* Glabellar treatment units are shown in white, and the nasoglabellar units in black.

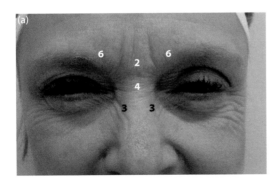
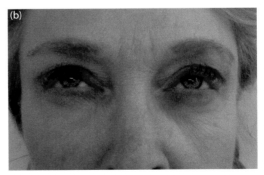

Figure 14.17 This 67-year-old patient is shown (a) before and (b) 2 weeks after an OnaBTX-A treatment. *Note:* Glabellar treatment units are shown in white, and the nasoglabellar units in black.

2. When nasoglabellar lines are produced as a result of compensatory contraction of the transverse nasalis after an OnaBTX-A treatment, they are referred to as the "BOTOX® sign."

3. Treat vertical nasoglabellar frown lines (i.e., those produced by the contraction of the transverse nasalis) along with horizontal glabellar frown lines (i.e., those produced by the contraction of the procerus) during the same treatment session.

4. Injections of OnaBTX-A should be performed intradermally or subcutaneously into the lateral aspect of the nasal bridge and radix.

5. Injections given too low and too deeply into the nasofacial sulcus may result in ecchymoses, hematoma, an asymmetric smile, or even upper lip ptosis and upper lip incompetence and functional difficulties of the sphincteric action of the mouth.

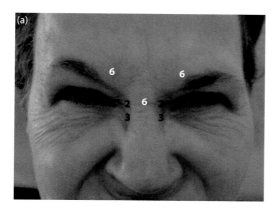
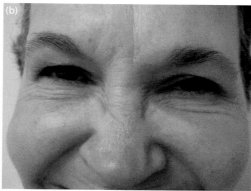

Figure 14.18 A 66-year-old patient frowning (a) before and (b) 1 week after a treatment with OnaBTX-A of both the glabellar and nasoglabellar lines (nasoorbicular and nasoalar). Note the diminished "bunny lines." Glabellar treatment units are shown in white, and the nasoglabellar units in black.

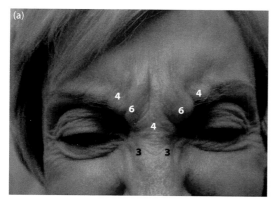
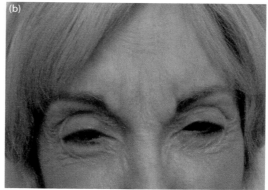

Figure 14.19 This 80-year-old patient is seen before (a) and 3 months after (b) an OnaBTX-A treatment of nasoglabellar or "bunny" lines. Note that the glabella was treated simultaneously. Glabellar treatment units are shown in white, and the nasoglabellar units in black.

6. Additional units of OnaBTX-A may be needed along the lateral aspect of the nasal radix and the proximal and distal nasal bridge in different patterns to efface all the nasoglabellar lines in ~60% of patients.
7. Patients with inelastic, lax skin who squint excessively may produce nasoglabellar lines that cannot be reduced by OnaBTX-A injections.

NASAL FLARE

Introduction: Problem Assessment and Patient Selection

Noses come in different forms and shapes (Figure 14.20). The size, shape, and proportions of the nose contribute to an individual's beauty or handsomeness, by virtue of its position in the center of the face. A broad classification of noses is based on the shape of the nasal or alar base. The *leptorrhine* or long and narrow nose is found on Causcasian

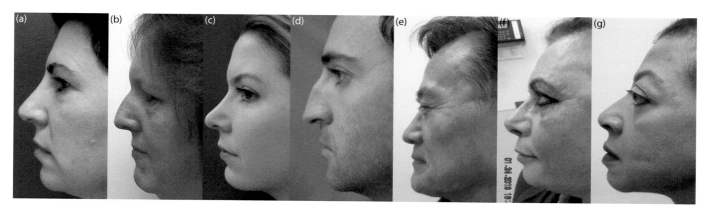

Figure 14.20 Different types and variations in nasal profile: (a) Grecian; (b) Roman; (c) Nordic; (d) Middle Eastern/Northern African; (e) Asian-Mongolian; (f) Asian-Indian; (g) sub-Saharan African.

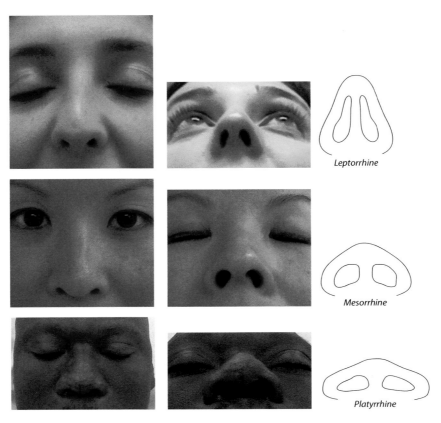

Figure 14.21 Examples of different nostril shapes seen frontally and from slightly below: *leptorrhine* (long and narrow), *mesorrhine* (medium), and *platyrrhine* (broad and flat).

faces, the *mesorrhine* or somewhat flat nose of medium length and width is found on the faces of the Oriental races and the *platyrrhine* or short, broad and flat nose is found on the faces of the Negroid races[22] (Figure 14.21). An individual's nose is one of the most distinguishing anatomical structures that identifies a person's race and differentiates one's ethnic group from another.[23] It is the shape of the nose that is a person's signature indicating one's race, ethnicity, age, and sex. Anthropometric differences also vary with age, sex, and ethnic and racial background. However, in this age of globalization with unrestricted travel and all-inclusive social exchanges, interracial mingling resulting in interindividual variations, has now become considerably more extensive among the different ethnic groups and races.[23–27] For example, in the West, particularly in the Americas, the "mestizo" population originates from three predominant races: the Indigenous Indian, the European Caucasian, and the African Negroid populations. Latin American mestizos do not have a specific phenotypical racial pattern, and their predominant facial features vary depending on the geographic zone from which they originate. People from Mexico, Peru, Bolivia, and many Central American countries exhibit stronger Indigenous Indian facial characteristics, whereas people from Argentina and Chile exhibit stronger European facial characteristics. People from Brazil, the Caribbean islands, and the coasts of Colombia and Venezuela exhibit a stronger African influence in their facial features. The same can be said of other cultures and ethnic groups in different parts of the East where the influences of globalization also have taken place (see Chapter 17, by Kyle Seo).

Mestizo facial charactersitics vary widely from the traditional western European Caucasian face, even though they are genotypically related. The mestizo face tends to be broad with thick skin and a nose that looks small, undefined, bulbous, and slightly flattened.

The underlying structural support of the mestizo or mesorrhine nose is less robust than a leptorrhine nose: bones are small and wide, although many have a deep radix and a small hump. Cartilaginous structures are thin and weak with a wide cartilaginous vault. Nasal tip support is weak because of a weak caudal septum, small nasal spine, and unsupportive alar cartilages. Externally, the mestizo mesorrhine nose can have a wide nasal bridge, low radix, wide nasal base, short columella, acute nasolabial angle, and nostrils that tend to have a more flaring and horizontal shape (Figure. 14.22).[25] It is not surprising that the Asian messorrhine nose also shares similar characteristics as the Mestizo mesorrhine nose, since more than 30,000 years ago people with Asian and Mongolian features crossed the Bering Straits and formed the different indigenous tribes that inhabited the regions of the New World when the Spanish and Portuguese sailed to the Americas in the fifteenth and sixteenth centuries.[22,25]

There are some individuals who, either naturally or when they are under physical or emotional stress, flare their nostrils and widen their nasal aperture repeatedly as they inspire. Noticeable movement of the nostrils with forced inspiration can impart to the casual observer a negative attitude, which may include anger, fear, exhaustion, concern, disapproval, or personal distress. For some, active dilation of the nostrils also occurs while they are speaking, smiling, laughing, or expressing an emotion (Figures 14.23 and 14.24). This unwanted predilection for inadvertently flaring the nostrils occurs more frequently in those who possess a broad nasal bridge with a wide nasal alar base. It can also occur in those individuals with a more leptorrhine shaped nose (Figures 14.23 and 14.24). Generally, however, it is those individuals with a more mesorrhine or platyrrhine shaped nose, whose alar lobules visibly contract uncontrollably during inspiration and facial animation

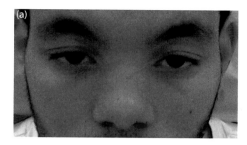
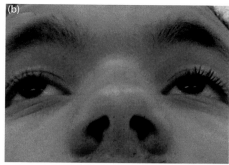

Figure 14.22 (a, b) A "Mestizo nose" has a wide nasal bridge, low radix, wide nasal base, short columella, acute nasolabial angle, and nostrils that are horizontal in shape and flare more readily.

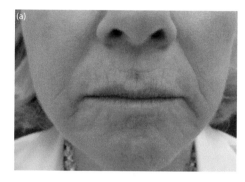
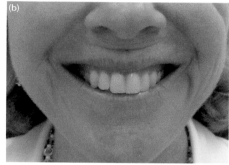

Figure 14.23 (a, b) This 63-year-old patient flares her nostrils and curls the upper lip forming a transverse upper lip crease with smiling. Note the downward rotation of the nasal tip with nostril flaring. Note the posterior gummy show and the difference between this older patient and the younger one of Figure 14.30.

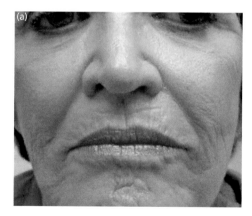
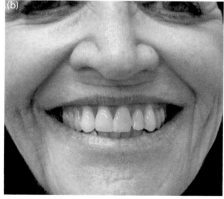

Figure 14.24 (a, b) This 72-year-old has a horizontal upper lip crease and actively dilates her nostrils when she smiles.

who seek relief from these embarrassing involuntary movements of their noses. This unconscious flaring of the nostrils occurs in some individuals because the overall mesorrhine and platyrrhine shape of their noses predisposes their alar musculature (i.e., dilator nares and levator labii superioris alaque nasi) to be more developed and active, because they are larger and stronger. These muscles also will allow such individuals to dilate their nostrils deliberately as well as involuntarily. Consequently, their noses possess a variety of additional nasal movements more so than noses of a leptorrhine shape and form.[27] For individuals who are troubled with involuntary nasal flaring, injections of OnaBTX-A may diminish this embarrassing, idiosyncratic synkinesis.

Functional Anatomy (See Appendix 2) of a Nasal Flare

Nasal flaring is the result of the involuntary contraction of the muscles of the nasal lobules, causing the alae nasi to dilate repeatedly during inspiration and facial animation, particularly while eating, drinking, speaking, laughing, and smiling[9,10] (Figures 14.23 and 14.24).

Before commencing with a decscription of nasal musculature, it is important for the reader to understand that there are significant inconsistencies, contradictions, and even inaccuracies in nomenclature of the different nasal muscles, depending on the date of a particular study and the prevailing terminology in use at the time of the publication. The age, race, and ethnic origins of the subjects studied and whether a given citation is an anatomic versus a surgical study all have some bearing on the names of the muscles identified and described. More importantly, not all muscles will be present in all individuals, and interindividual variation may be substantial for those muscles which are present, depending on the age, sex, race, and ethnic background of the study subjects.[12,28,29] It is even more confounding when either anatomic or physiologic criteria are emphasized in a given study. Consequently, comparative referencing can lead to some misinterpretation and confusion when defining the three-dimensional functional anatomy of the nose.[12,13]

The nose, even more so than the ear, is a distinctively three-dimensional structure that projects off the anterior surface of the face. The mimetic muscles of the upper face can visibly function both as separate and distinct muscles and as interdependent grouped agonists or antagonists, and thus contract synergistically as co-depressors (corrugator supercilii, depressor supercilii, procerus, orbicularis oculi) or independently as a levator (frontalis). However, only a few if any of the mimetic muscles of the nose can function independently from one another, but generally function synergistically during respiration, phonation, and expression of an emotion in a noncompetitive, complementary manner as compressors and dilators.[12] The nasal muscles possess different directional movements needed to maintain a patent passageway for air, and to sustain a functional external and internal nasal valve for unobstructed breathing through the nostrils.[30] In addition, the nose has the unique ability to assist in the formation of distinctive sounds as when one speaks, hums, or sings. If the normal passage of air through the nasal vault is compromised in the slightest amount, for example, because of a negligible deviation in the nasal cartilagenous supporting structures or even because of edematous nasal mucosa and turbinate hypertrophy caused by seasonal allergies or an upper respiratory ailment, normal nasal muscle movements can be altered. The result is an impairment of the nasal airway patency, an increase in air flow resistance and an interference with one's ability to resonate air and clearly enunciate words or sing a tune. In addition, the overall appearance of one who is not feeling well can be easily identified as one who "looks sick," conspicuously expressed by the involuntary and voluntary writhing movements of one's mimetic facial muscles, including the muscles of the nose. Therefore, the different nasal muscles must be appreciated for their divergent movements functioning in a unified manner that are complementary to one another. They maintain the integrity and consistency of inspiration and expiration, as well as the unique activities of animation, verbal and non-verbal communication.

The musculature of the non-cartilaginous portion of the alar lobule contains two similarly functioning identifiable muscles that complement each other: the alar nasalis, also called the "*posterior* dilator naris," which is an extension of the more superiorly positioned transverse nasalis, and the "*anterior* dilator naris" (Figure 14.25). In live or cadaveric dissections, it is usually difficult to separate completely the individual fibers of the *posterior* from the *anterior* dilator nares.[29]

The *posterior* dilator naris originates from the maxilla just above the lateral incisor and canine teeth, slightly lateral to the bony origin of the depressor nasi septi and medial to the bony attachment of the *transverse nasalis*, with which it partially merges (hence its other name, *alar nasalis*) under the nasolabial fold (Figure 14.25). The muscle fibers of the alar nasalis or *posterior* dilator naris travel superiorly and anteriorly to insert into (a) the skin of the alar lobule above the posterior circumference of the lateral crus of the greater nasal cartilage (also known as the lower lateral cartilage), (b) the accessory alar (sesamoid) cartilages in the hinge area, and (c) the alar facial crease or groove at the margin of the nasal aperature. It also inserts into the posterior part of the mobile septum Figure 14.26).[14] The alar nasalis also contributes to the formation of the upper ridge of the philtrum and nostril sill (Figure 14.26).

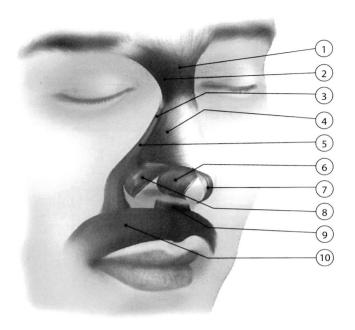

Figure 14.25 The non-cartilaginous portion of the alar lobule contains the alar nasalis (also called the "posterior dilator naris"), an extension of the transverse nasalis, and the anterior dilator naris. The muscles complement one another in function. The compressor narium minor (when present) arises from the intermediate crus of the lower lateral cartilage, interdigitates with some muscle fibers of the anterior dilator naris and inserts into the skin of the nasal dome near the margin of the nostrils and travels vertically down the columella to insert into the nasal spine. When present, the "dilator apicis nasi" (also called the "small dilator muscle of the nose") is found attached to the lateral crus of the lower lateral cartilage and encircles the distal lobule tip and nasal dome. 1, procerus; 2, depressor supercilii; 3, anomalus nasi; 4, transverse nasalis; 5, levator labii superioris alaeque nasi and levator alae nasi; 6, anterior dilator naris; 7, compressor narium minor; 8, posterior dilator naris (alar nasalis); 9, depressor septi; 10, orbicularis oris.

Laterally, alar fibers of the *posterior* dilator naris interdigitate with muscle fibers of the LLSAN and LLS. Medially, fibers of the alar nasalis (i.e., *posterior* dilator naris) also interdigitate with muscle fibers of the "*anterior* dilator naris" and the depressor septi nasi (Figure 14.26). The *posterior* dilator naris draws the hinge area of the ala laterally, and it can move the ala and the posterior part of the columella downward, thereby assisting in elongating the nose and widening the nasal aperture.

The *anterior* dilator naris is a fan-like muscle that originates from the upper edge of the lower lateral cartilage in front of the alar nasalis (*posterior* dilator naris) and the caudal margin of the lateral crus of the lower lateral cartilage (Figure 14.25). It encircles the naris occupying most of the lateral wall of the external nose (alar lobule) that lacks cartilaginous support and interdigitates with the compressor narium minor when it is present in the nasal dome[13] (Figure 14.25). The *anterior* dilator naris inserts into the rim of the lateral alar skin and nasal spine. Its muscle fibers are arranged in a typical crisscross pattern similar to the intrinsic muscles of the tongue.[29] The primary function of the *anterior* dilator naris is to stabilize this most flaccid portion of the lateral nasal wall, assist in dilating the nostrils and prevent the ala nasi from collapsing, especially during inspiration, thereby maintaining the competency of the external nasal valve.[9,10,14–17] However, it is the primary muscle responsible in causing nasal flaring, which results in an increase in nostril diameter and widening of the nasal vestibule.

Ducut and colleagues found in their cadaver dissection study of Asian noses that there was a significant difference in the characteristics of some nasal muscles which have a direct effect on the alar lobule and nostril shape.[27] The more horizontally shaped nostrils (of mesorrhine or

(a)

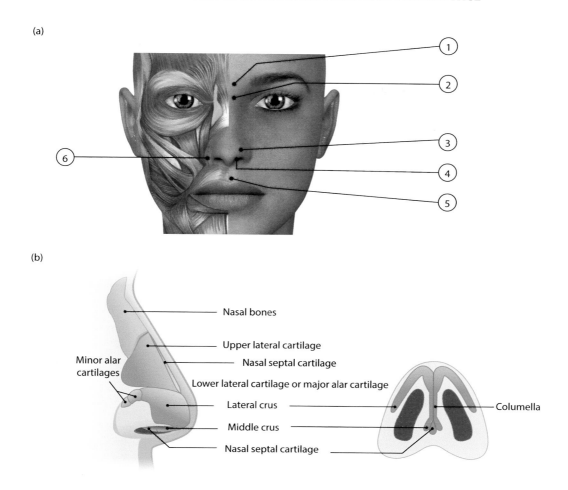

(b)

Figure 14.26 (a) The external surface and skeletal anatomy of the nose: 1, nasal root (frontal bone); 2, nasal bridge (nasal bone); 3, ala; 4, naris; 5, philtrum; 6, alar nasalis. (b) The cartilages and muscle origins of the nose. The alar nasalis (posterior dilator naris) originates from the maxilla and inserts in the skin of the alar lobule above the posterior edge of the lateral crus of the lower lateral cartilage, accessory (sesamoid) alar cartilages, and the alar facial crease, and into the upper ridge of the philtrum. Laterally it interdigitates with the levator labii superioris alaeque nasi and the levator labii superioris. Medially it interdigitates with the depressor septi nasi and the anterior dilator naris.

platyrrhine noses) have larger and more developed *anterior* and *posterior* dilator nares and depressor septi nasi than those of a more vertical leptorrhine nose.[27] In fact, in horizontally shaped nostrils the insertion of the *posterior* dilator naris extended to the midpoint between the alar base and the nasal tip, whereas the *posterior* dilator naris of a vertically shaped nose was limited to the alar base. The origin of the *anterior* dilator naris was also easily identified in horizontally shaped nostrils as emerging from the upper lateral cartilage and inserting into the caudal margin of the lower lateral crus and alar lobular skin, whereas the *anterior* dilator naris of the more vertically oriented nostrils was even difficult to identify. The *anterior* dilator naris is the primary dilator of the nose, widening the ala as it contracts. Contraction of the *posterior* dilator naris on the other hand draws the ala and the posterior aspect of the columella downward, which also widens the nasal aperture and can elongate the nose. Hyperkinetic *anterior* and *posterior* dilator nares in mesorrhine and platyrrhine noses tend to maintain the nostrils in an enlarged and widened state by constantly pulling them downward and pushing them outward.[27]

In addition, Ducut et al. found that in the horizontally shaped nostrils of mesorrhine and platyrrhine noses, the depressor septi nasi was more developed and prominently attached to the footplate of the medial crus of the lower lateral cartilage, extending and inserting into the columella, the membranous septum and the skin of the columellar and medial nasal vestibule. This anatomical configuration permits the depressor septi nasi

to pull in a downward direction the columella, the tip of the nose and the dorsal border of the nostril. On the other hand, in vertically shaped nostrils of leptorrhine noses, they found that the muscle attachment of the depressor septi nasi barely reached the footplate of the medial crus or it terminated just into the skin of the columellar base.[27]

Isometric contraction of the *posterior* dilator naris (alar nasalis) is initiated with inspiration, and its dilator effect stabilizes the airway lumen and maintains a fine control of air flow resistance by preventing the sidewalls of the internal nasal valve from collapsing. Furthermore, it was this muscle, the *posterior* dilator naris (alar nasalis), that Ducut et al. surgically severed at its attachment to reduce the alar flare and create a more vertically directed nostril.[27] With the reduced dilating effect and lateral pull of the *posterior* dilator naris, the alar lobule shifted medially, producing a more leptorrhine shape to the previously mesorrhine or platyrrhine shaped nose.[26] It is possible to produce a similar effect with a less invasive "chemical myotomy" using OnaBTX-A injected into the appropriate areas of the nose of a properly selected patient (Figure 14.27).

A secondary dilator of the nares is the medial alar portion of the LLSAN also known as the *levator alae nasi*. The LLSAN originates from the upper part of the frontal process of the maxilla and travels downward obliquely and laterally, dividing into medial and lateral slips of muscle. The medial fascicles of the LLSAN continue down along the

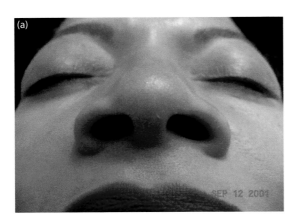
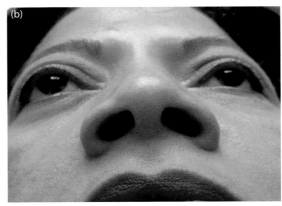

Figure 14.27 A 57-year-old patient at rest (a) before and (b) 4 weeks after a treatment with OnaBTX-A. A slight reduction of a nasal flare was achieved with 5 U of OnaBTX-A injected into the posterior dilator naris (alar nasalis) bilaterally. Note the more vertical orientation of the nasal base after treatment.

nasal sidewall and attach into the perichondrium of the lateral crus of the lower lateral cartilage and insert into the overlying skin. In some individuals, the levator alae nasi pulls the lateral crus superiorly displacing the circumalar furrow laterally and modifying its curvature. It also assists in dilating the nostrils. Because the levator alae nasi at times can function together with the nasal tip muscle fibers of the depressor septi nasi to retract the tip of the nose and help dilate the nostrils, both muscles are considered secondary nasal dilators, but they have little or no direct influence on the external nasal valve[31] (see below).

In addition to the standard nasal musculature discussed above, there are different accessory muscles of the nose which are not always found in all people. The presence of these accessory muscles varies widely between individuals, and their muscle function depends on the age, sex, race, and ethnic background of a person and the size and shape of his or her nose.[9]

The "anterior dilator naris," at times has been misleadingly associated with the "dilator apicis nasi" or the "small dilator muscle of the nose"[14] (Figure 14.26). This very small muscle, like the anterior dilator naris, is also found attached to the lateral crus of the lower lateral cartilage, hence the confused association. However, in most reports, the apicis nasi is not always present or identifiable and frequently considered too small to be functionally significant.[12,13] When present, however, the dilator apicis nasi was found to encircle the distal part of the nose and lobule tip, allowing the nasal tip to have barely perceptible circular movements that are concentric or convergent and eccentric or divergent. Since subtle expressions of pleasure and friendliness can be detected by involuntary circular movements of the nasal tip, these circular movements have been attributed to the contractions of the apicis nasi.[9,13,16,17,29]

In contradistinction, expressions of displeasure, dislike, and aversion are seen as vertical movements of the nasal tip. These vertical movements can be attributed to yet another small muscle not always present in the vicinity of the nasal tip called the compressor narium minor (Figure 14.25). It arises from the intermediate crus of the lower lateral cartilage and also interdigitates with some muscle fibers of the anterior dilator naris. It inserts into the skin of the dome of the nose near the margin of the nostrils and travels vertically down the columella to insert into the nasal spine. From the anatomical position and location of its fibers, this muscle is thought to be able to contract concentrically and slightly compress and narrow the nasal aperture.[9,12–14]

Dilution (See Appendix 3) When Treating a Nasal Flare
Moderate diffusion of OnaBTX-A can be advantageous when treating the lower dilators of the nose. Therefore, reconstituting a 100 U vial of OnaBTX-A with 1–2.5 mL of normal saline to inject into this area is acceptable.

Dosing: How to Correct the Problem (See Appendix 4), (What to Do and What Not to Do) When Treating a Nasal Flare
Treat the patient in the sitting or semireclined position with subcutaneous injections of 2–3 U of OnaBTX-A at each injection point into the center of each ala nasi equidistant from the alar groove and rim, along the lateral fibers of the alar nasalis (*posterior* dilator naris) and *anterior* dilator naris for a total of 4–10 U. This will weaken involuntary muscle contractions of the nostrils.[3,32] Such results can be useful in ethnic groups who possess a mesorrhine or platyrrhine shaped nose with the characteristic broad nasal bridge and wide alar base that flares easily because of hyperkinetic dilator nares (*anterior* and *posterior*). Only those patients who can deliberately and actively flare their nostrils are candidates for OnaBTX-A injections in this area (Figure 14.27). However, the physician injector should always be aware of the possible differences in strength and activity between the *anterior* and *posterior* dilator nares when treating a person with a platyrrhine shaped nose as opposed to someone with a mesorrhine or leptorrhine shaped nose. When well selected, obvious candidates do not experience a substantial improvement after a treatment with OnaBTX-A, the physician should reassess the appropriateness of the placement of the injections. Modification in technique, injection location, and unit dosing might be necessary, depending on which dilator muscle or muscles are more influential on that particular patient's nasal flare: the *anterior* or *posterior* dilator naris, the levator alae nasi (i.e., the medial alar portion of the LLSAN), or the depressor septi nasi. Injecting any one or all of these muscles at varying low doses will have a positive influence in diminishing an involuntary, dynamic nasal flare and reducing a horizontally oriented nostril aperture to a more vertically oriented one. Patients of African, Latino, and Asian descent or other individuals with either a mesorrhine or platyrrhine shaped nose, who may have a characteristically broad nasal bridge and wide alar base, but who cannot deliberately flare their nostrils will not experience any appreciable diminution in the involuntary, dynamic nasal flaring or even narrowing of their nasal aperature with injections of OnaBTX-A, and therefore should not be treated. Conversely, patients with a leptorrhine shaped nose who are afflicted with an involuntary dynamic nostril flare will reap some benefit from injections of OnaBTX-A. For these patients, carefully placed injections of OnaBTX-A into the primary nasal dilators (*anterior* and *posterior* dilator nares) and secondary nasal dilators (levator alae nasi, i.e., the medial alar portion of the LLSAN and the depressor septi nasi) will diminish a dynamic nasal flare, but will not appreciably alter the vertical orientation of the nostril aperture (Figure 14.28). However, an overzealous treatment with OnaBTX-A in a leptorrhine nose may more easily result in an adynamic nose than an overdose in

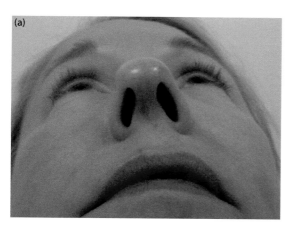 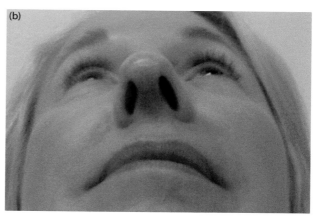

Figure 14.28 A 47-year-old patient with a leptorrhine shaped nose at rest (a) before and (b) 2 weeks after 6 U of OnaBTX-A was injected into each ala. A slight reduction of an involuntary dynamic nasal flare was achieved.

a mesorrhine or platyrrhine shaped nose (see nasal tip ptosis below). For some patients in whom the secondary nasal dilator, the depressor septi nasi may be strong and very active, their nasal flaring may be accompanied by a dynamic downward and upward movement of the nasal tip while they pronounce certain words, especially those containing W, O, U, and Q. In these patients, an injection of 2–4 U of OnaBTX-A into the center of the columella along with the injections of the primary nasal dilators is appropriate and at times necessary to sufficiently relieve their troublesome nasal flaring.

Outcomes (Results) (See Appendix 5) When Treating a Nasal Flare
For those individuals who are plagued with an involuntary propensity for dilating their nostrils when they breathe, speak, smile, or animate, or if they can flare or dilate their alae nasi willfully, injections of OnaBTX-A will decrease the frontal diameter of their nostrils and give their nose a narrower, more vertically leptorrhine appearance, without interfering with inspiration (Figure 14.28). Results can last up to 3–4 months and sometimes longer with repeat treatments. For patients who do not have well-developed muscle fibers of the *anterior* and *posterior* dilator nares and levator alae nasi (medial alar portion of the levator labii superioris alaeque nasi) and depressor septi nasi, and cannot dilate their nostrils at will, no amount of OnaBTX-A will relax these muscles enough to reduce their dynamic alar flaring or narrow their nostril aperature (see nasal tip ptosis below).

Complications (Adverse Sequelae) (See Appendix 6) When Treating a Nasal Flare
If patients are not selected properly, injections of OnaBTX-A might not be effective; then time, effort, and money will have been wasted. Otherwise, these patients experience no other adverse sequelae, except the usual ones that occur with transcutaneous injections, including pain, edema, erythema, and possible ecchymoses. Transcutaneous injections of the taut skin of the ala nasi with any injectable can be particularly painful. There have been no reports of difficulty with inspiration, nasoalar collapse, or nasal valve obstruction in those patients who have been treated successfully or unsuccessfully with OnaBTX-A to narrow an excessively wide nasal base or diminish dynamic alar flaring. However, the physician injector must not dismiss the potential or ignore the possibility for an adynamic nose and nostril collapse with forced inspiration inadvertently caused by either overzealous dosing or by misplaced injections of OnaBTX-A or both, especially when injecting someone who can only weakly dilate and flare their nostrils. Only precise amounts of low dose, low volume OnaBTX-A should be accurately injected in the mid and lower face (see nasal tip ptosis below).

Treatment Implications When Injecting the Nose for Nasal Flare
1. Treat only those individuals who can actively and willfully flare their nostrils.
2. Dynamic nasal flaring is predicated upon the particular shape of the nose and the different configuration and strength of the muscles present in the nose.
3. Not every nose has the same morphology of muscles configured in the same way with the same amount of strength.
4. Broader based noses with wide alae nasi and horizontally oriented nostrils have stronger anterior and posterior dilator nares and secondary nasal dilators with a predisposition for voluntary and involuntary dynamic nasal flaring.
5. Injections of a total of 4–10 U of OnaBTX-A along the alar rim and in the center of each ala nasi will relax the *anterior* and *posterior* dilator nares and diminish the involuntary flaring of the nostrils.
6. Treating hyperkinetic dilator nares with OnaBTX-A can produce an overall narrower nasal aperture without interfering with normal or forced respiration.
7. No adverse side effects have been identified with injections of OnaBTX-A in the nose.

NASAL TIP PTOSIS
Introduction: Problem Assessment and Patient Selection
With age, the nasal tip in some individuals naturally rotates downward, decreasing the angle between the upper lip and the columella. This occurs partly because of the pull of gravity and partly because of the pull of a hyperkinetic muscle of the nasal septum (i.e., depressor septi nasi). When this occurs, a person may possess the appearance of senility, feebleness, and decrepitude, projecting a pathetic and even sinister demeanor. There are others who, because of idiosyncratic skeletal morphology, possess a downwardly rotated nasal tip since birth (Figure 14.29). Still there are others whose nasal tip will noticeably and dynamically rotate downward in an up and down motion as they speak or pucker their lips, regardless of age (Figure 14.30). For those whose nasal tip actively moves and rotates downward when depressing the upper lip or when speaking, OnaBTX-A injections have provided a noninvasive means to elevate and project the nasal tip upward. Injections of OnaBTX-A will also stop the repeated up and down dynamic movement of the nasal dome while speaking, smiling, or drinking.

However, for an adynamic, static, inferiorly pointing nasal tip, only soft tissue fillers or surgical rhinoplasty can be corrective (Figure 14.31). An adynamic, ptotic, or an otherwise dynamic,

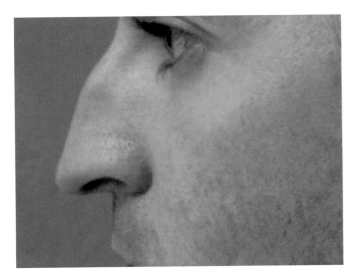

Figure 14.29 A naturally, downwardly rotated nasal tip in this 37-year-old patient.

plunging nasal tip and its nasolabial angle must be evaluated on lateral view[28,33] (Figures 14.29 through 14.31). The nasolabial angle is the relationship of the nasal base to the upper lip (Figure 14.31). The literature is replete with various methods of measuring this angle and its defining anatomical components. Customarily, the nasolabial angle is reported to range from 90 to 120 degrees allowing the treating physician to determine what the "ideal" nasolabial angle might be for the individual patient seeking treatment.[33] Armijo et al. recently studied 10 post-rhinoplasty men and 10 post-rhinoplasty women and concluded that the norms for the "ideal" nasolabial angle are changing and the ideal ranges for both men and women are not only more acute but similar in comparative angles to one another than previously reported. In their study, they found that the ideal nasolabial angle for men ranged from 93.4 to 98.5 degrees, and for women it ranged from 95.5 to 100.1 degrees.[33]

Dynamic nasal tip ptosis can be accompanied by excessive upper lip shortening and occasionally, the presence of a gummy smile and a transverse crease across the upper lip and philtrum, referred to as the "rhinogingivolabial syndrome" in the surgical literature (Figure 14.30).[34–37] This horizontal upper lip crease can be exaggerated in

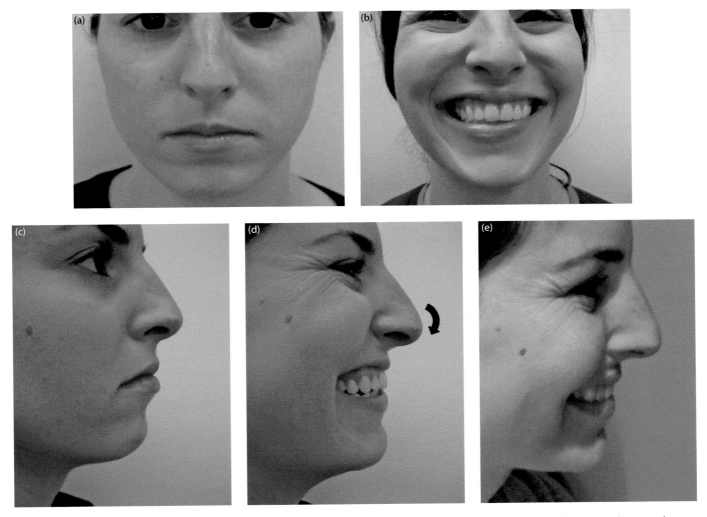

Figure 14.30 (a, b) This 26-year-old has a dynamic nasal tip ptosis, an upper lip shortening, an asymmetric posterior gummy smile, and a transverse line across her upper lip when smiling before OnaBTX-A. (c, d) View of the profile of the same patient. Note the dynamic nasal tip ptosis, gummy smile, narrowing of the nasolabial angle and downward turn of the nose when actively smiling. (e) Same patient seen 1 week after OnaBTX-A treatment. Note the reduction in the gummy smile and nasal tip ptosis with smiling. (See Figure 14.32.)

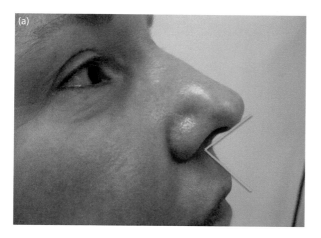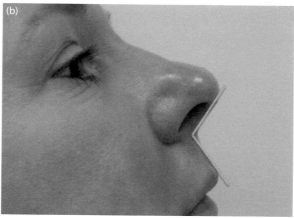

Figure 14.31 This 48-year-old patient has an adynamic, static, inferiorly rotated nasal tip, which could only be treated with a soft tissue filler. She is seen here (a) before and (b) 2 weeks after treatment with an intracolumella injection of calcium hydroxylapatite. Note the retracted base of columella; the acute columella-labial angle (<90°) and the inferiorly rotated and dropped nasal tip before treatment; and the anterior projection of base of columella; the obtuse columella-labial angle (~110°) and the superiorly rotated and enhanced nasal tip projection after the intracolumella injections of calcium hydroxylapatite.

older patients with dermatochalasis and skin laxity Figures 14.23 and 14.24). It also is found in younger patients when there is retraction and curling of a short upper lip with smiling (Figures 14.30 and 14.32).[35,38] These patients typically will also exhibit an excessive amount of maxillary alveolar gingiva when smiling or laughing, known as a "gummy smile" (Figure 14.30b,d) (see below). Nasal tip ptosis is not a rare problem and it can be seen in different ethnic noses worldwide.[36] Depending on a person's idiosyncratic anatomy and strength of the relevant muscles involved, not all the upper lip components (gummy smile and midphiltral transverse crease) associated with nasal tip ptosis are present in all patients concomitantly.[37]

Functional Anatomy (See Appendix 2) of Nasal Tip Ptosis

The depressor septi nasi is a short, relatively thick, paired muscle located on either side of the nasal septum that may be absent up to 20% of the time[10] (Figure 14.33). It is considered a component part of the *anterior* dilator naris by some. The depressor septi nasi originates at the center of the incisive fossa of the maxilla deep within the orbicularis oris (Figure 14.33).[9,10,35] Its fibers interdigitate with the superficial muscle fibers of the orbicularis oris and course upward within the mucous membrane of the upper lip to insert into (a) the superior aspect of the maxilla close to the medial crura of the lower lateral cartilage, (b) into the anterior nasal spine, (c) into the mobile cartilaginous nasal septum, and (d) the mucous membrane undersurface of the ala nasi. A few muscle fibers may even continue upward between the medial crura and into the nasal tip (Figure 14.33).[9,10] Rohrich et al. identified three types of depressor septi nasi from their cadaver dissections. Type I depressor septi nasi, the most prevalant (62%), was visible, identifiable, and interdigitated completely with the orbicularis oris at its origin and then terminated in the medial crural footplates. Type II depressor septi nasi, the second most commonly seen (22%), was also visible and identifiable but revealed little or no interdigitation with the orbicularis oris (Figure 14.33c, left). Type III depressor septi nasi, seen least often (16%), was only rudimentary or even absent[38] (Figure 14.33c, right). Even when present, however, the strength and direction of pull of the depressor septi nasi varied from patient to patient.[39]

When a person smiles the depressor septi nasi contracts. Depending on its size, strength, and the extent of its muscle fibers interdigitating with muscle fibers of the orbicularis oris, the depressor septi nasi can lower the tip of the nose, shorten the upper lip, pull the nasal septum downward, draw the ala nasi inferiorly, and narrow the nostril transversely.[9,10] In some individuals, fibers of the dilator nares (both anterior and posterior) have also been found to interdigitate with those of the depressor septi nasi. Consequently,

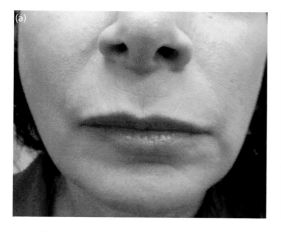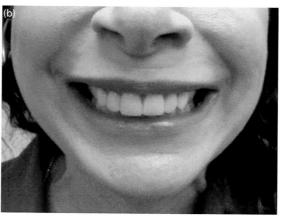

Figure 14.32 A 52-year-old patient curls the upper lip with smiling. Note the visible upper lip transverse crease and downward rotation of the nasal tip. Also note the difference between this older patient and the younger one of Figure 14.30.

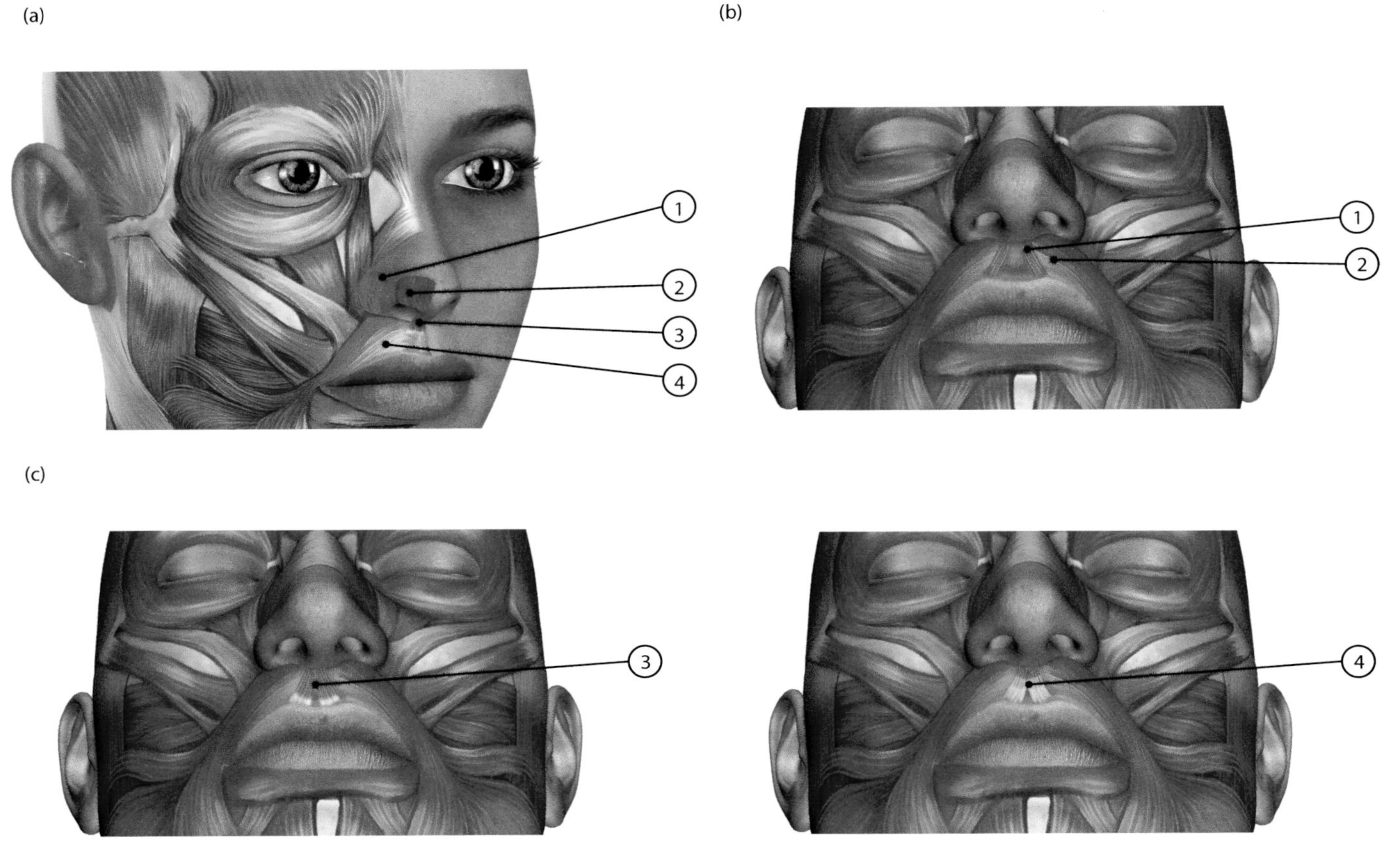

(a)

(b)

(c)

Figure 14.33 (a) Depressor septi nasi may intermingle with the anterior dilator naris and superficial fibers of the orbicularis oris. 1, posterior dilator naris (alar nasalis); 2, anterior dilator naris; 3, depressor septi nasi; 4, orbicularis oris. (b) There are three types of depressor septi muscles: the most common (in an estimated 62% of population) is type I (shown here), visible, identifiable, and traceable to full interdigitation with the orbicularis oris from the medial crural foot plate. Type I is thought to be responsible for producing a horizontal crease above the upper lip when an individual animates, especially when smiling. (See further Reference 37) 1, depressor septi Type I; 2, orbicularis oris. (c) Type II muscles (left side here; 22 percent) are visible and identifiable but, unlike Type I group, demonstrate little or no interdigitation with the orbicularis oris; and Type III (right side here; 16%) includes cases where no, or only a rudimentary, depressor septi muscle is visible. 3, depressor septi Type II; 4, depressor septi Type III.

when the depressor septi nasi contracts in unison with the dilator nares as the upper lip is set in motion (e.g., when smiling or pursing the lips to whistle, kiss, or pronounce words containing W, O, U, J, M, G, B, P, Q sounds), a concomitant widening of the nasal aperture will then occur and the nasal tip will actively rotate downward and upward and often repeatedly while one is speaking (see Figures 14.30 and 14.32) (see nasal flare above).

Yet in some other individuals, the lip and alar insertions of the depressor septi nasi are also comingled with lateral labial fibers of the LLSAN.[35] Consequently, during animation when the nasal tip is pulled downward while the upper lip is pulled upward in a curling motion, a horizontal upper lip crease appears and a maxillary gummy show is the result (Figures 14. 23, 14.24 and 14.30) (see below, gummy smile,). There is also another subset of individuals that produces an ominous and unfriendly sneer when they smile, as their nasal tip rotates downward from the pull of their particular depressor septi nasi and the nostrils and alar base are simultaneously pulled upward by their LLSAN[35,40] (Figure 14.30d). Because of individual variability in the anatomy of the depressor septi nasi, orbicularis oris, anterior and posterior dilator nares, accessory nasal tip musculature (apicis nasi and compressor narium minor) and the medial alar portion of the LLSAN (or levator alae nasi), along with the multifactorial etiology of a dynamic nasal tip ptosis with or without upper lip and nasal base retraction, injections of OnaBTX-A to elevate and project the tip of the nose usually is not as easy to perform as one might think.

Dilution (See Appendix 3) When Treating Nasal Tip Ptosis

In the paranasal area, minimum amounts of OnaBTX-A should be used so as not to accidentally affect the levators of the upper lip by the inadvertent spread of OnaBTX-A. Therefore, a 100 U vial of OnaBTX-A should be reconstituted with only 1 mL of normal saline.

Dosing: How to Correct the Problem (See Appendix 4) (What to Do and What Not to Do) When Treating Nasal Tip Ptosis

For those patients who can intentionally depress and rotate the tip of their noses downward by puckering or lowering their upper lip, noninvasive injections of OnaBTX-A now can be helpful in raising and projecting their nasal tip instead of resorting to the more invasive types of different surgical resections.[36–39,41] To effectively treat a dropped nasal tip, first identify the concave curvature that demarcates the junction between the columella with the center of the upper lip. Then ask the patient to smile and a more pronounced groove or crease becomes more apparent at the point in question (Figure 14.34). Next, with the patient in a sitting or semireclined position have the patient depress their upper lip downward, widening that junction between the base of the columella and the upper lip. This maneuver elongates the depressor septi nasi, separating it functionally and anatomically away from the orbicularis oris in those 30%–40% of individuals whose depressor septi nasi does not interdigitate with muscle fibers of the orbicularis oris and whose nasal tip ptosis does not simultaneously retract and shorten the

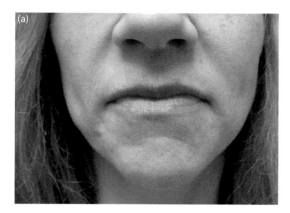
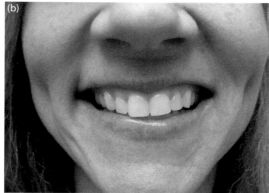

Figure 14.34 The concave curvature that demarcates the junction between the columella with the center of the upper lip (a) becomes a more pronounced groove or crease when a person smiles (b).

upper lip when they smile. This allows one to place the needle precisely into the depressor septi nasi at the base of the columella, and not into fibers of the orbicularis oris, before injecting OnaBTX-A. Then grasp the columella between the thumb and index finger of the nondominant hand at the same time the patient is forcing the upper lip downward and underneath their incisors and canines (Figure 14.35). Another technique is to lift the tip of the nose superiorly and gently push it posteriorly with the thumb of the nondominant hand (Figure 14.35).

Depending on the strength of the depressor septi nasi, 2–4 U of OnaBTX-A can be injected just superior (1–2 mm) to the labiocolumella boundary line crease (Figure 14.35). If the strength of the depressor septi nasi is visibly excessive causing it to be hyperfunctional, an additional 2–4 U of OnaBTX-A can be injected into the middle of the columella and even into the nasal tip to neutralize any additional downward pull of the compressor narium minor or the dermocartilaginous ligament of Pitanguy[36] (Figure 14.35c and d). Stronger muscles will require higher doses of OnaBTX-A.[42] In some patients whose depressor septi nasi also interdigitates with the anterior dilator naris, an additional injection of 2–6 U of OnaBTX-A on both lateral aspects of the nasal tip, that is, into the center of the ala nasi just behind the alar rim, will be necessary to effectively elevate and project the nasal tip.[42]

To reduce the depth of the horizontal upper lip crease, injections of OnaBTX-A should be placed lateral to the alae nasi and into the lateral labial fibers of the LLSAN. This actually is the treatment for an exaggerated maxillary gummy smile and is discussed in detail below.

Outcomes (Results) (See Appendix 5) When Treating Nasal Tip Ptosis

Injecting OnaBTX-A into the depressor septi nasi will relax the muscle, lifting and projecting the nasal tip upward (Figure 14.36). The combination of injecting both the columella and the alae nasi just lateral to the nasal tip with OnaBTX-A will relax the lower end of the nostrils and base of the nose, producing additional lifting of the nasal tip and lateral widening of the nostrils by the medial (alar) fibers of the LLSAN provided this muscle remains functional (Figure 14.37).[42] If one can see obvious movement and a downward rotation of the nasal tip when a patient smiles, speaks, depresses the upper lip, puckers or purses the lips, then injections of OnaBTX-A will be effective (Figures 14.38 and 14.39). Results can last 3–4 months and slightly longer with repeat treatments. If there is no movement of the nasal tip when the upper lip is depressed or while the patient smiles, speaks, puckers, depresses the upper lip, or purses the lips, OnaBTX-A injections should not be given.

Perez-Atamoros has devised a therapeutic dosing scheme whereby he can predict the height change in the nasal tip elevation and projection in patients he treats with OnaBTX-A.[42] Injecting 2 U of OnaBTX-A deeply into each of the right and left sides of the nasal tip into the *anterior* dilator naris and 2 U of OnaBTX-A into the depressor septi nasi (total of 6 U of OnaBTX-A) produces a slight elevation of the nasal tip. Approximately 4 U of OnaBTX-A injected into each of the right and left side of the nasal tip and the depressor septi nasi (total of 12 U of OnaBTX-A) produce a medium elevation of the nasal tip. For a high elevation and projection of the nasal tip, 6 U of OnaBTX-A into each of the right and left *anterior* dilator nares and depressor septi nasi (total of 18 U of OnaBTX-A) may be needed (Figures 14.37 and 14.40).[42] Results can last as long as 4–5 months. This is due presumably to the compensatory upward contraction of the secondary nasal dilator, the levator alae nasi, that is, the medial (alar) fibers of the LLSAN.

When a horizontal upper lip midphiltral crease is accentuated with smiling, with or without a downward rotation of the nasal tip, an additional 1–3 U of OnaBTX-A can be placed into each lateral portion of the LLSAN as described below in the section on a gummy smile. Injecting the depressor septi nasi and the lateral (labial) fibers of the LLSAN with a very small amount of OnaBTX-A not only can diminish the transverse line of the upper lip, but, when done appropriately, it also can provide an apparent increase in the vertical distance between the columella and vermillion border. This occasionally can create a fuller, more voluminous upper lip for some patients. However, for many others, especially for older patients, similar injections can adversely further elongate a thin and low-hanging upper lip and vermillion.[43] Dayan and Kempiners[35] also found that with 5 U of OnaBTX-A placed into each depressor septi nasi and 3 U placed into each LLSAN, on lateral view the nasal tip became less ptotic, the alar facial insertion remained in a more neutral position, and the nasolabial angle widened from 110 to 115 degrees. In addition, on frontal view there was a relative elongation and a relaxation in the curling of the upper lip with smiling and laughing that accompanied a diminution of the mid philtral horizontal crease, a more horizontal orientation to the alar base insertion, and an attenuation in the appearance of a snarl (Figure 14.30). Consequently, the depressor septi nasi is one of the muscles that also might need to be weakened when treating a patient for an exaggerated upper gummy smile (see "Gummy Smile" below). When there still is evidence of a horizontal upper lip crease after an appropriate treatment of OnaBTX-A, injections of a strategically placed soft tissue filler may be the only solution for its complete elimination (see Gummy Smile below) (Figure 14.41). The

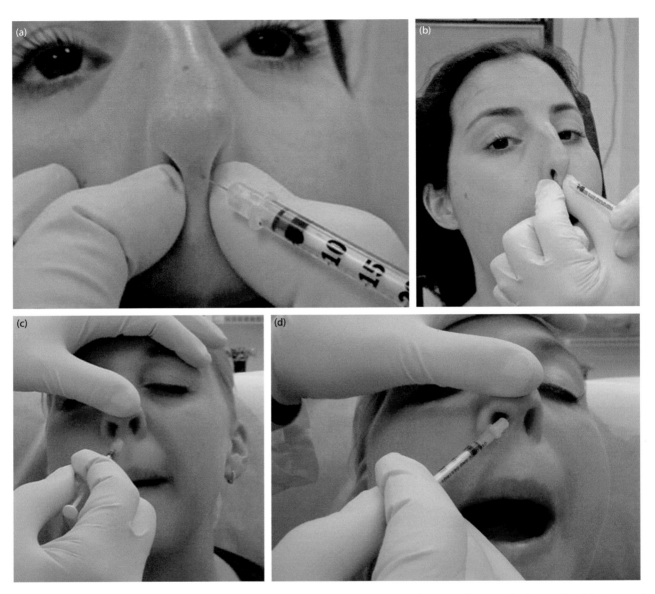

Figure 14.35 (a, b) Injection of the depressor septi nasi in the center of the columella. Note how the patient depressing their upper lip downward and the injector pinching the columella facilitate the injection. (c, d) Injection of the depressor septi nasi at the base of the columella. Note the placement of the needle, above the orbicularis oris, while the thumb of the nondominant hand gently pushes the nasal tip upward and backward.

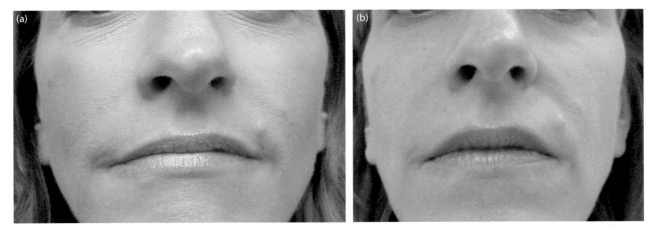

Figure 14.36 This 41-year-old at rest (a) before and (b) after 4 U of OnaBTX-A were injected at the base and midsection of the nasal columella. Note the slight elevation of the ptotic nasal tip after treatment. Dynamic tip rotation with speaking and lip puckering was also reduced.

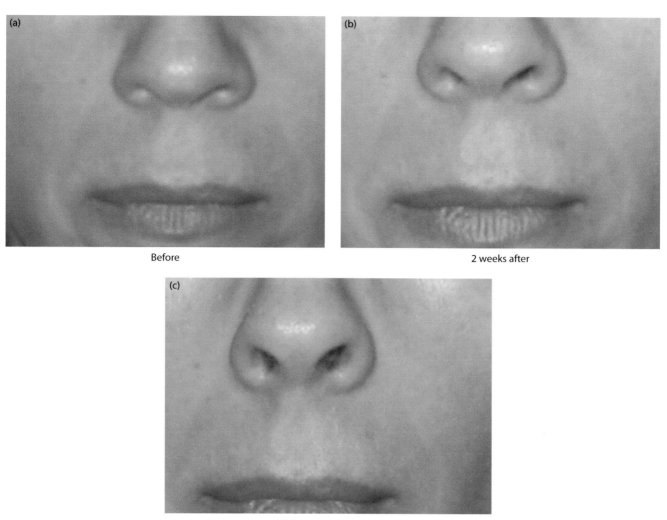

Figure 14.37 Exaggerated elevation of the nasal tip, flattening of the tip projection and excessive widening of the nostrils can be seen in this patient who was injected with a total of 18 U of OnaBTX-A (6 U into each anterior and posterior dilator nares equally divided per side and 6 U into the depressor septi nasi in the base and mid columella). (Courtesy of Dr. Francisco Perez-Atamoros.)

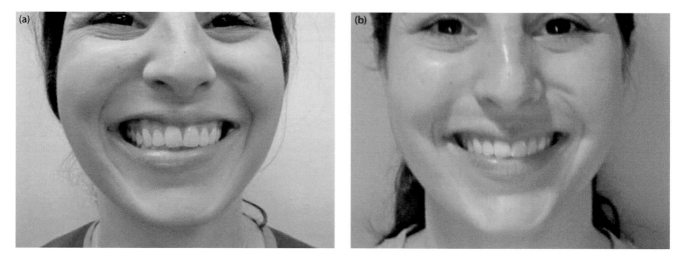

Figure 14.38 (a) The nasal tip of this 26-year-old patient actively rotated downward with speaking, smiling, and laughing before 4 U of OnaBTX-A: 2 U at the base and 2 U in the center of the columella. (b) Same patient 1 week after OnaBTX-A treatment.

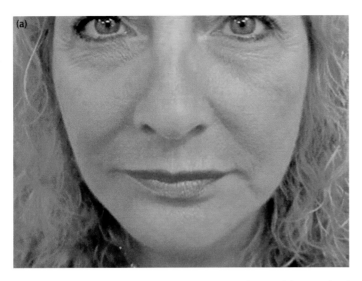
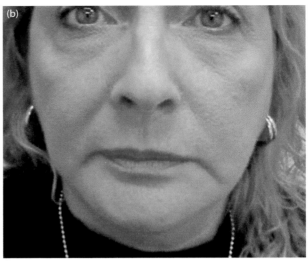

Figure 14.39 (a) The nasal tip of this 52-year-old patient actively rotated downward with speaking, smiling, and laughing before 4 U of OnaBTX-A: 2 U at the base and 2 U in the center of the columella. (b) Same patient 2 weeks after OnaBTX-A treatment. Note the slight nasal tip elevation and projection.

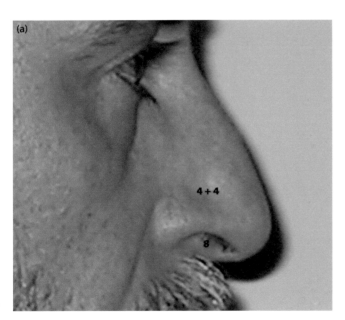
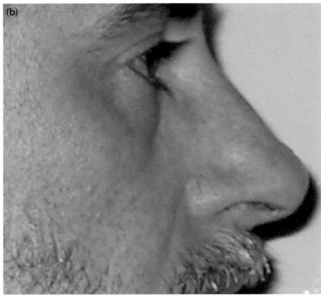

Figure 14.40 Nasal tip (a) before and (b) 1 month after a treatment with OnaBTX-A. An overall total of 16 U of OnaBTX-A were injected: 8 U into the anterior dilator nares (4 U on each side) and 8 U (4 U at the base and 4 U into the mid portion of the columella) into the depressor septi nasi to achieve these results. (From Atamoros, PF. Botulinum toxin in the lower one–third of the face. Editor AV Benedetto. *Clin Derm* 2003; 21: 505–12, by courtesy of Dr. Francisco Perez-Atamoros.)

effect of the injected OnaBTX-A in this area sometimes lasts for only 2–3 months, and even less in some patients.

Complications (Adverse Sequelae) (See Appendix 6) When Treating Nasal Tip Ptosis

When treating nasal tip ptosis, it is extremely important for the physician injector to assess accurately a patient's nasal morphology, the structure and composition of the muscles that are actively functioning in that particular person's nose. Not every muscle in every patient's nose functions exactly the same way, with the same strength or in exactly the same direction. The existing functional anatomy of an individual patient depends on the size, shape, sex, age, and racial and ethnic background of that patient. Overzealous injections with high doses of OnaBTX-A only into the interdigitating fibers of the depressor septi nasi and *anterior* dilator nares without relaxing the *posterior*

dilator nares or the medial alar fibers of the LLSAN can result in an unattractive, exaggerated widening of the nostrils along with the projection and elevation of the nasal tip (Figure 14.37). This forced widening of the nostrils in some patients is accompanied by persistent pain and soreness over the nasal tip that can last for over 2 weeks.[42] Therefore, it is extremely important to treat each person individually with the appropriate technique of dosing and injection placement.

Weakening only the depressor septi nasi may just elevate the nasal tip. However, if the OnaBTX-A diffuses laterally from the midpoint of the base of the nasal columella and into the central upper lip levators (i.e., LLSAN, levator labii superioris, or zygomaticus minor), then the upper lip can become elongated and thinned, obliterating the depth of the philtrum and the contour of the philtral columns. Asymmetry of the lips and alterations in functional buccal sphincteric control may also result, producing difficulty

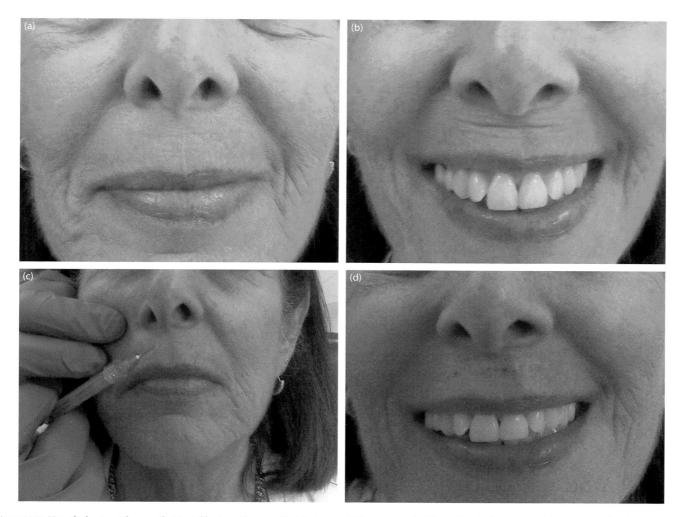

Figure 14.41 Note the horizontal crease that is visible above the upper lip (a) at rest and (b) accentuated while smiling in this 69-year-old patient 3 weeks after a treatment with OnaBTX-A. (c) Proper injection technique for eliminating the transverse crease of the upper lip. (d) The same patient seen in (a, b) immediately following treatment with a cohesive polydensified matrix type of hyaluronic acid-based injectable filler. Note the complete effacement of the transverse upper lip crease.

with eating, swallowing, and speaking. Unless there is an obvious downward displacement of the anterior aspect of the nose and nasal tip when a patient forcibly puckers or lowers his or her upper lip, speaks, or smiles, injections of the depressor septi nasi should not be attempted.

Treatment Implications When Injecting the Nose for Nasal Tip Ptosis
1. The tip of the nose may rotate downward because of muscle contraction, age, and gravity.
2. When the depressor septi nasi visibly depresses the tip of the nose when one smiles, speaks, puckers, or purses the lips, OnaBTX-A injections will elevate and project the nasal tip.
3. In some patients, additional deep injections of OnaBTX-A into the anterior dilator naris along the alar rim toward the nasal tip as well as the depressor septi nasi may be necessary to elevate and project the tip of the nose.
4. Inject OnaBTX-A on a case by case basis into all the nasal muscles which contribute to a particular person's nasal tip ptosis. Injecting OnaBTX-A into the columella (depressor septi nasi) and along the alar rim (*anterior* dilator naris) can cause an amplified widening of the nostrils if the *posterior* dilator naris and medial alar portion of the levator labii superoris alaque nasi are not weakened.

5. Misplaced and overzealous treatment with OnaBTX-A can cause excessive nostril widening, prolonged pain, an exaggerated elevation, and a flattening of the nasal tip projection.
6. Diffusion of OnaBTX-A lateral to the base of the columella can affect the upper lip levators, elongating the upper lip, blunting the contour of the philtrum, and causing lip asymmetry.
7. Upper lip asymmetry and oral sphincter weakness can result from injecting too high a dose of OnaBTX-A too superficially at the base of the columella which can diffuse into the central upper lip levators and superficial fibers of the orbicularis oris.

NASOLABIAL FOLDS
Introduction: Problem Assessment and Patient Selection
Chronological aging and a downward shift of soft tissue in the mid cheek area can deepen a nasolabial sulcus, which, in turn, augments its fold. Accentuated by side lighting and shadows, the nasolabial fold is enhanced by the overall diminution of structural skeletal and muscular support and intensified by the incessant effects of aging and the pull of gravity. The descent of cheek soft tissue mass occurs in the infraorbital and submalar area at different depths and stages in an inferiomedial direction and varies with each individual.[41,44–46] The redistribution of facial soft tissue and fat increases with time and leads to the development of a characteristic vertical

groove and fold that extend from the alar facial sulcus to the lateral labial commissures.[43] The appearance of these so-called nasolabial folds probably is more frequently seen in genetically predisposed individuals, but more than likely they also can be acquired by those whose mid facial movements are constant, excessive, and intense.[47] Usually absent in children, nasolabial folds emerge around the age of 25 years in those individuals who continuously display constant expressions of emotion, laughter, fatigue, pain, and so on. By age 35, the nasolabial folds become more fixed in those so predisposed and exhibit a great deal of morphologic variability.[47,48] Deep, diagonal folds that form at the sides of the nose and continue downward toward the angle of the mouth, and at times even lower into marionette lines, project an attitude of disgust and dismay and are a characteristic sign of advanced age. These deep furrows and folds remain as one of the more difficult and still barely correctable harbingers of senescence in the treatment of the aging face. In the past, different surgical procedures have attempted to efface the outline and depth of the nasolabial groove, thereby flattening the fold. These procedures are fraught with scars and failure.[40] Recently, injections of different soft tissue fillers have been most beneficial in achieving a modicum of success in effacing a deep nasolabial fold and restoring lost soft tissue support in the center of the face. The minimally invasive injection of fillers probably is still the best method for elevating and diminishing the inescapable, recalcitrant evidence of impending senescence, the deep nasolabial sulci, and folds. Nevertheless, injections of OnaBTX-A also have been employed in an attempt to reduce the depth and obtrusive appearance of nasolabial folds. Unfortunately, intramuscular injections of OnaBTX-A appear not to be the long sought-after panacea for this problem and they too have proven to be fraught with complications and failure in this area of the mid face.

Functional Anatomy (See Appendix 2) of Nasoloabial Folds
There is significant variation in the anatomy that creates the nasolabial fold, which extends from a point lateral to the nasal ala to a point lateral to or lower than the oral commissure. The etiology of a prominent nasolabial fold is the result of multiple contributing alterations occurring with advancing age, including varying degrees of soft tissue atrophy involving the skin, fat, and muscles along with ptosis and downward migration of fat and its retaining ligaments, in conjunction with atrophy of facial bones resulting in widening of the orbits, nasal pyriform aperture, and retrusion of the maxilla and mandible.[8,41,45,49] The cutaneous insertions of the different mimetic facial muscles along this fold may promote the early appearance and deepening of the nasolabial fold and furrow or sulcus, starting in those so predisposed persons in their mid to late twenties.[47] In older patients, a combination of any of the following also may contribute to a prominent nasolabial fold:

- Loss of skin thickness over the sulcus
- Redundant skin lateral to the sulcus
- Excessive fat deposits lateral to the sulcus that are fixed in place by retaining ligaments, with or without Ptosis of the malar and submalar fat laterally because of a weakening of the SMAS in the mid upper cheek

Aging and frequent mimetic action by the causative facial muscles can deepen the vertical sulcus that runs from the upper border of the nasofacial angle downward and laterally toward the commissures of the mouth. Depending on the unique morphologic variations of an individual's facial anatomy, it is the resultant idiosyncratic movements of a combination of any one of the mid face mimetic muscles (zygomatic complex, the central upper lip levators, and the levator anguli oris and

risorius) that are responsible for elevating the upper lip and producing a person's characteristic smile.[47,48,50] They also contribute significantly either individually or as a group to the initial formation and the progressive intensification of the nasolabial folds (Figure 14.42).

Nasolabial folds can appear convex (60%), straight (30%), or concave (10%)[48] (Figures 14.43 and 14.44). The length of a nasolabial fold also can vary from being one that is extended (42%), short (38%), or continuous (20%) from the alar base to the mandible[47,48] (Figure 14.45). With respect to an individual's idiosyncratic facial morphology, the nasolabial fold can be divided into three sections: the upper or medial, middle, and lateral or lower sections (Figure 14.46).[50] However, no significant correlation was found by Pessa et al. between the muscles present and their patterns of perioral attachments, and the length and contour of the nasolabial crease and fold.[48]

In many patients, according to some authors, it is the LLSAN that is the muscle most responsible for producing the upper *medial* portion of the nasolabial fold and the LLS for deepening the *middle* of the nasolabial fold.[3,4,47,50–52] It is the zygomatic major, levator anguli oris, risorius and, at times, the LLS which contribute primarily to deepening and extending the lower lateral aspect of the nasolabial fold when they laterally retract and elevate the upper lip to produce a smile.[4] In some individuals, however, the LLSAN is less important in the formation of a smile, especially if elevating the medial aspect of the upper lip is minimal when they do smile (see Gummy Smile below) In many other individuals, the zygomaticus complex, along with a contribution from the LLS and levator anguli oris, can deepen the middle as well as the lower lateral portions of the nasolabial fold.

In addition, aging and redundant inelastic skin cause certain individuals to exaggerate lateral canthal wrinkles, extending crow's feet downward over the surface of the mid and lateral cheeks when they smile enthusiastically (Figure 14.47). This seems to occur in certain individuals because their decussated zygomaticus complex muscle fibers (zygomaticus major and zygomaticus minor) also interdigitate with the lower medial and lateral aspects of the *orbital* orbicularis oculi.[53] In most individuals, the zygomaticus major and levator anguli oris help to elevate the corner of the mouth and move it laterally and

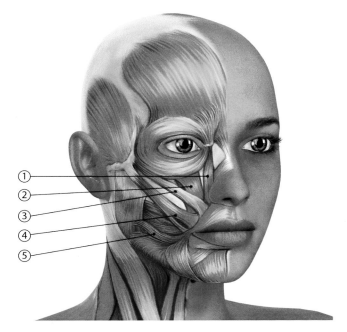

Figure 14.42 Muscles that contribute to the formation of the nasolabial fold. 1, levator labii superioris alaeque nasi; 2, levator labii superioris; 3, zygomaticus minor; 4, zygomaticus major; 5, risorius.

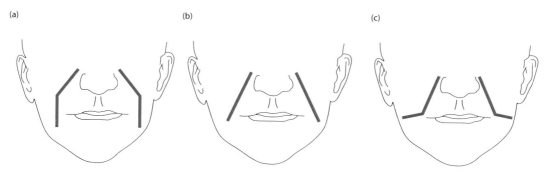

Figure 14.43 The three different morphological types of nasolabial folds: (a) convex; (b) straight; (c) concave. (See further Reference Zufferey J. *Plast Reconstr Surg* 1992; 89(2): 225–31.)

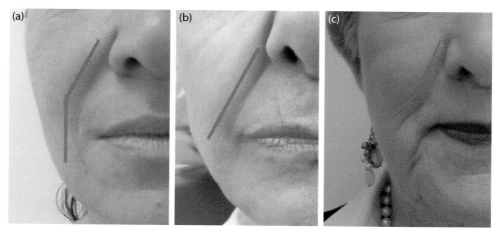

Figure 14.44 Clinical examples of the types of nasolabial folds: (a) convex; (b) straight; (c) concave. (See further References Zufferey J. *Plast Reconstr Surg* 1992; 89(2): 225–31 and Pessa JE et al. *Plast Reconstr Surg* 1998; 102(6): 1888–93.)

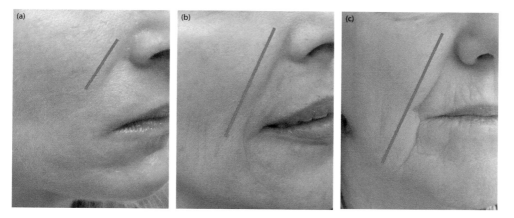

Figure 14.45 Different lengths of the nasolabial folds in relationship to the corner of the oral commissures: (a) short; (b) extended; (c) continuous. (See further Reference Pessa JE et al. *Plast Reconstr Surg* 1998; 102(6): 1888–93.)

slightly upward with smiling. In so doing, they also can mobilize mid cheek skin upward and laterally, extending the lower crow's feet down the face, especially in individuals who have inelastic, loose, redundant skin (Figure 14.47).

The zygomaticus major originates on the lower aspect of the zygomatic bone, just anterior to the zygomaticotemporal suture line (Figure 14.42). It then continues downward obliquely toward the angle of the mouth and joins other muscle fibers just lateral to the commissure, interdigitating with them as they all interlace with each other to form a muscular node, called the modiolus. Then the zygomaticus major exits the modiolus and inserts its fibers into the corner of the mouth. In the modiolus the zygomaticus major co-mingles with fibers of the levator anguli oris, depressor anguli oris, risorius, buccinator, platysma, and superficial and deep fibers of the orbicularis oris.[54] In a study by Pessa et al., the zygomaticus major was present as a single muscle in 66% of the 50 cadavers examined.[48] In the other 34% of the cadavers studied, the zygomaticus major appeared bifid with two separate muscle bundles, which was more commonly found in the female cadavers (65%). The larger main bundle decussated into the modiolus and then inserted into or above the corner of the mouth, while the more superficial and narrower bundle inserted into the deep dermis below the corner of the mouth.[47,48] When pulled on separately, the superficial bundle created a

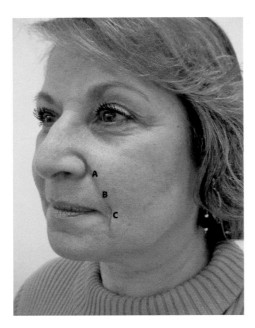

Figure 14.46 Sections of the nasolabial fold: (A) medial (or upper) nasolabial fold; (B) middle nasolabial fold; (C) lateral (or lower) nasolabial fold. (See further Reference Pessa JE, Brown F. *Aesth Plast Surg* 1992; 16: 167–71.)

concave nasolabial fold, and the main bundle created a convex nasolabial fold. On occasion, additional dermal insertions were found along the course of the smaller, more superficial bundle. This was thought to represent the reason for the presence of parabuccal dimples.

The zygomaticus minor, on the other hand, when present, originates more medially on the zygoma than the zygomaticus major, just behind the zygomaticomaxillary suture line, and more anteriorly and inferiorly to the origin of the zygomaticus major. At its origin, the zygomaticus minor is lateral to the LLSAN, superficial to the LLS, and deep to and interdigitates with the *orbital* orbicularis oculi[53,55] (Figure 14.42).

Pessa et al. found the zygomaticus minor present only in 36% of their Caucasian cadavers studied, while Youn et al. found the zygomaticus minor present in 95% of their Korean cadavers[48,53] One of the reasons why the zygomaticus minor was found so much more frequently in Korean cadavers was because Youn and colleagues were able to identify the elusive zygomaticus minor at its origin, that is, by the presence of muscle fibers on the zygoma and not by trying to identify separate muscle fibers of the zygomaticus minor from those of the zygomaticus major. When they initially attempted to locate the zygomaticus minor without identifying it at its bony origin, their identification of the zygomaticus minor was just as low in frequency and had similar morphology as those of other studies, that is, 34.4% (21 of 61 of the cadavers studied). However, after determining the origin of the zygomaticus minor on the zygomatic bone, its nonexistence in the Youn et al. study dropped to only 4.9% (3 of 61). They then concluded that the presence or abscence of the zygomaticus minor should be based on its bony origin and the direction of the projection of its muscle fibers and not on its differentiation from the zygomaticus major. Interestingly, they also found muscle fibers of the zygomaticus minor could not be distinguished from those of the zygomaticus major in 34.4% (21 of 61) of the cadavers examined. When the two muscles could be identified as separate muscle bundles, the zygomaticus minor interdigitated with the inner lower aspect of the *orbital* orbicularis oculi in 34 of 61 (56%) cadavers examined and continued downward parallel with the upper lip levators (LLSAN and LLS) into the upper lip. More strikingly, they also found 54 of 61 (88.5%) cadavers in which muscle fibers of the lateral aspect of the *orbital* orbicularis oculi interdigitated with the zygomaticus minor before it inserted into the upper lip[53] (Figure 14.48a) (see Chapter 13, "Lateral Canthal Lines"). The usual course of the zygomaticus minor, when it is present, is to travel downward to insert more medially than the zygomaticus major and directly into the upper lip, interdigitating with fibers of the LLSAN, orbicularis oris, and zygomaticus major, after the zygomaticus major exits the modiolus (Figure 14.48b and c).

Choi et al. after their Korean cadaver dissection study classified the zygomaticus minor into three different types, according to anatomic morphology and muscle insertion patterns.[55] The most commonly encountered pattern type of zygomaticus minor found in 34 of the 54 (63%) cadavers studied was where the muscle attached directly into the upper lip either by a straight course in 17 (31.5%) of the specimens or in a curved course also in 17 (31.5%) of the cadavers dissected (Figure 14.48c1 and c2).

The second most frequently seen pattern of insertion, 15 of 54 (28%) cadavers studied, was where the zygomaticus minor attached to either fibers of the orbicularis oris within the upper lip or at the lateral ala nasi. As the zygomaticus minor passed from its origin on the zygoma toward its insertion within the upper lip or ala nasi, many of its transverse and descending muscle fibers could not be separated from those

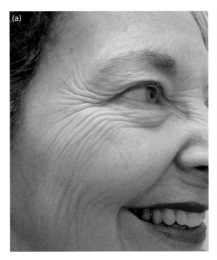
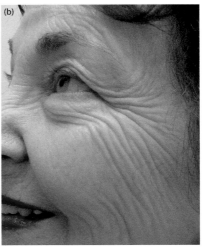

Figure 14.47 (a, b) Lower crow's feet, lateral cheek rhytides and deep nasolabial folds creating "accordion-like" wrinkles down the cheeks. Note also the horizontal wrinkle across the philtrum on the upper lip.

of the inner lower aspect of the *orbital* orbicularis oculi, similar to what was reported in the Youn study[53] (Figure 14.48c3).

The third and least encountered insertion pattern of the zygomaticus minor was seen in 5 of 54 (9.3%) cadavers where there were no or just some very rudimentary muscle fibers of the zygomaticus minor (Figure 14.48c4).

Youn et al. also found that the origin of the zygomaticus minor had two different muscular origins on the zygoma. The more superficial origin of the zygomaticus minor that interdigitated with the *orbital* orbicularis oculi passed downward and medially into the

upper lip. Whereas the deeper muscle fibers from their origin on the zygomatic bone attached to the lateral ala nasi possibly creating a tell-tale small bulge or protrusion on the lateral aspect of the ala nasi visible in some individuals during facial animation (Figure 14.48d). These fibers, attached to the lateral ala nasi, also could be seen as supplementing the actions of the LLSAN, LLS, and *anterior* and *posterior* dilator nares in flaring the nostrils and producing a gummy smile (see Nasal Flare above and Gummy Smile below). This could be an obvious revealing landmark used to identify those patients who will benefit from treatments of a nasal flare or a gummy smile.

(a)

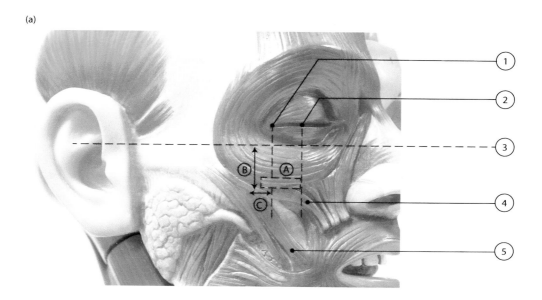

(b)

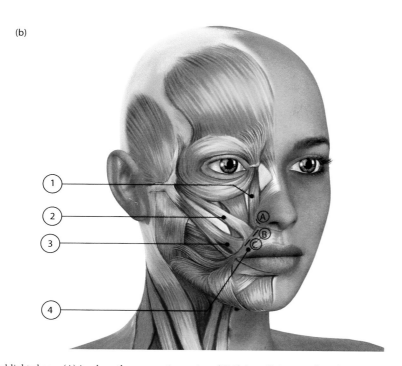

Figure 14.48 (a) The highlighted area (A) is where the zygomaticus minor (ZMi) interdigitates with and is inseparable from the *orbital* orbicularis oculi (OOc) and is located (B) approximately 17.8 mm inferior to the Frankfort plane and (C) laterally at 8.9 mm from the vertical line that perpendicularly connects the lateral canthus and the Frankfort plane. The inseparable interlacing of the two muscles extends medially for a distance of 16 mm. 1, lateral canthus; 2, midpoint of the palpebral fissure; 3, Frankfort plane; 4, zygomaticus minor; 5, zygomaticus major. (b) The zygomaticus minor inserts (A) into the lateral aspect of the ala nasi; (B) into the lower aspect of the levator labii superioris alaeque nasi; and (C) in the area where the medial margin of the zygomaticus major and the orbicularis oris join. 1, levator labii superioris alaeque nasi; 2, zygomaticus minor; 3, zygomaticus major; 4, orbital orbicularis oris.

(Continued)

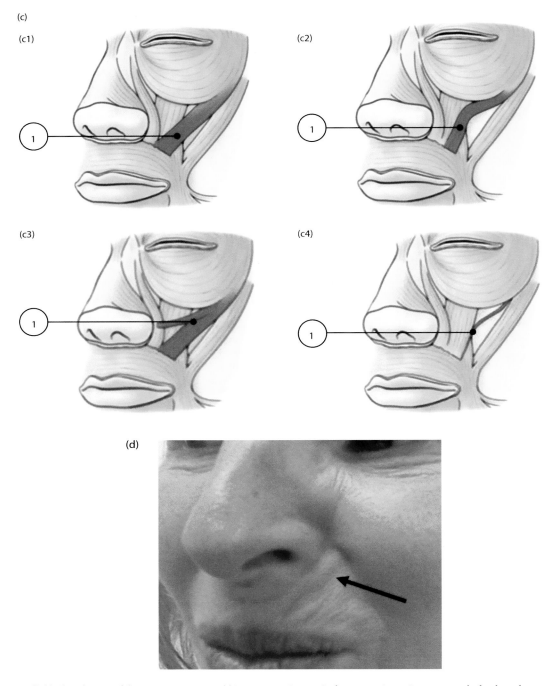

Figure 14.48 (Continued) (c) Classification of the zygomaticus minor (1) into 3 types. In type A, the zygomaticus minor was attached only to the upper lip, but the type is subdivided into 2 subtypes: straight (A-1) (c1) and curved (A-2) (c2). In type B (c3), the zygomaticus minor attached to both the upper lip and the alar portion of the nose with many of its transverse and descending muscle fibers closely interdigitated with fibers of the inner lower aspect of the *orbital* orbicularis oculi. In type C (c4), there was either no or only underdeveloped zygomaticus minor fibers. (See further reference 54) (d) Small protrusion adjacent to ala nasi (arrow) may represent the insertion of zygomaticus minor muscle fibers. (From Choi DY et al. 2014. *Dermatol Surg* 40(8):858–63. With permission.)

The cadaver dissection studies of Youn and Choi versus that of Pessa underscore the structural consistency, but also the diversity of the morphological composition of the human face and the importance of the phenotypic influences that race and ethnicity have on the functional differences of facial mimetic anatomy. In other words, the width, height and depth of an Asian versus a Caucasian facial skeleton make it more conducive to having a more robust and significantly more functional zygomaticus minor in an Asian face than in a Caucasian face. These and other similar anatomical studies confirm that there are indeed inter- and intra-racial variations of muscle morphology and movement which are dependent on the overall skeletal shape and inherent muscle composition of a particular person's face, which may vary according to the different anatomical characteristics of that person's ethnic and racial background. There also seems to be a particularly high degree of variability in mid face musculature according to the anatomic studies in the literature currently available.[48,50,53–55] This high degree of mid face anatomical variability is embodied in different individuals' ability to express the same emotions in a wide range of different but similarly subtle facial movements with the same or possibly different muscles. These spontaneous, subconscious, or at times intentional facial mimetic movements can span a gamut of different emotions from a smile of happiness or pleasure to the laughter of enjoyment or embarassment; from a grimace of sadness or disappointment to a sneer of scorn or contempt; from a smirk of arrogance or disdain to a grin of agreement or displeasure. All of these facial expressions are centered in the mid face and are dependent on the slightest mimetic movement of the available facial muscles, whose presence and actions ostensibly are a reflection of one's character, personality and inner feelings, all of which are easily interpreted by casual observers. Because of the different vectors of movement which intrinsically occur consistent with the types of zygomaticus minor anatomical configurations, one can easily appreciate that different types of muscular movements can take place to express the same emotion, expressed by different individuals in their own unique way. Generally, the zygomaticus minor along with the LLS and the zygomaticus major pull the upper lip superolaterally, while the LLSAN pulls the upper lip superomedially, exposing the maxillary teeth and deepening the nasolabial sulcus and enlarging the fold. Both muscles of the zygomaticus complex can deepen the nasolabial fold when they contract to produce a smile. In most individuals, when the zygomaticus minor contracts together with the central upper lip levators (i.e., LLSAN and LLS), they will cause the upper lip to curl when expressing smugness, contempt, or disdain. Likewise, when a person contracts the lateral and medial aspect of the lower eyelid as in a wink or squint, most of the time the mid to lateral aspect of the upper lip and cheek also contracts upward.[53]

Symmetry of the zygomaticus minor was calculated in regard to its morphology and vectors of movement by Choi et al.[55] They found that the zygomaticus minor was asymmetric in 12 of the 18 (66.6%) cadavers studied, one of the identifiable probable causes of upper lip asymmetric smiles (see Asymmetric Smiles below).

The LLSAN is a long thin rectangular muscle that originates from the superior part of the frontal process of the maxilla close to the side of the nose (Figure 14.49). Covered by the orbital orbicularis oculi, the facial angular vessels can be found traversing along the nasojugal fold between the two muscles. As the LLSAN travels obliquely downward and laterally, it divides into two separate muscle bundles. The one smaller bundle inserts medially into the perichondrium of the lateral

crus of the greater alar cartilage and skin of the nose, while interdigitating with fibers of the posterior and anterior dilator nares. The other larger lateral muscle bundle continues downward toward the medial aspect of the upper lip and crosses over the front of the LLS, merging its fibers with those of the LLS and orbicularis oris. It inserts under the dermis and into the overlying skin of the ipsilateral upper lip near the upper medial part of the nasolabial sulcus and fold. The lateral labial muscle bundle raises and everts the upper lip and raises, deepens, and increases the curvature of the upper aspect or medial nasolabial sulcus. The medial nasal muscle bundle of the LLSAN, also known as the levator alae nasi, pulls the lateral cartilaginous crus laterally and upward to dilate the nostrils. It also displaces the circumalar facial sulcus laterally, modifying its curvature and elevating the nasolabial sulcus and fold.[10]

The LLS is the widest of all the upper lip levators. It originates from the maxilla at the lower margin of the orbit, just above the infraorbital foramen, deep to the *orbital* orbicularis oculi (Figure 14.49). Coursing downward between the lateral labial bundle of the LLSAN, the zygomaticus minor, and the levator anguli oris, some of the fibers of the LLS insert directly into the skin overlying these muscles in the central and lateral aspect of the upper lip and other fibers interdigitate with those of the orbicularis oris. While still in some individuals the LLS can interdigitate with the depressor septi nasi. The function of the LLS is to raise and evert the central aspect of the upper lip. In conjunction with other muscles, it moves and deepens the middle of the nasolabial sulcus, especially during expressions of seriousness and sadness.

The levator anguli oris originates more deeply in the canine fossa of the maxilla, just below the infraorbital foramen (Figure 14.49). It lies deeply beneath the upper lip levators and the zygomaticus complex. Its muscle fibers travel downward into the modiolus and then interdigitate with those muscle fibers of the zygomaticus major while wrapping around the oral commissure also to interdigitate with the fibers of the orbicularis oris and the depressor anguli oris. The levator anguli oris then inserts into the overlying skin at and just below the angle of the mouth and the lower portion of the nasolabial sulcus. It raises the lateral aspect of the upper lip, and the corners of the mouth when smiling or laughing. In some patients, it also deepens and shifts the contour of the lower nasolabial sulcus.

The preceding group of four upper lip levators was previously identified as the *quadratus labii superioris*, which, when contracted, was felt to cause the nasolabial sulcus to deepen. The quadratus labii superioris was described as comprising four muscle heads: the *angular head* or the LLSAN, the *infraorbital head* or the LLS, the *zygomatic head* or the zygomaticus minor, and the *canine head* or the levator anguli oris (Figure 14.50). Because of the intricacies of the mid face functional anatomy necessary for complex deliberate and subtle involuntary and spontaneous fine facial mimetic movement, injecting OnaBTX-A anywhere in the mid face must be performed with absolute precision and accuracy.

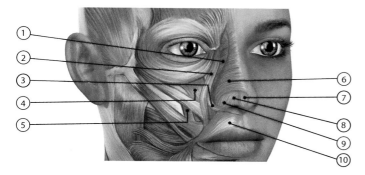

Figure 14.49 The levator labii superioris alaeque nasi is divided into two separate bundles of muscles distally; the medial bundle inserts into the skin over the ala nasi and interdigitates with the fibers of the anterior and posterior dilator naris, and the lateral bundle inserts into the skin and mucosa of the center of the upper lip interdigitating with fibers of the orbicularis oris. The levator labii superioris, widest of all the lip levators, is a deeper muscle originating from the maxilla at the lower margin of the orbit, just above the infraorbital foramen and under the *orbital* orbicularis oculi and inserts directly into the skin of the central and lateral aspect of the upper lip, interdigitating with the orbicularis oris. The levator anguli oris lies deep to all the muscles of the midface, originates in the canine fossa of the maxilla, travels downward into the modiolus, interdigitating with the other modiolar muscles, and inserts into the overlying skin at and just below the angle of the mouth and the lower portion of the nasolabial sulcus. 1, Anomalus nasi; 2, levator labii superioris alaeque nasi; 3, levator alae nasi; 4, levator labii superioris; 5, levator anguli oris; 6, transverse nasalis; 7, compressor narium minor; 8, anterior dilator naris; 9, posterior dilator naris; 10, orbicularis oris.

Dilution (See Appendix 3) When Treating Nasolabial Folds

Injecting minimal volumes of OnaBTX-A in this area is of paramount importance so as not to have unintended diffusion of the OnaBTX-A affect the surrounding muscles of the midface. Therefore, a 100 U vial of OnaBTX-A should be reconstituted with only 1 mL of normal saline.

Dosing: How to Correct the Problem (See Appendix 4) (What to Do and What Not to Do) When Treating Nasolabial Folds

Injecting 1 U and not more than 2 U of OnaBTX-A into the middle of the nasofacial angle just lateral to the upper border of the ala nasi will weaken the lateral fibers and some of the medial fibers of the LLSAN and flatten the upper medial aspect of the nasolabial fold

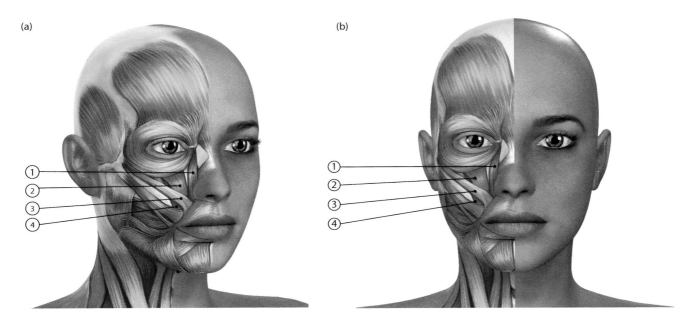

Figure 14.50 Quadratus labii superioris, (a) viewed from the side and (b) viewed from the front. 1, levator labii superioris alaeque nasi; 2, levator labii superioris; 3, zygomaticus minor; 4, levator anguli oris.

(Figures 14.51 and 14.52). While sitting or in a semi-reclined position, ask the patient to sneer or lift the upper lip forcibly in an upward direction to expose the upper central teeth as one does when sneering or expressing abhorrence, disgust, or repugnance (Figure 14.53). With the index finger of the nondominant hand directly over the nasofacial angle and palpating the area gently, one will feel the contracture of muscle fibers as the patient repeats the sneer maneuver. With the needle pointed perpendicularly to the surface of the skin, advance it approximately 3–5 mm deep and just before contacting bone as not to inflict additional undue pain on the patient. Inject only 1 or 2 U of OnaBTX-A directly into the thickest bulge of muscle contraction (Figure 14.54). Depending on the position and depth of the nasolabial sulcus and the height of the nasolabial fold, the bulge of muscle contracture palpated may actually correspond to the interdigitating lower fibers of the LLS and zygomaticus minor together with the lower lateral labial fibers of the LLSAN[55] (Figure 14.55). This also is the same technique used to inject OnaBTX-A to reduce a gummy smile (see Gummy Smile below). These injection techniques should be performed only by the very experienced physician whose patient possesses nasolabial folds that are deep and become exaggerated with a simple upward movement of the upper lip, as in sniffing, sneering, and smiling (Figure 14.56). Proper patient selection is of paramount

importance because untoward sequelae resulting in a lack of control of essential buccal sphincteric functions can occur very easily and be devastating to the patient. The use of electromyographic guidance when treating this area can be helpful to the novice injector.[1]

For those patients who produce innumerable wrinkles of the mid cheek with smiling or squinting, an *intradermal* injection of 1–2 U of OnaBTX-A near the origins of the zygomaticus complex along the inferior lateral margin of the zygomatic arch at the inferior border of the *orbital* orbicularis oculi of the lower eyelid can achieve an additive effect of diminishing lower lateral canthal rhytides along with effacing nasolabial folds (Figure 14.57).[56] Depending on the idiosyncratic anatomy of a particular individual, the shape of the face, and the strength of the muscles, it might be necessary to administer one, two, or multiple injections of OnaBTX-A, each over the mid to lateral malar prominence, to obtain the consistent results desired (see Chapter 17 by Kyle Seo on intradermal injections).[5,56,57] This technique always is accompanied by a drop of the upper lip or a reduction in the lateral excursion of the oral commissures especially when smiling, laughing, or speaking.

Shao-Ping et al. injected a total of 20–25 U of OnaBTX-A intradermally into the entire face lateral to the nasolabial fold, including the temples and cheeks from the infraorbital area to the jawline at 1 cm

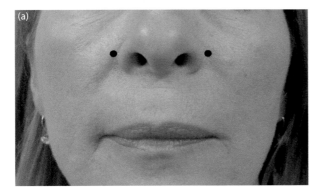

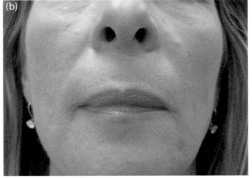

Figure 14.51 (a, b) ● marks the point where 1 U of OnaBTX-A was injected into this 53-year-old to diminish the depth of the nasolabial sulcus. Note the elongation of the upper lip, flattening of the philtrum and thinning of the vermillion in this patient at rest.

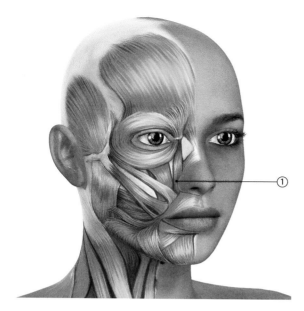

Figure 14.52 • marks the point where 1–2 U of OnaBTX-A can be injected to weaken the lateral labial and some of the medial nasal fibers of the levator labii superioris alaeque nasi to diminish the depth of the nasolabial fold.

intervals.[10,58] A 100 U vial of OnaBTX-A was reconstituted with 10 mL of normal saline to achieve a concentration of 10 U of OnaBTX-A for each 1 mL of solution. Each site on the face was injected with 0.02 mL of OnaBTX-A solution. This technique of microBOTOX (also known as mesoBOTOX) injections is very popular in Far East Asia where a subtle lifting and diminution of the fine facial wrinkling is in demand (see Chapter 17 by Kyle Seo on micro-intradermal injections of BoNT-A).

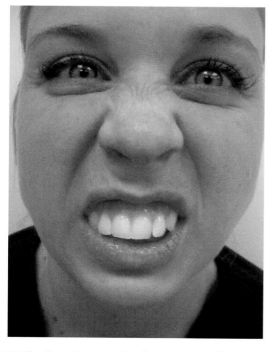

Figure 14.53 Elevation of the upper lip when sneering, sniffing, or smiling will contract the levator labii superioris alaeque nasi as well as the levator labii superioris and the zygomaticus minor in most patients. Note the deep nasolabial fold and gummy smile.

Outcomes (Results) (See Appendix 5) When Treating Nasolabial Folds

There have been a few attempts to establish a fail-safe technique in which some of the upper lip levators could be treated with OnaBTX-A to reduce a deep nasolabial sulcus and fold without attendant adverse effects on lip function and symmetry. If one considers the LLSAN the principal muscle that creates the upper medial aspect of the nasolabial fold, and the other central and lateral lip levators (the LLS, zygomaticus complex, levator anguli oris, and risorius) responsible for deepening the mid and lower nasolabial sulcus when they contract, then precisely placed low-volume injections of concentrated OnaBTX-A should be able to reduce the appearance of the nasolabial fold and the depth of its sulcus. Because this is not the only or primary function of these muscles, injections of OnaBTX-A can unwittingly produce secondary changes that interfere with and diminish the primary functions of these muscles, that is, elevating the upper lip and laterally abducting the corners of the mouth, which are necessary movements when one speaks, smiles, laughs, yawns, eats, drinks, or forcibly breathes by mouth. Nasolabial fold effacement and its accompanying side effects can last up to 3 months or as long as the OnaBTX-A treatment is effective.

Petchngaovila describes an intradermal injection technique of highly diluted OnaBTX-A, which relaxes what she considers the major depressors of the face (i.e., platysma and lateral *orbital* orbicularis oculi) and allows the levators of the mid face (zygomaticus complex, LLSAN, LLS and levator anguli oris) and lateral frontalis to reverse the sagging and wrinkling of the upper and mid face.[57] According to Petchngaovila, this intradermal mid face lifting realigns the imbalance of the muscles of the midface by weakening the downward pull of the depressors (platysma, lateral fibers of the *orbital* orbicularis oculi) and allowing the levators of the mid face and lateral frontalis to contract and lift the skin in a compensatory fashion. This treatment requires not only multiple repeat injections before obvious results are produced, but also frequent maintenance injections every 2–3 months. This procedure is best done for sheet-like muscles rather than for individual muscle bundles, and when muscles are flaccid and poorly defined. This technique also is best suited for older patients with loose, lax skin who want to realign and uplift their mid face, diminish the wrinkling of their cheeks, and soften the nasolabial folds (Figures 14.58 through 14.60) (see Chapter 17 by Kyle Seo on intradermal injections). With the possible future introduction of topical preparations of BoNT-A, intradermal microinjections of BoNTs may eventually wane in popularity. (see Chapter 4 by Richard Glogau).

Complications (Adverse Sequlae) (See Appendix 6) When Treating Nasolabial Folds

Just 1–3 U of OnaBTX-A into each lip levator complex in the lower nasofacial sulcus will collapse the upper extent of the nasolabial fold and also elongate the upper lip, with fairly long-lasting results.[1] However, injecting this area can result in a flat mid face with elongation of the upper lip, effacement of the philtrum, diminution of the fullness and narrowing of the upper lip vermillion (see Figure 14.51). This is an appearance that is not well accepted by most individuals, especially those who already have a naturally longer, thinner upper lip (Figure 14.61). Overzealous treatment of this area can result in an asymmetric smile and a ptotic upper lip, causing drooling and fluid incontinence when drinking from a glass or cup. It also can result in biting the upper lip when chewing. In most patients, these nasolabial lines are best treated with soft tissue fillers, implants, or surgical rhytidectomy, and not with OnaBTX-A.[3] (See Chapter 7 by Alastair and Jean Carruthers).

Injecting OnaBTX-A any lower than the upper alar facial border, that is, closer to the alar labial sulcus or along the nasal sill, can

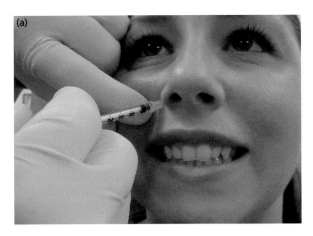
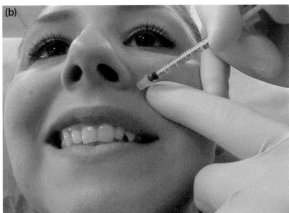

Figure 14.54 (a, b) Injecting OnaBTX-A should be performed intramuscularly with the needle perpendicular to the skin surface.

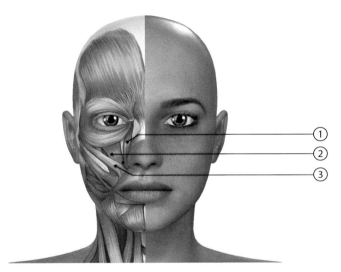

Figure 14.55 • marks the point where 1–2 U of OnaBTX-A can be injected to weaken the levator labii superioris and zygomaticus minor along with the levator labii superioris alaeque nasi to diminish the nasolabial fold. 1, levator labii superioris alaeque nasi; 2, levator labii superioris; 3, zygomaticus minor.

produce a weakening of the central upper lip levators and the orbicularis oris resulting in an inability to elevate the upper lip, elongating its overall dimensions. This is a common technique used to drop the upper lip and correct a gummy smile, but is not appropriate in most patients just seeking a reduction in the depth and fullness of their nasolabial folds (see Gummy Smile below).

Usually, injecting only 1–2 U of OnaBTX-A intradermally away from the mouth, and near the origins of the zygomaticus major and minor and LLS at the inferior border of the lateral *orbital* orbicularis oculi, can help both diminish the nasolabial fold and efface the lower lateral canthal wrinkles and lower lateral cheek rhytides. This technique usually is accompanied by a reduction in the strength of the upper lip sphincter competence and smile symmetry.[3,5] It is extremely important, however, that minimal volume of OnaBTX-A is injected deeply and precisely into the fibers of the targeted muscles, to lightly weaken and not paralyze them. Even with a light weakening of the LLS and the zygomatic complex, a certain amount of lip ptosis will occur, and is actually expected. This should be discussed with the patient before treatment, and should not be considered a true adverse outcome or complication (Figures 14.51 and 14.61)[2,59] (see Dr. Seo's Chapter 17 for similar results with the microinjection technique).

In older patients who have a large amount of excessive fat deposition or ptotic malar fat along with redundant skin lateral to the nasolabial sulcus, weakening the central upper lip levators will have no effect on

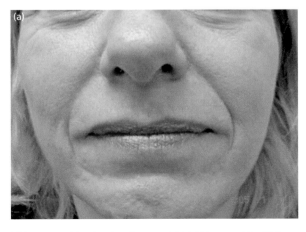
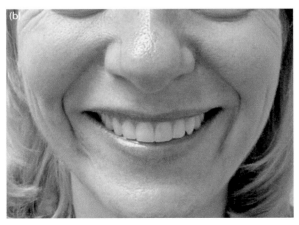

Figure 14.56 This 51-year-old patient has deep nasolabial folds at rest (a), which are exaggerated by smiling (b). Note the inversion and foreshortening of the upper lip with smiling.

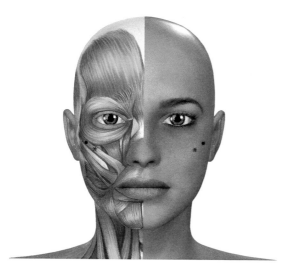

Figure 14.57 Intradermal injection of 1–2 U of OnaBTX-A (•) at the lateral zygomatic arch near the origin of the zygomaticus complex can diminish lower crow's feet lines, mid cheek wrinkles and help efface the upper and mid nasolabial sulcus and fold. Depending on the individual's anatomy, shape of face and strength of the muscles, a second injection point (*) might be necessary to produce the same results. See Chapter 17 on microinjections of BoNTA.

the extent and depth of the nasolabial folds. The nasolabial folds might even be enhanced if the lateral upper lip levators are weakened, causing a reduction in the lateral muscle support, which in turn will allow the ptotic fat and redundant skin to sag even more so. On the other hand, in younger patients (i.e., those in their early thirties to late fifties) with good cutaneous elasticity and soft tissue support, much of the appearance of the nasolabial fold is caused by mimetic muscle contraction, the bulk of which can be attributed to the LLSAN. When this muscle is weakened in younger persons, the nasolabial fold is diminished, usually uneventfully. Attempting to weaken some of the other upper lip levators may cause undesirable sequelae, for example, upper lip ptosis, buccal asymmetry, and even oral sphincter incompetence. For example, also weakening the zygomaticus muscles can soften the nasolabial folds, but the smile may be changed, reducing the extent of

the upward and lateral excursion of one's smile. However, for those patients displaying an excessive amount of gingiva when smiling or laughing, weakening of the central upper lip levators may actually be desirable because it can reduce the full upward movement of the upper lip that overexposes the crown and gums of the upper incisors and canines (see Gummy Smile below).

Injecting OnaBTX-A in the mid face in an attempt to diminish the nasolabial folds and to eliminate the random wrinkling of the lateral aspect and center of the cheeks produced by squinting or smiling should only be attempted by the most experienced physician injector.[6] Selecting the right patient can be more important than any other aspect of an OnaBTX-A injection technique. Understanding how certain facial and cheek wrinkles and folds are produced, and how to palpate and identify the correct target muscles for injection, is the key to success or failure. Attempting to reduce midcheek wrinkling and nasolabial folds with injections of OnaBTX-A can result in not only a flattening of the nasolabial fold, but also an overall flattening of the cheek and an elongation of the upper lip, an eclabion or lip ptosis as well as lip asymmetry and lack of oral sphincter control.[57] For these reasons, it is probably most advisable not to treat this area of the mid face with OnaBTX-A unless the patient is willing to endure unconditionally the expected and inadvertent sequelae. Subcising deeply adherent nasolabial sulci, injecting them with a soft tissue filler and resurfacing the cheeks by chemical peeling, dermabrasion, fractionated laser ablation or deep tissue nonablative laser remodeling is probably a more reliable way to address these problems and produce consistent, longer lasting results.[5]

Treatment Implications When Injecting Nasolabial Folds
1. Successful treatment of the nasolabial fold is absolutely dependent on proper patient assessment of what is physically causing, and what muscles, are actually creating and exaggerating the nasolabial fold and deepening the sulcus.
2. The levator labii superioris alaeque nasi is usually the muscle primarily responsible for the creation and enhancement of the upper, medial portion of the nasolabial sulcus and fold.
3. Nasolabial folds are best reduced by injections of soft tissue fillers, subcision, implants, and surgical rhytidectomy rather than with injections of OnaBTX-A.

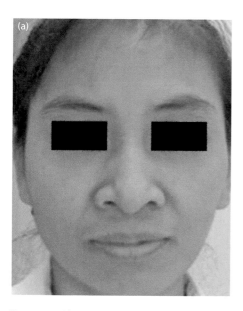
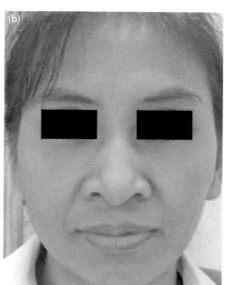
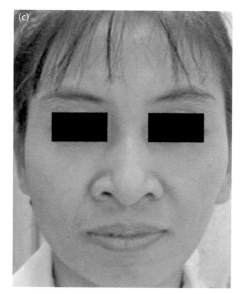

Figure 14.58 This 40-year-old patient is seen (a) before, (b) 2 weeks after intramuscular treatments, and (c) 10 weeks after intradermal injections of BoNTA, giving her a slight lift of the total face. (Courtesy of Chariya Petchngaovila, MD)

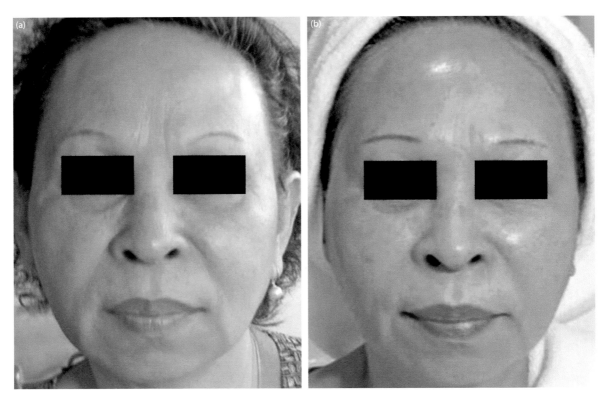

Figure 14.59 This 61-year-old patient is seen (a) before and (b) 2 weeks after intradermal injections of OnaBTX-A. Note the overall appearance of a "face lift." (Courtesy of Chariya Petchngaovila, MD)

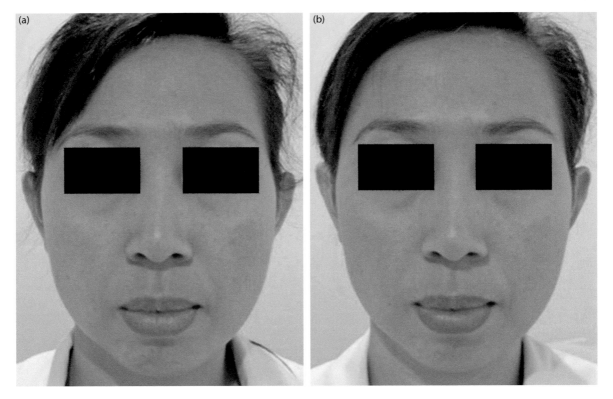

Figure 14.60 This 33-year-old patient is seen (a) before and (b) 10 days after intradermal injections of OnaBTX-A, giving her the appearance of a "facial lift." (Courtesy of Chariya Petchngaovila, MD)

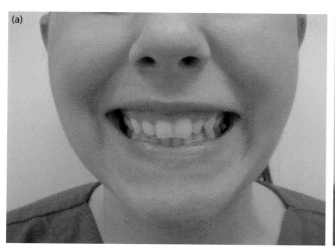
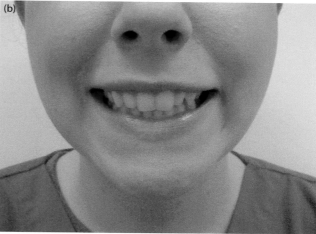

Figure 14.61 A 29-year-old patient smiling (a) before and (b) 2 weeks after a treatment with OnaBTX-A to efface a deep nasolabial fold. Note the slight upper lip ptosis that is unavoidable with this treatment. Note the upward direction of the commissures, which is created by the untreated and unopposed action of the zygomaticus major, levator anguli oris, and risorius.

4. In the properly selected patient injections of 1–2 U of OnaBTX-A can be given in the upper alar facial sulcus in an attempt to flatten the nasolabial fold.

5. Injections of OnaBTX-A too low along the alar facial angle will produce an elongation or ptosis of the upper lip, an asymmetric smile, and functional incompetence of the oral sphincter.

6. Injections of OnaBTX-A too lateral to the nasofacial angle will produce an overall flattening of the midcheek and a drop in the soft tissue support of the malar fat pad.

7. In the properly selected patient, a combination of injections of OnaBTX-A and either soft tissue fillers or some form of surgical intervention or both will produce longer lasting results than if the nasolabial folds were to be treated solely with either alone.

EXCESSIVE MAXILLARY GINGIVAL DISPLAY (GUMMY SMILE)

Introduction: Problem Assessment and Patient Selection

Some individuals tend to reveal an excessive amount of their maxillary gingival mucosa when they smile or laugh, which is euphemistically known as a "gummy smile." This commonly is seen as a familial trait, which can be particularly disconcerting in women or men who display this type of smile. Most of the time, since this is a source of considerable embarrassment, one can observe these individuals concealing with their fingertips or hands the appearance of their gums and teeth when they smile or laugh. Also, while speaking in an animated fashion which causes them to smile or laugh during conversation, they can be seen covering their mouths in whatever way possible. No matter how hard they try, it is impossible for these individuals to smile or laugh without revealing their maxillary gingiva. Consequently, they attempt only to smile partially when being photographed or during social interactions which creates a certain amount of anxiety for those who are more self-conscious.[60] These individuals also tend to have sharply defined nasolabial folds with deep furrows (see Figure 14.53) (see Nasolabial Folds above).

Some patients, in conjunction with the inadvertent shortening of their upper lip causing an exaggerated gingival smile, also are plagued with exhibiting an involuntary lowering of the tip of their nose (see nasal tip ptosis above). There are still others who also form a transverse furrow across the philtrum of their upper lip when they speak, laugh, or smile. Occasionally, the same person exhibits a combination of all these idiosyncratic anatomical changes which has been identified by Cachay-Velasques as the *rhinogingivolabial* syndrome[34,61] (see nasal tip ptosis above). A horizontal furrow across the upper lip usually is seen in older individuals or in those whose photodamaged skin has reduced elasticity and soft tissue bulk, causing the lax upper lip skin to fold easily into a deep horizontal upper lip furrow (Figure 14.62). Circumoral vertical wrinkles that radiate away from the vermilion with every movement of their lips are also frequently seen in individuals who have a long history of smoking tobacco (see perioral lip lines in Chapter 15).

Functional Anatomy (See Appendix 2) of an Excessive Maxillary Gingival Display (Gummy Smile)

The essential components of a smile are the teeth, the gingiva, and the lips that surround them.[62] The aesthetics of an "ideal smile" vary according to idiosyncratic structural and topographic peribuccal anatomy predicated on a person's gender, familial traits (genotypic and phenotypic characteristics), race, and ethnicity. An atttractive smile is influenced by the color, shape (silhouette), and the position of the teeth in the mouth, along with the symmetrical architecture and periodontal health of the gums and the free gingival margin. The lips frame a smile and the outline of the scalloped gingival margins should be parallel to both the incisal edges of the teeth and the curvature of the lower lip. An attractive smile possesses symmetrical gingival margins of the central incisors while the more lateral teeth can have a certain amount of asymmetry.[63] When analyzing a smile, a certain amount of gingival exposure can be considered aesthetically pleasing and even youthful. The length of a normal upper lip measured from the subnasale to the lower border of the upper lip is 20–24 mm in young adults and increases in length with age (Figure 14.63). A maxillary central incisor display at rest averages 3–4 mm in young women and 2 mm in young men, and decreases with age (Figure 14.64).

In general, an attractive smile has been identified by many authors as having the following characteristics:[63]

1. Minimal gingival exposure
2. Symmetrical display and harmony between the maxillary gingival line and the upper lip
3. Healthy gingival tissue filling the entire interproximal spaces
4. Harmony between the anterior and posterior segments (gradation principle)
5. Teeth in correct anatomical form, proportion, and position
6. Proper color and shade of the teeth

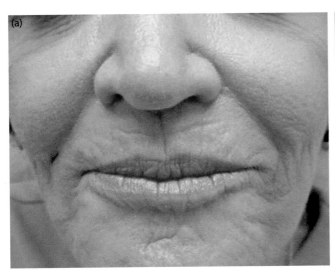

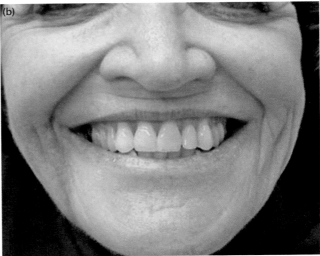

Figure 14.62 (a, b) A transverse rhytide is seen across the philtrum of the upper lip at rest, which is intensified with smiling in this 68-year-old non-smoker with extensive photodamage. Note the minimal gummy show, deep nasolabial folds and furrows, widening of the alar base, and the slight nasal tip downward rotation with smiling. Her shallow vertical lip lines are due to sun damage and aging and not to tobacco smoking.

7. Lower lip parallel to the incisal edges of the maxillary anterior teeth and to the imaginary line passing through the contact point of these teeth

A smile is formed in two dynamic stages.[64] In the first dynamic stage of a smile the upper lip is lifted toward the nasolabial fold by the contraction of the levator muscles originating in the fold and inserting into the upper lip. The fibers of the *medial* levators (LLSAN, LLS, zygomaticus minor, central orbicularis oris, and in some individuals, the depressor septi nasi) raise the lip upward over the anterior teeth while the fibers of the *lateral* levators (LLS, zygomaticus major, levator anguli oris, and lateral orbicularis oris, and in some individuals, the risorius) raise the lip laterally and slightly upward above the posterior teeth. There is then self-limiting resistance at the nasolabial fold because of cheek fat.

The second dynamic stage of a smile involves further lifting of the lip and the nasolabial fold by three bundles of muscle: (1) the LLS of the upper lip, originating at the infraorbital region; (2) the zygomaticus major, and (3) superior fibers of the buccinators. Often, squinting accompanies the final stage of smiling. It represents the contraction of the perioral musculature (zygomaticus major and minor, LLSAN, and LLS) that interdigitates with the muscle fibers of the lower *orbital* orbicularis oculi that supports maximum upper-lip elevation through the fold[63,64] (see nasolabial folds above).

The "smile line" is the position of the upper lip to the maxillary incisors and gingiva reached during a naturally full smile. Someone with a "low smile line" exposes less than 75% of the crown height of the maxillary anterior teeth. Those with an "average smile" display 75% to 100% of the maxillary crown height and no more exposure than 1–2 mm of upper gum mucosa.[65] Someone with a "high smile line" reveals the entire crown of the tooth and usually over 2 mm of contiguous maxillary gingiva[64,66] (Figure 14.65). Generally, men exhibit a lower smile line and less interlabial excursion than women who characteristically exhibit a higher smile line.[64,67,68]

There are three main reasons for a high "gingival smile," also known as a "gummy smile"; they include vertical maxillary excess, altered or delayed passive eruption, and hyperkinetic upper lip levators.[62] It is extremely important to correctly assess and diagnose clinically why a

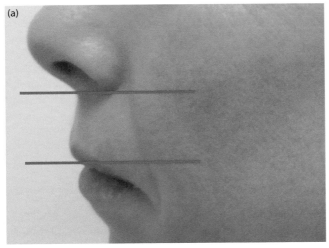

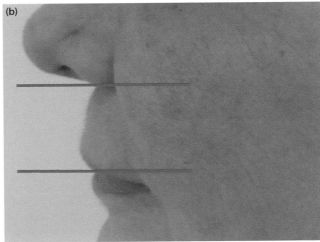

Figure 14.63 The length of a normal upper lip measured from the subnasale to the lower border of the upper lip is 20–24 mm in young adults (a) and increases in length with age as seen in this 67-year-old patient (b).

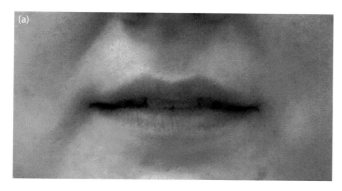

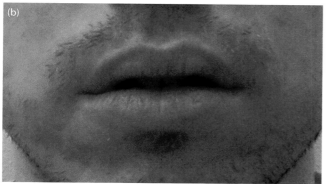

Figure 14.64 Maxillary central incisor display with someone at rest is 3–4 mm in young women as seen in a 31 year old patient (a), and 2 mm in young men as seen in a 34-year-old patient (b), and decreases with age.

person may possess a gummy smile before deciding on, and initiating any treatment. Incorrect diagnoses and treatment plans are frought with failure, disappointment, and adverse sequelae.

"Vertical maxillary excess" is identified clinically as an elongation of facial height created by a hyperplastic overgrowth of the maxillary skeleton resulting in an excessive vertical length of the maxilla, otherwise known as "long face syndrome".[63,66,69,70] An increase in facial height appears mainly in the lower half of the face. This skeletal dysplasia causes the teeth to be positioned farther away from the skeletal maxillary base, exposing the gingiva below the inferior border of the upper lip. It also causes the lower lip to cover the incisal edges of the maxillary canines and premolars. Most often the length of the upper lip is normal even though clinically it may appear relatively shorter.[63] Depending on the amount of skeletal hyperplasia and gingival display present, which can reach over 8 mm of gingival exposure, the only corrective solution might be cephalometric analysis and possible bone resection, or orthognathic surgical realignment with or without periodontal and restorative therapy.[1] Hence, referral to the appropriate dental and maxillofacial specialists is advisable.

Another frequently encountered dental condition to be identified when determining the reason for someone's gummy smile is the short square tooth with a short crown height (visible tooth length) with or without malpositioning of the incisors.[63] The difference between the *anatomical* crown height of a tooth and its *clinical* crown height will help determine whether the short crowns of the anterior maxillary teeth are a result of the natural wearing of the incisal surface of a tooth or the position of the gingival margin over the coronal aspect of the teeth; the *anatomical* crown height is the distance between the incisal edge of a tooth to the cementoenamel junction, whereas the *clinical* crown height is the distance from the incisal edge of a tooth to the free gingival margin[63] (Figure 14.66). When the gingival margin recedes at the apical aspect of a completely erupted tooth to the level of the

cementoenamel junction, this is known as "passive eruption." It is the natural physiologic progression of the growth and development of a normal tooth and it can continue well into the third decade of life. When the gingival margins are delayed or completely fail to recede to the level of the cementoenamel junction this is called "altered" or "delayed passive eruption," which can be found in 12% of the general population (Figure 14.67). Altered passive eruption is an aberration in normal tooth development, and may involve one or many teeth where a large portion of the dental crown remains covered in an overgrowth of gingiva. Characteristically, the gingival margin above the tooth appears flat with a minimal degree of scalloping or arching. Affected teeth appear short and square, instead of elliptical and ovoid in form. When this excess amount of gingiva is observed below the inferior border of the upper lip, the result is an "excessive maxillary gingival display" or a "gummy smile." If a physician is unaware of this condition when evaluating someone with a gummy smile during the pre-injection assessment, the physician injector can be easily misled into misdiagnosing a "high smile line" when in reality the presenting patient has a normal lip line or an otherwise "medium smile line"' which does not require treatement with a BoNT but instead will benefit from a referral to a periodontist a referral to a periodontist for gingivoplastic treatment.

The third most common cause for a gummy smile is the excessive contraction of the upper lip levators, producing an exaggerated exposure of the maxillary gingiva on smiling or laughing.[67,68] This can occur in conjunction with or without an increase in the interlabial space at rest. Prior to the advent of the BoNTs, various perioral muscular resection procedures (myotomies and myectomies of specific mimetic muscles) were devised to eliminate or at least diminish the causative muscular contractions that excessively elevated the upper lip and produced a gummy smile. Now various injection techniques of BoNT have superseded and replaced the need for the more invasive and morbid surgical procedures of treating gummy smiles due to hyperkinetic muscular activity.[71] Another not so common cause of a gummy smile is a genetically short upper lip that is less than 15 mm in height measured from the subnasale to the lower border of the upper lip (Figure 14.68). Even though the same treatment used for hyperactive lip levators causing a gummy smile can be used to treat a gummy smile that results from a congenital short upper lip, in reality the only suitable treatment for this type of a congenital defect is an appropriate surgical intervention.

Functionally, according to Rubin, there are three different patterns of smiles that can be identified when a person smiles.[72,73] The first and most commonly encountered type of smile (67% of the patients studied) is when the zygomaticus major dominates the movement of the lips. This is called the "Mona Lisa" or "commissural" smile and is initiated with a sharp elevation and outward pull of the corners of the mouth and then a soft elevation of the center of the upper lip, revealing approximately 80% of the incisors (Figure 14.69). This type of smile is produced predominantly by the pull of the zygomaticus major.

The "canine" or "cuspid" smile is the second most commonly identified smile pattern (35% of the patients studied) and is characterized by a high elevation of the center of the upper lip, exposing the canine teeth first before the rest of the upper lip is elevated (Figure 14.70). The canine smile can produce anywhere from a partial central dental reveal to an exaggerated full denture show with a certain amount of gingival exposure. This pattern of smile is produced predominantly by the contraction of the LLS elevating the upper lip. When the contraction of the LLS is intense and severe, a gummy smile results (Figure 14.71).

The third and least commonly seen smile pattern is the "full denture" or "complete" smile, which was seen in about 2% of the patients studied. The full denture smile is characterized by the simultaneous separation of both the upper and lower lips in which both the upper

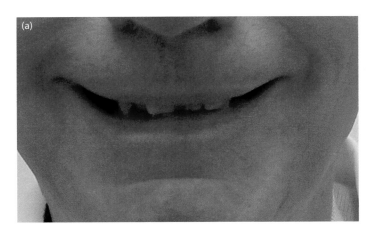

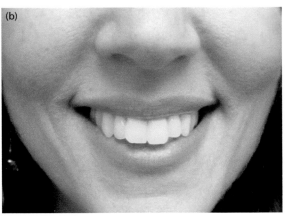

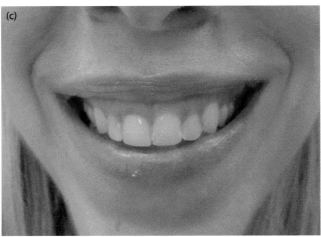

Figure 14.65 The smile line is the position of the upper lip and its relationship, when smiling, with the maxillary anterior incisors and gingiva. There are three types of smiles. (a) A person with a low smile line reveals less than 75% of the crown height when smiling; (b) a person with a medium or average smile line reveals 75%–100% of the maxillary crown height; (c) a person with a high (or "gingival") smile line reveals 2–3 mm or more of upper gum when smiling and is often referred to as having a "gummy smile."

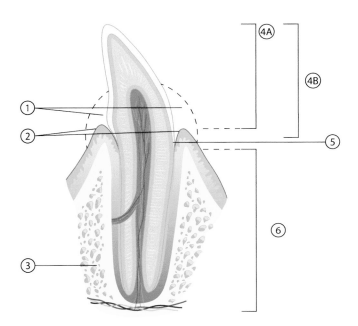

Figure 14.66 Anatomy of a "gummy smile": 1, excess amounts of gingiva in delayed or passive eruption; 2, normal gingival margins; 3, alveolar bone; 4A, clinical crown; 4B, anatomical crown; 5, cementoenamel junction; 6, root.

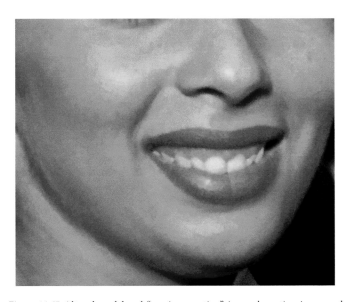

Figure 14.67 Altered or delayed "passive eruption" is an aberration in normal tooth development, involving many teeth where a large portion of the dental crown remains covered in an overgrowth of gingiva and the gingival margin above the tooth appears flat with a minimal degree of scalloping or arching. Affected teeth appear short and square, instead of elliptical or ovoid in form. This excess amount of gingiva seen below the inferior border of the upper lip, results in an "excessive maxillary gingival display" or a "gummy smile."

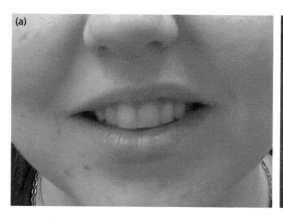
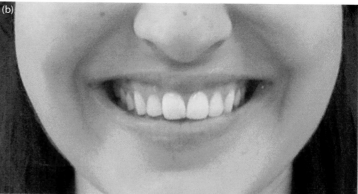

Figure 14.68 (a, b) Both these patients have a genetically short upper lip, measuring less than 15 mm in height measured from the subnasale to the lower border of the upper lip.

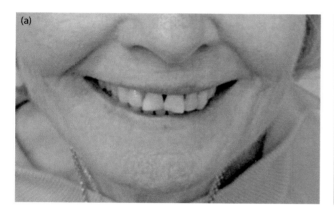
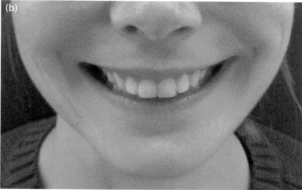

Figure 14.69 (a) The most common type of smile, the Mona Lisa smile, is produced primarily by the pull of the zygomaticus major. (b) Patients with a Mona Lisa or commissural smile after being treated with OnaBTX-A for a high lip line have found themselves with a "joker-like" smile, because the central lip levators were weakened while the lateral lip levators were not.

maxillary and lower mandibular dentures have partial or full exposure. This type of smile is the result of the contraction of all the upper lip levators and lower lip depressors around the mouth all at the same time (Figure. 14.72).

Commonly found accompanying a naturally occurring or an exaggerated canine smile (i.e., a "gummy smile") are individuals with deep nasolabial furrows and highly mounded nasolabial folds (Figures 14.61, 14.65c, 14.68b and 14.71b). These two conditions usually are found together. Contraction of the LLSAN creates an ascending steep medial nasolabial fold while lifting the central upper lip a few extra millimeters in conjuction with the LLS. The result is a high smile line and exposure of the alveolar gingiva (i.e., a gummy smile). Generally, an unattractive "gummy smile" reveals more than 2–3 mm of ginigiva above the central maxillary incisors. Most orthodontists and dentists prefer to see the lip elevation stop at the gingival margins of the maxillary incisors with a posed smile, but minimal amounts of gingiva can show with an exaggerated smile, depending on the individual's physiognomy. The aesthetics of a natural smile thus can vary from person to person depending on many different perceived subtle factors, including overall skeletal shape, ethnic proportions, and muscle configuration and variations in facial soft tissue and mimetic muscle composition and activity.[60]

Gummy smiles have been classified by Mazzuco and Hexsel as anterior, posterior, mixed or asymmetric.[74] They identified an *anterior* gummy smile as displaying more than 3 mm of maxillary gingiva over the area between the upper canine teeth and attributed it

to the action of the LLSAN. A *posterior* gummy smile was identified as displaying more than 3 mm of gingiva over the area posterior to the upper canine teeth, but with normal anterior maxillary gingival exposure of less than 3 mm. It was attributed to the action of the zygomaticus muscles. A *mixed* gummy smile displays excessive amounts of gingiva both in the anterior and posterior aspects of the maxillary gingiva. This was attributed to the variable actions of any one of a combination of the different levator muscles which produce a smile: the LLSAN, zygomaticus major and minor, as well as the LLS, levator anguli oris, and possibly the risorius. When individual central maxillary retractors (e.g., the LLSAN or the zygomaticus major) are hyperkinetic, *asymmetric* gummy smiles usually are not uncommon (Figures 14.73 and 14.74).

Dilution (See Appendix 3) When Treating Excessive Maxillary Gingival Display (Gummy Smile)

Injecting minimal amounts of low-volume OnaBTX-A in the mid face is of paramount importance. The least amount of unintended diffusion of OnaBTX-A in the stratified lamellae of the different muscle bundles of the perioral area can be disastrous to the overall therapeutic success and cosmetic appearance of the patient. The reputation of a physician injector who treats the mid face is tenured in the aesthetic outcomes of his or her skillful injection techniques. Therefore, the most experienced and qualified physicians treating this area of the face will reconstitute a 100 U vial of OnaBTX-A with only 1 mL of normal saline.

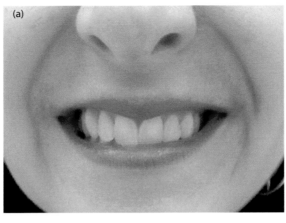

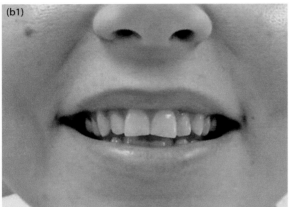
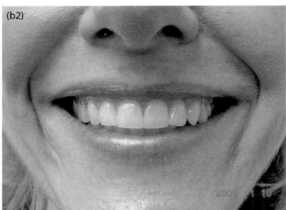

Figure 14.70 (a) The canine smile exposes the canine teeth before the rest of the upper lip is elevated. (b1,b2) An exaggerated canine smile in a younger and older patient.

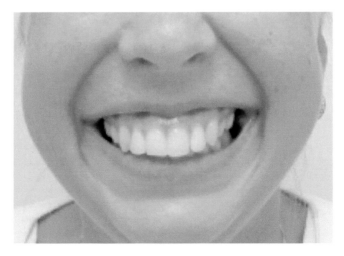

Figure 14.71 An exaggerated gummy canine smile in this 23-year-old patient. Note the deep nasolabial folds and furrows that often accompany a gummy smile.

Dosing: How to Correct the Problem (See Appendix 4) (What to Do and What Not to Do) When Treating Excessive Maxillary Gingival Display (Gummy Smile)

As one ages, the upper lip becomes flaccid and lengthens with time, making noninvasive treatments of a gummy smile with OnaBTX-A a more preferred option over the morbidity, long recovery time, and high cost of more invasive bone or muscle resection surgery that is frought with scar contracture and protracted regeneration of muscle activity. However, when deciding on an injection pattern for a patient with a gummy smile, it is of utmost importance to select the proper candidate prior to treatment. Of all the patients Kane treated for an excessive maxillary gingival display, he discovered that only those patients with a canine or cuspid type smile were the most appropriate candidates for injections of OnaBTX-A.[51,52] These patients had the best outcomes and were the most satisfied with their reults.[71]

To nonsurgically elongate the upper lip, especially during a smile, the central upper lip retractors (LLSAN and LLS) need to be gently relaxed (not paralyzed) with injections of OnaBTX-A. This can be

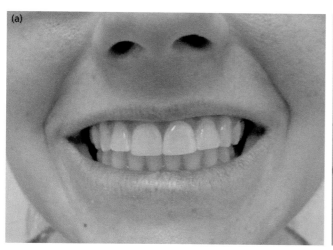 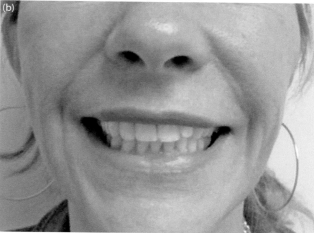

Figure 14.72 (a) The full denture smile is a result of the contraction of all the upper lip levators and lower lip depressors around the mouth, all at the same time, and is characterized by the simultaneous partial or full exposure of both upper and lower dentures. (b) Note a slight ptosis of the upper left quadrant.

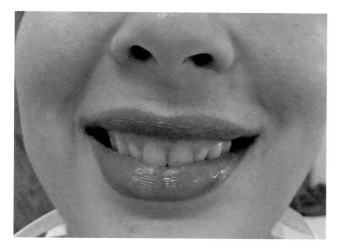

Figure 14.73 Hyperkinetic central upper lip levators create a slight gummy commissural or "Mona Lisa" smile that is asymmetrically higher in the upper right quadrant of this 29-year-old. Note the deep nasolabial folds.

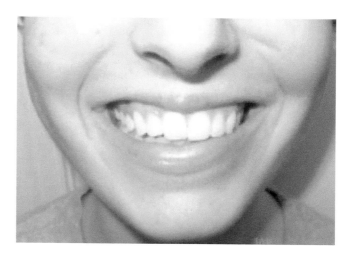

Figure 14.74 Hyperkinetic lateral upper lip levators create a slight gummy canine smile that is asymmetrically higher in the upper right quadrant of this 20-year-old. Note the deep nasolabial folds.

accomplished with the patient in a sitting or semireclined position. Then palpate the nasomaxillary groove with the fingertip of the index finger of the nondominant hand, until the fingertip pad straddles the lower lateral aspect of the alar facial sulcus and the superior edge of the maxillary alveolar process. Excessive pressure with palpation in this area can cause some discomfort to the patient, so this maneuver should be done as gently and expeditiously as possible. As the patient smiles and with the index finger in this position, contraction of the LLSAN can be felt. At the point of maximum thickness of the muscle, insert the needle perpendicularly to the surface of the skin and deeply into the nasofacial groove for about 3–5 mm. Inject 1–2 U of OnaBTX-A intramuscularly and just above the periosteum of the canine fossa (Figure 14.75). An additional unit of OnaBTX-A may be required if the central lip levators are very strong and the center of the upper lip is lifted extremely high. Remember to reserve this injection technique only for those patients with a canine or cuspid type smile who have an exaggerated gingival display, and in whom the upper lip retractors can be palpated.[51,52,60,75] The direct upper lip retractors are the LLSAN, the LLS, and, according to different live patient and cadaver dissection studies, the zygomaticus minor and central orbicularis oris. Depending on the overall facial shape and the variations

of muscular activity, the indirect upper lip retractors—that is, those which pass through the modiolus first before inserting into the lips—may also play a role in an excessive maxillary gingival display. They include the zygomaticus major, levator anguli oris, lateral orbicularis oris, and risorius.[76] It is the subtle variations in muscle location and activity that account for the variations in individual idiosyncratic facial expressions and the differences in treatment response and final outcome with OnaBTX-A even when the injection technique is impeccable. Also, remember that injecting OnaBTX-A at this site may reduce the height and extent of the nasolabial fold by weakening the LLSAN as well as the LLS and zygomaticus minor (Figure 14.76). When correcting only a central gummy smile, it is best to avoid weakening the more laterally located lip levators, that is, zygomaticus major, levator anguli oris, and risorius; otherwise, either an adynamic or asymmetric smile can result. Weakening only the central upper lip levators without affecting these lateral upper lip levators allows the lateral levators full and uninhibited movement during a smile. Focused central upper lip weakening can be enhanced by also treating the depressor anguli oris with OnaBTX-A, thereby removing any additional antagonistic lateral lower lip depressor action against unnecessary and unintentional weakening of the lateral upper lip levators.

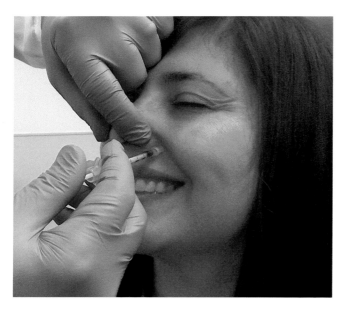

Figure 14.75 Place the needle perpendicular to the skin surface and inject 1–2 U of OnaBTX-A deeply into the belly of the muscle at the nasomaxillary groove while the patient smiles excessively.

The depressor septi nasi at times may require treatment with 1–2 U of OnaBTX-A at the base or along the length of the columella when the depressor action of the muscle is hyperkinetic. This additional maneuver will help produce a more natural smile. By lowering the central aspect of the upper lip, not only is the extent of an exaggerated gummy smile reduced, but also the depth of a horizontal upper lip crease can be diminished (see nasal tip ptosis above). However, if migration of OnaBTX-A extends into the central superficial fibers of the orbicularis oris, an inability to fully pucker the lips also will occur. An alternative technique is to inject 1–2 U of OnaBTX-A intraorally into the bellies of the two central upper lip levators. By passing the needle on either side

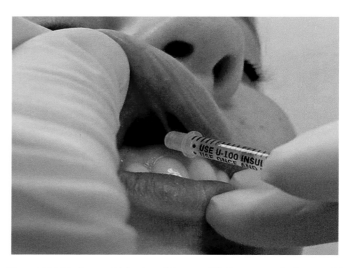

Figure 14.77 The intraoral injection of the central lip levators may be less painful to the patient, but a less precise way of injecting OnaBTX-A.

of the phrenulum through the gingivo-labial sulcus above the alveolar ridge at the same point in the nasofacial groove and canine fossa as described above (Figure 14.77).[68] A minimum dose of low-volume OnaBTX-A should just barely relax the central upper lip levators so that the upper lip cannot fully retract upward. If the excessive gummy show persists and is at its highest point in the center of the upper lip with or without evidence of a transverse horizontal line across the upper lip and philtrum, then an additional 1 U of OnaBTX-A can be injected into the depressor septi nasi at the base of the columella (Figures 14.33 and 14.78).

When treating a gummy smile with OnaBTX-A, most studies target the LLS and the LLSAN as the main muscles to weaken and reduce the height of a high lip line. In a study of 14 (13 female and 1 male) Caucasian patients ages 23–48 years old by Suber and colleagues, the

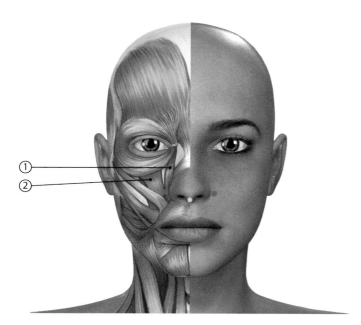

Figure 14.76 The central lip levators (i.e., direct retractors): levator labii superioris alaeque nasi and levator labii superioris can be treated with 1 or 2 U of OnaBTX-A ● to diminish a gummy smile. The indirect retractor, depressor septi nasi, also may be treated with 1–2 U of OnaBTX-A ● when upper lip retraction is extreme. 1, levator labii superioris alaeque nasi; 2, levator labii superioris.

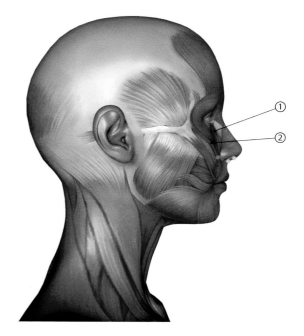

Figure 14.78 The central lip levators (i.e., direct retractors): levator labii superioris alaeque nasi and levator labii superioris can be treated with 1 or 2 U of OnaBTX-A ● to diminish a gummy smile. The indirect retractor, depressor septi nasi, also may be treated with 1–3 injection points along the columella with 1–2 U of OnaBTX-A ● when upper lip retraction elevation is extreme.

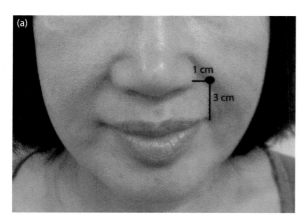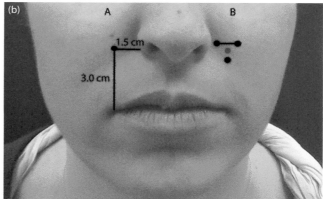

Figure 14.79 (a) Hwang and colleagues determined that the ideal injection point, the "Yonsei" point, is found at the intersection of two lines, one approximately 1 cm–1.5 cm lateral to the most lateral aspect of the ala nasi and the other approximately 3 cm up from the oral commissure. (b) According to Suber et al., the preferred injection treatment points on the surface of the face corresponded to an inverted triangle with one injection point 2 mm lateral to the alar-facial groove at the level of the nasal passage, the other injection point 2 mm lateral to the first point in the same horizontal plane and a third injection point 2 mm inferior and between the first 2 injection sites. This is almost identical to the "Yonsei" point.

topographical landmarks encompassing the preferred three injection treatment points on the surface of the face corresponded to an inverted triangle with one injection point 2 mm lateral to the alar-facial groove at the level of the nasal passage, the other injection point 2 mm lateral to the first point in the same horizontal plane, and a third injection point 2 mm inferior and between the first two injection sites[71] Figure 14.79b). This location adjacent to the ala nasi is the preferred site for injecting OnaBTX-A and has been identified by many authors as the area of intersecting muscle fibers of the LLS, LLSAN, and in some individuals, the zigomaticus minor, when present.[53,55,60,71,74–77]

In a study of 50 hemi-faces of 25 (12 female and 13 male) Korean cadavers between the ages of 47 and 88 years of age, Hwang and colleagues identified the ideal location lateral to the ala nasi for injecting BoNT to treat a gummy smile.[76] This ideal injection point is found at the intersection of two lines, one approximately 1 cm–1.5 cm lateral to the most lateral aspect of the ala nasi and the other approximately 3 cm up from the oral commissure (Figure 14.79a). They described how the zygomaticus minor and the LLSAN were located in a superficial plane that covered the medial and lateral margins of the LLS and how all three muscles converged on a small triangular area lateral to the ala nasi. They named the center of this triangle the "Yonsei point." This single injection point was located easily and felt to target effectively the LLSAN, LLS, and zygomaticus minor with just a single injection of OnaBTX-A, as opposed to Suber et al.[71] and Polo[60,77] who injected each muscle separately. There was no statistically significant difference in location measurements between males and females in the Hwang study.[76] Because the shape of the faces between Caucasians and Asians may vary, an exact injection point for treating a gummy smile may not be clinically obvious by ruler measurements; consequently, the best way to identify the ideal injection point is to palpate the general area lateral to the ala nasi and ask the patient to raise the upper lip and make sneering motions as described above. When the contracting muscle fibers can be palpated, then injecting OnaBTX-A into this location is probably safe and effective, provided only 1–2 units of concentrated, low volume OnaBTX-A are injected.[51,52,60,71,74–76]

Mazucco and Hexsel treated with abobotulinumtoxinA (AboBTX-A) 16 patients with a maxillary gingival display of over 3 mm. They used a dose equivalency of 2.5:1 IU of AboBTX-A to OnaBTX-A and injected subcutaneously. There were 3 patients with an *anterior* gummy smile. They were injected at a standard location 1 cm lateral and 1 cm below the nasal ala to weaken the LLSAN. They were injected with either 2.5 or 5 units of AboBTX-A depending on the amount of gingiva exposed. There were 7 patients with a *posterior* gummy smile and they were injected at two locations in the malar region that followed a lateral and superior path corresponding to the path of the zygomaticus major and zygomaticus minor. The first injection point was located in the nasolabial fold at the point of greatest lateral pull during a full smile. The second injection point was 2 cm lateral to the first point at the level of the tragus. At each injection point, 2.5 units of AboBTX-A was injected.[74] There were 3 patients who had an anterior and posterior or "*mixed*" component to their gummy smile. They were injected at all 6 points, 3 on each side of the midline, in the locations just described; however, at the site closest to the nasal ala, the dose was reduced by 50%, that is, only 2.5 units of AboBTX-A were given, while the malar injections remained the same at 2.5 units. There were 3 patients with asymmetric gummy smiles, who received bilateral but asymmetric injections of AboBTX-A with a higher dose on the hyperkinetic side according to the pattern of their asymmetry. The contralateral side was also treated but with minimal doses of AboBTX-A (2.5 units) at the more inferior location adjacent to the oral commissure where the lateral pull was highest. The bilateral injections were performed to avoid the possibility of reverse asymmetry caused by compensatory muscle contraction of the untreated side.[74]

Outcomes (Results) (See Appendix 5) When Treating Excessive Maxillary Gingival Display (Gummy Smile)

Treating patients with an exaggerated gingival smile can produce a variety of anatomic and functional changes. By limiting the exaggerated upward movement of the upper lip with injections of OnaBTX-A, an obvious reduction in the amount of upper gingival and dental show will result, along with elongation of the upper lip, some flattening of the philtrum, thinning of the vermillion, and effacement of the medial aspect of the nasolabial fold and sulcus (Figure 14.51).

Patients who experienced the best results with the least amount of adverse events were those individuals who primarily possessed a canine or cuspid type smile and were successfully treated with 1 or 2 units of concentrated, low volume OnaBTX-A.[51,52] They usually are the ones who gladly return for repeat maintenance treatments with OnaBTX-A because their low dose, low volume treatments gave them the most natural appearing results with the least troublesome side effects.[51,52]

Even for those patients with a full type of gummy smile with anterior and posterior components with or without asymmetry, minimal doses of concentrated low volume OnaBTX-A is the best injection technique. Start with low doses that can be augmented with another 1 or 2 units of OnaBTX-A after 2 or 3 weeks if necessary, when the patient returns for a follow-up visit.

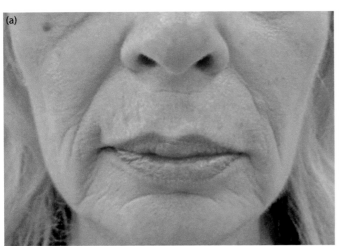
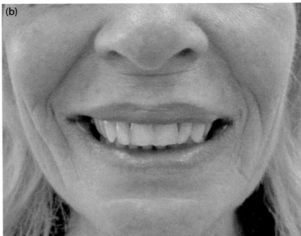

Figure 14.80 Note the transverse rhytide across the upper lip in this light complexioned 68-year-old individual both at rest and when smiling.

Polo conducted a study to determine the doses required and the injection sites preferred to correct gummy smiles, while providing consistent, statistically significant and aesthetically pleasing results.[60] Thirty patients (29 females, 1 male) with an upper gummy smile caused by hyperfunctional upper lip levators received 2.5 U of OnaBTX-A at two sites per side (a total of four sites) into two distinct points lateral to the alar facial angle. The one injection point was more medial and at the alar facial angle where the LLSAN overlaps the LLS. The other injection point was more lateral and where the LLS overlaps the zygomaticus minor. The injection sites were determined only by palpation of contracting musculature while the patient smiled. No electromyographic guidance was used like in his previous study.[77] A gummy smile was defined as an excessive gingival display above the tooth crown of at least 3.0 mm on unrestricted, nonposed, "full-blown," spontaneous smiling. The pretreatment gingival display averaged 5.2 mm (±1.4 mm). Two weeks after treatment, the mean gingival display declined to 0.09 mm (±1.06 mm). This was a mean reduction in gingival display for all 30 patients of 5.1 mm. Along with the anticipated relative lengthening of the upper lip on smiling, Polo also reported a marked reduction of the nasolabial fold as the most frequently observed accompanying side effect. Other attendant sequelae included a reduction in the hypercontractibility of the transverse nasalis when smiling and an effacement of lower periocular rhytides of the *orbital* orbicularis oculi. This was thought to be caused in these particular individuals by the attendant relaxation of the interdigitating muscle fibers of their LLSAN, LLS, and zygomaticus minor which might have been in close proximtity to the transverse nasalis and muscle fibers of the lower portion of the *orbital* orbicularis oculi. Polo believes a successful treatment with OnaBTX-A depends on a multitude of factors, including the physician injector's appreciation of an individual's particular facial aesthetics and the injector's ability to discern correctly which muscles are responsible for the particular movements causing the wrinkles in question. There is a great deal of variability among different individuals and the strength of their facial mimetic muscles and how they move and produce wrinkling. However, injections of OnaBTX-A are most successful when they are given into those muscles that move in a perpendicular direction from the direction of the wrinkles being treated. Polo also concluded that the dose of 5 U per side was best for patients who had at least a 5.0 mm gingival display. For those who had less than a 5.0 mm gingival display, lower doses of OnaBTX-A were more appropriate. The results lasted 24–30 weeks.[60]

In addition, it may be possible to diminish the appearance of an idiosyncratic horizontal rhytide when it is present across the upper lip (Figure 14.80). An additional 1–2 U of OnaBTX-A at the base of the columella into the depressor septi nasi by the technique described above may be necessary to further diminish the depth of the central aspect of this horizontal upper lip rhytide (Figure 14.35). Most of the time, however, injections of a soft tissue filler are the only reliable way to completely efface a deep, transverse upper lip wrinkle, especially when it persists after an OnaBTX-A treatment of the central levators of the upper lip (see Figure 14.41). Most patients who develop the transverse rhytide across their upper lip seem to be those over the age of 60 who are of light complexion (usually of skin type II and III), have spent a lot of time outdoors, and may or may not have a history of smoking tobacco (Figures 14.62 and 14.80).

Suber et al. treated with OnaBTX-A 14 patients (13 females and 1 male) who only possessed a cuspid type (canine) smile with a 2 mm or more gingival display.[71] Between 4 and 6 units of OnaBTX-A were injected at three sites on both sides of the nose lateral to the alae nasi and into the LLS and LLSAN. Before the injections of OnaBTX-A the gingival show over the central incisors averaged 4.89 mm (range, 3–7 mm) and 4.25 mm (range, 1–7 mm) above the canines. Approximately 2 weeks after the OnaBTX-A injections, the gingival show decreased on an average of 4.14 mm (range, 1–8 mm) over the central incisors and 3.51 mm (range, 1–5 mm) above the canines. No major complications were observed.[71]

All patients in the Mazzucco and Hexsel series experienced a decrease in their exaggerated gingival display of over 75%.[74] The average improvement of patients with an anterior gummy smile was 96%; with a posterior gummy smile, 61.06%; with a mixed gummy smile, 90.1%; and with asymmetry, 71.93%. Adverse effects were mild and minimal. One patient with a posterior gummy smile developed asymmetry after the initial treatment, and was corrected with 2.5 units of AboBTX-A into the nasolabial fold on the side of greater gingival exposure at a follow-up visit. Another patient with a posterior gummy smile had difficulty with smiling. The physical examination revealed a slight lowering of the commissures creating a "sad smile," which was attributed to hyperactivity of the depressor anguli oris on both sides of the mouth. This was successfully treated with 5 units of AboBTX-A bilaterally into the depressor anguli oris. None of the patients in this study reported any difficulty with any lip movement or with speaking.[74]

Treating exaggerated maxillary gingival exposure with BoNTs provides affected patients with a quick and affordable solution that is safer and less traumatic than any surgical procedure currently available. Results can last anywhere from 3 to 6 months and sometimes even longer when treatments are executed properly.

Complications (Adverse Sequelae) (See Appendix 6) When Treating Excessive Maxillary Gingival Display (Gummy Smile)

Because of the anatomy of the different codependent levator muscles and their attachments in both the upper lip skin and orbicularis oris, the risk–benefit ratio of treating a patient with a gingival smile is high and the potential comorbidity is significant. When attempting to treat an exaggerated maxillary gummy smile with injections of OnaBTX-A, assistance with an electromyograph (EMG) might ensure more accurate needle placement and avoid untoward results.[77] The upper lip levators (i.e., levator labii superioris alaeque, levator labii superioris, the zygomaticus complex, risorius, levator anguli oris, and orbicularis oris) (Figure 14.81) can easily be affected by the least amount of inadvertent diffusion of OnaBTX-A. Inaccurate needle placement or overzealous dosing in this area is subject to upper lip ptosis, buccal sphincter incompetence, and an asymmetric smile. This in turn leads to an inability of the upper lip to appose the lower lip completely and tightly or to move in a full smile or pucker. This can lead to dysarthria, and difficulty with producing particular sounds and articulating certain words. Buccal sphincter incompetence can result in an embarrassing public display of functional compromise, especially when incontinence of liquid or solids is an unexpected and unavoidable consequence.

Patients with a Mona Lisa or commissural smile after being treated with OnaBTX-A for a high lip line found themselves with a "joker-like" smile, because the central lip levators were weakened while the lateral lip levators were not.[51,71] This allowed the commissures of the mouth to move higher laterally and the center of the lip to remain low without elevation (Figure 14.69b).

Patients with a full denture or complete smile have a reverse type of result to those with a Mona Lisa or commissural smile. Because a full denture smile recruits both the upper lip levators and lower lip depressors when a smile is activated, it can create a range of different anterior and posterior gummy smile profiles, depending on the variable strength of the muscles producing it. When either the center of the upper lip or the zygomatic component of the posterior maxillary gingival overexposure are treated with OnaBTX-A to reduce the maxillary gingival display, the normally functioning unopposed lower lip lateral depressor, that is, the depressor anguli oris will pull down vigorously on the lateral commissures. With the upper lip central and especially lateral levators weakened and the lower lip depressors contracting in full compensatory activity, a grimace is produced or even a look of dismay or horror when a smile is attempted. This was identified as a "sad smile" when a posterior type of gummy smile was treated by Mazzuco and Hexsel.[74] They remarked that if the depressor anguli oris is observed as hyperactive prior to treating a gummy smile, then it should be treated at the same time along with the other muscles which are being treated for a gummy smile.

When reviewing the present literature on treating gummy smiles it is important to keep in mind that all the studies used fixed doses to weaken the upper lip retractors no matter how strong or weak they were or how high the maxillary gingival reveal was. However, the patients with the stronger muscles and the highest gingival exposure did better than those with weaker muscles and lesser gingival displays because the dose was not reduced to accommodate their weaker muscles. In clinical practice, on the other hand, it is of paramount importance to tailor the dose of BoNT in proportion to the strength of the muscles being treated, especially in the midface. Because the deep and superficial mimetic muscles of the midface are contiguous and even interdigitate with each other, any amount of BoNT injected in any area no matter how directly localized to a muscle the injection is given, the toxin will easily and freely spread into the adjacent muscles that might have similar or not so similar actions. In the mid face, one only needs to weaken a muscle lightly with minimal amounts of OnaBTX-A to get a significant response, unlike treating the upper face where large doses of OnaBTX-A are necessary to realize the expected outcome. Consequently, because of diffusion characteristics, ease of dosing, and outcome reliability, many physician injectors will prefer OnaBTX-A over AboBTX-A when treating patients in the mid and lower face.[76] Because of their overall small size and reduced strength, as is indicative of most mid face muscles, their response to treatment with OnaBTX-A can still be precariously variable in the mid and lower face than it is with the larger muscles of the upper face. Mid and lower facial muscles frequently respond differently to the first and subsequent injections of OnaBTX-A. With each subsequent injection, the muscles remain weakened for a longer period of time and require less dosing, probably because of disuse atrophy. Other reported adverse events after OnaBTX-A injections for a gummy smile are usually due to either inexperienced injectors' overzealous or misplaced injections or both, causing ptosis or elongation of the upper lip; grossly asymmetric, "funny-looking" and dysfunctional smiles; as well as difficulty with chewing and attendant severe drooling; an inability to pucker the lips or enunciate certain words or sounds, and "stroke-like" animation.[1,78] In a response to Niamatu, Polo confirms the importance of understanding the functional anatomy of all the mimetic muscles of the face, and knowing exactly where the limits of the muscles are before injecting them, being conservative in treating the mid face musculature with low doses of concentrated OnaBTX-A and keeping meticulous clinical and photographic records so that repeat treatments are reproducible with the same outcomes.[79]

Treatment Implications When Injecting a Gummy Smile

1. Injecting OnaBTX-A into the central upper lip retractors (levator labii superioris alaeque nasi, the levator labii superioris, and zygomaticus minor) at a particular point lateral to the alae nasi can reduce an exaggerated gingival show by elongating the upper lip.
2. Inject the central upper lip retractors only when they definitely can be palpated as they contract lateral to the alae nasi; otherwise, adjacent, nontargeted muscles will be affected, and lip competence and symmetry will be compromised.

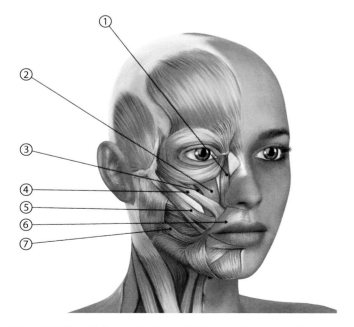

Figure 14.81 Properly functioning levator labii superioris alaeque nasi, zygomaticus major and minor, levator labii superioris, levator anguli oris, risorius, and orbicularis oris are essential for buccal sphincter competence. 1, levator labii superioris alaeque nasi; 2, levator labii superioris; 3, levator anguli oris; 4, zygomaticus minor; 5, zygomaticus major; 6, orbicularis oris; 7, risorius.

3. Patients with a canine smile are the best candidates to receive OnaBTX-A injections for an exaggerated maxillary gingival smile.

4. Injecting OnaBTX-A into the levator labii superioris alaeque nasi also will efface the upper medial aspect of the nasolabial sulcus and fold and flatten the philtrum and attenuate the vermillion.

5. Inject only low volumes of low doses of concentrated OnaBTX-A in the perinasal area. The depressor septi nasi also may need to be injected with OnaBTX-A to diminish the depth of the transverse horizontal furrow in the center of the upper lip if it persists after injections for a gummy smile. Complete effacement is usually only accomplished with injections of a soft tissue filler.

6. Treat with injections of OnaBTX-A a hyperactive depressor anguli oris along with the upper lip levators when reducing an exaggerated posterior maxillary gingival display of someone with a canine, or a complete full-denture type smile otherwise, a sad smile grimace will result.

7. Photographic to any treatment with OnaBTX-A, inform the patient of the potential risks, benefits, comorbidities, and inherent functional and cosmetic changes expected when perioral mimetic muscles are weakened.

REFERENCES

1. Carruthers J, Carruthers A. Aesthetic botulinum A toxin in the mid and lower face and neck. *Dermatol Surg* 2003; 29: 468–76.
2. de Sa Earp AP, Marmur ES. The five D's of botulinum toxin: Doses, dilution, diffusion, duration and dogma. *J Cosmet Laser Therapy* 2008; 10: 93–102.
3. Rohrich RJ, Janis JE, Fagien S et al. The cosmetic use of botulinum toxin. *Plast Reconstr Surg* 2003; 112(Suppl): 177s–87s.
4. Fagien S, Rasplado H. Facial rejuvenation with botulinum neurotoxin: An anatomical and experiential perspective. *J Cos Laser Th* 2007; 9(Suppl 1): 23–31.
5. Carruthers JD, Glogau RG, Blitzer A et al. Advances in facial rejuvenation: Botulinum toxin type A, hyaluronic acid dermal fillers, and combination therapies–consensus recommendations. *Plast Reconstr Surg* 2008; 121: 5s–30s.
6. Fagien S. Botulinum toxin type A for facial aesthetic enhancement role in facial shaping. *Plast Reconstr Surg* 2003; 112(Suppl 1): 6s–18s.
7. Fagien S. BOTOX® for the treatment of dynamic and hyperkinetic facial lines and furrows: Adjunctive use in facial aesthetic surgery. *Plast Reconstr Surg* 1999; 103: 701–7.
8. Ahn BK, Kim YS, Kim HJ et al. Consensus recommendations on the aesthetic usage of botulinum toxin type A in Asians. *Dermatol Surg* 2013; 39: 1843–60.
9. Standring S, (ed). *Gray's Anatomy: The Anatomical Basis of Clinical Practice*. Philadelphia: Elsevier; 2016.
10. Lamilla GC, Ingallina FM, Poulain B, Trevidic P. *Anatomy and Botulinum Toxin Injections. Master Collection Volume 1.* Paris, France: Expert 2 Expert SARL; 2015.
11. Hur MS, Hu KS, Park JT et al. New anatomical insight of the levator labii superioris alaeque nasi and the transverse part of the nasalis. *Surg Radiol Anat* 2010; 32: 753–56.
12. Letourneau A, Daniel RK. The superficial musculoaponeurotic system of the nose. *Plast Reconstr Surg* 1988; 82(1): 48–57.
13. Figallo EE, Acosta JA. Nose muscular dynamics: The tip trigonum. *Plast Reconstr Surg* 2001; 108: 1126.
14. Clark MPA, Greenfield B, Hunt N et al. Function of the nasal muscles in normal subjects assessed by dynamic MRI and EMG: Its relevance to rhinoplasty surgery. *Plast Reconstr Surg* 1998; 101: 1945–55.
15. Ju-Young Lee JY, Hur MS. An anatomical description of the anomalous nasi muscle. *Korean J Phys Anthropol* 2017; 30(3): 109–112.
16. Hexsel C, Hexsel D, Porto MD et al. Botulinum toxin type A for aging face and aesthetic uses. *Dermatologic Therapy* 2011; 24: 54–61.
17. Carruthers J, Carruthers A. Botulinum toxin (BOTOX®) chemodenervation for facial rejuvenation. *Facial Plast Surg* 2001; 9: 197–204.
18. Blitzer A, Binder WJ. Current practices in the use of botulinum toxin in the management of facial lines and wrinkles. *Facial Plast Surg* 2001; 9: 395–404.
19. Tamura BM, Odo MY, Changi B et al. Treatment of nasal wrinkles with botulinum toxin. *Dermatol Surg* 2005; 3: 271–75.
20. Matarasso SL. Complication of botulinum A exotoxin for hyperfunctional lines. *Dermatol Surg* 1998; 24: 1249–54.
21. Goldwyn R, Rohrich R. Consensus recommendations on the use of botulinum toxin type A in facial aesthetics. *Plast Reconstr Surg* 2004; 114(Suppl): 1s–22s.
22. Aung SC, Foo CL, Lee ST. Three dimensional laser scan assessment of the Oriental nose with a new classification of Oriental nasal types. *Br J Plast Surg* 2000; 53(2): 109–16.
23. Romo T, Abraham MT. The ethnic nose. *Facial Plast Surg* 2003; 19(3): 269–78.
24. Uzun A, Ozdemir F. Morphometric analysis of nasal shapes and angles in young adults. *Braz J Otorhinolaryngol* 2014; 80(5): 397–402.
25. Cobo R. Hispanic/Mestizo rhinoplasty. *Facial Plast Surg Clin N Am* 2010; 18: 173–88.
26. Cobo R. Rhinoplasty in the Mestizo nose. *Facial Plast Surg Clin N Am* 2014; 22: 395–415.
27. Ducut EG, Han SK, Kim SB et al. Factors affecting nostril shape in Asian noses. *Plast Reconstr Surg* 2006; 118: 1613.
28. Anderson KJ, Henneberg M, Norris RM. Anatomy of the nasal profile. *J. Anat* 2008; 213: 210–6.
29. Bruintjes TD, van Olphen AF, Hillen B, Huizing EH. A functional anatomic study of the relationship of the nasal cartilages and muscles to the nasal valve area. *Laryngoscope* 1998; 108: 1025–32.
30. Aksoy F, Veyseller B, Yildirim YS et al. Role of nasal muscles in nasal valve collapse. *Otolaryngol Head Neck Surg* 2010; 142(3): 365–9.
31. Arregui JS, Elejalde MV, Regalado J et al. Dynamic rhinoplasty for the plunging nasal tip: Functional unity of the inferior third of the nose. *Plast Reconstr Surg* 2000; 106: 1624–29.
32. LeLouran C. Botulinum toxin A and facial lines: The variable concentration. *Aesthet Plast Surg* 2001; 25: 73–84.
33. Armijo BS, Brown M, Guyuron B. Defining the ideal nasolabial angle. *Plast Reconstr Surg* 2012; 129: 759.
34. Cachay–Velásquez H. Rhinoplasty and facial expression. *Ann Plast Surg* 1992; 28: 427–33.
35. Dayan SH, Kempiners JJ. Treatment of the lower third of the nose and dynamic nasal tip ptosis with Botox. *Plast Reconstr Surg* 2005; 115: 1784.
36. Tellioglu AT, Inozu E, Ozakpinar R et al. Treatment of hyperdynamic nasal tip ptosis in open rhinoplasty: Using the anatomic relationship between the depressor septi nasi muscle and the dermocartilaginous ligament. *Aesth Plast Surg* 2012; 36: 819–26.
37. Benlier E, Balta S, Tas S. Depressor septi nasi modification in rhinoplasty: A review of anatomy and surgical techniques. *Facial Plast Surg* 2014; 30: 471–6.
38. Rohrich RJ, Huynh B, Muzaffar AR et al. Importance of the depressor septi nasi muscle in rhinoplasty: Anatomic study and clinical application. *Plast Reconstr Surg* 2000; 105: 376–83.
39. Kosins AM, Lambros V, Daniel RK. The plunging tip: Analysis and surgical treatment. *Aesthet Surg* 2015; 35(4): 367–77.
40. Pessa JE. Improving the acute nasolabial angle and medial nasolabial fold by levator alae muscle resection. *Ann Plast Surg* 1992; 29: 23–30.

41. Gierloff M, Stoehring C, Buder T et al. Aging changes of the Midfacial fat compartments: A computed tomographic study. *Plast Reconstr Surg* 2012; 129: 263–73.

42. Atamoros PF. Botulinum toxin in the lower one–third of the face. Editor AV Benedetto. *Clin Derm* 2003; 21: 505–12.

43. Trindade de Almeida AR. Nose. In: Hexsel D, Trindade de Almeida AR, (eds). *Cosmetic Use of Botulinum Toxin.* Porto Allergre, Brazil: AGE Editora; 2002: 158–63.

44. Rohrich RJ, Pessa JE. The fat compartments of the face: Anatomy and clinical implications for cosmetic surgery. *Plast Reconstr Surg* 2007; 119: 2219–27.

45. Donofrio L, Weinkle S. The third dimension in facial rejuvenation: A review. *J Cosmet Dermatol* 2006; 5(4): 277–83.

46. Fitzgerald R, Rubin AG. Filler placement and the fat compartments. *Dermatol Clin* 2014; 32: 37–50.

47. Zufferey J. Anatomic variations of the nasolabial fold. *Plast Reconstr Surg* 1992; 89(2): 225–31.

48. Pessa JE, Zadoo VP, Adrian VK et al. Variability of the midfacial muscles: Analysis of 50 hemifacial cadaver dissections. *Plast Reconstr Surg* 1998; 102(6): 1888–93.

49. Kahn DM, Shaw RB. Overview of current thoughts on facial volume and aging. *Facial Plast Surg* 2010; 26: 350–5.

50. Pessa JE, Brown F. Independent effect of various facial mimetic muscles on the nasolabial fold. *Aesth Plast Surg* 1992; 16: 167–71.

51. Kane MAC. The effect of botulinum toxin injections on the nasolabial fold. *Plast Reconstr Surg* 2003; 112(5): 66s–72s.

52. Kane MAC. The functional anatomy of the lower face as it applies to rejuvenation via chemodenervation. *Fac Plast Surg* 2005; 21: 55–64.

53. Youn KH, Park JT, Park DS et al. Morphology of the zygomaticus minor and its relationship with the orbicularis oculi muscle. *J Craniofac Surg* 2012; 23: 546–8.

54. Shim KS, Hu KS, Kwak HH et al. An anatomical study of the insertion of the Zygomaticus major muscle in humans focused on the muscle arrangement at the corner of the mouth. *Plast Reconstr Surg* 2008; 121: 466–73.

55. Choi DY, Hur MS, Youn KH et al. Clinical anatomic considerations of the zygomaticus minor muscle based on the morphology and insertion pattern. *Dermatol Surg* 2014; 40(8): 858–63.

56. Fagien S. Botox for the treatment of dynamic and hyperkinetic facial lines and furrows: Adjunctive use in facial aesthetic surgery. *Plast Reconstr Surg* 2003; 112: 40s–52s.

57. Petchngaovila C. Midface lifting with botulinum toxin intradermal technique. *J Cosmet Derm* 2009; 8: 312–16.

58. Chang SP, Tsai HH, Chen WY et al. The wrinkles soothing effect on the middle and lower face by intradermal injection of botulinum toxin type A. *Dermatol Surg* 2008; 47: 1287–94.

59. Matarasso SL, Matarasso A. Treatment guidelines for botulinum toxin type A for the periocular region and a report on partial upper lip ptosis following injections to the lateral canthal rhytides. *Plast Reconstr Surg* 2001; 108: 208–14.

60. Polo M. Botulinum toxin type A (Botox) for the neuromuscular correction of excessive gingival display on smiling (gummy smile). *Am J Orthod Dentofacial Orthop* 2008; 133(2): 195–203.

61. Benlier E, Top H, Aygit AC. A new approach to smiling deformity: Cutting of the superior part of the orbicularis oris. *Aesthet Plast Surg* 2005; 29(5): 373–8.

62. Garber DA, Salama MA. The aesthetic smile: Diagnosis and treatment. *Periodontology 2000* 1996; 11: 18–28.

63. Silberberg N, Goldstein M, Smidt A. Excessive gingival display—etiology, diagnosis, and treatment modalities. *Quintessence Int* 2009; 40: 809–18.

64. Peck S, Peck L, Kataja M. The gingival smile line. *The Angle Orthodontist* 1992; 62: 91–100.

65. Sarver DM. The importance of incisor positioning in the esthetic smile: The smile arc. *Am J Orthod Dentofac Orthop* 2001; 120: 98–111.

66. Ezquerra F, Berrazueta MJ, Ruiz–Capillas A. New approach to the gummy smile. *Plast Reconstr Surg* 1999; 104: 1143–50.

67. Kokich V, Nappen D, Shapiro P. Gingival contour and clinical crown length: Their effects on the esthetic appearance of maxillary anterior teeth. *Am J Orthod* 1984; 86: 89–94.

68. Arnett GW, Bergman RJ. Facial key to orthodontic diagnosis and treatment planning. *Am J Orthod Dentofac Orthop* 1993; 103 (part 1): 299–312, (part 2) 395–411.

69. Schendel, SA, Eisenfeld J, Bell WH et al. The long face syndrome: Vertical maxillary excess. *Am J Orthod* 1976; 70(4): 398–408.

70. Angelillo JC, Dolan EA. The surgical correction of vertical maxillary excess (long face syndrome). *Ann Plastic Surgery* 1982; 8(1): 64–70.

71. Suber JS, Dinh TP, Prince MD, Smith PD. OnaBTX-A for the treatment of a "gummy smile." *J Aesthet Surg* 2014; 34(3): 432–7.

72. Rubin LR. The anatomy of a smile: Its importance in the treatment of facial paralysis. *Plast Reconstr Surg* 1974; 53: 384–87.

73. Rubin LR. The anatomy of the nasolabial fold: The keystone of the smiling mechanism. *Plast Reconstr Surg* 1999; 103: 687–91.

74. Mazzuco R, Hexsel D. Gummy smile and botulinum toxin: A new approach based on the gingival exposure area. *J Am Acad Dermatol* 2010; 63: 1042–51.

75. Jaspers GWC, Pijpe J, Jansma J. The use of botulinum toxin type A in cosmetic facial procedures. *Int J Oral Maxillofac Surg* 2011; 40: 127–33.

76. Hwang WS, Hur MS, Hu KS et al. Surface anatomy of the lip elevator muscles for the treatment of gummy smile using botulinum toxin. *Angle Orthod* 2009; 79: 70–7.

77. Polo M. Botulinum toxin type A in the treatment of excessive gingival display. *Am J Orthod Dentofacial Orthop* 2005; 127: 214–8.

78. Niamtu J. Botox injections for gummy smiles. *Am J Orthod Dentofac Orthop* 2008; 133: 782–3.

79. Polo M. Author's response. *American Journal of Orthodontics and Dentofacial Orthopedics* 2008; 133(6): 783–4.

80. Chun KW, Kang HJ, Han SK. Anatomy of the alar lobule in the Asian nose. *J Plast Reconstr Aesth Surg* 2008; 61: 400–7.

81. Sinno S, Chang JB, Saadeh PB, Lee MR. Anatomy and surgical treatment of the depressor septi nasi muscle: A systematic review. *Plast Reconstr Surg* 2015; 135: 838e–48e.

82. Gosain AK, Amarante MTJ, Hyde JS, Yousif NJ. A dynamic analysis of changes in the nasolabial fold using magnetic resonance imaging: Implications for facial rejuvenation and facial animation surgery. *Plast Reconstr Surg* 1996; 98: 622–36.

15 Cosmetic uses of botulinum toxin A in the lower face, neck, and upper chest
Anthony V. Benedetto

INTRODUCTION

Anatomic delineation of the lower face for our purposes encompasses the perioral region, chin, and jaw line, which is the area that includes the remainder of the superficial muscles of facial expression. One of those muscles is the sheet-like neck muscle, the platysma. Even though it originates in the mid to upper chest, most of its insertions are in the lower and mid face. The platysma functions as one of the essential mimetic muscles of the lower face, and therefore is included in this chapter.

It is advisable to remind patients prior to any treatment, that injecting onabotulinumtoxinA (OnaBTX-A) for cosmetic purposes in the lower face or anywhere else on the face or body except in the forehead, glabella and lateral canthi is done off-label and without FDA approval.

The orbicularis oris, the major peribuccal muscle, functions as a sphincter providing a combination of circular as well as levator and depressor movements to the upper and lower lips, including the corners of the mouth. The other supplementary perioral muscles consist mostly of separate individual levators of the upper lip and depressors of the lower lip. These perioral levator and depressor muscles do not always move antagonistically to each other, especially when they contract involuntarily, but often function synergistically with one another in a spontaneous manner. This is in direct contrast with the upper face where levators and depressors function in a more antagonistic fashion, and move in direct opposition to each other. The perioral muscles open and close the mouth and perform essential buccal functions in unison with the orbicularis oris, such as maintaining the sphincter control and lip competence that is necessary when the mouth is filled with solid material, liquid, or air. Additional vital functions of the orbicularis oris acting as an agonist muscle together with its ancillary levators and depressors include the ability to make sounds and articulate them into speech, or chew and swallow solids and liquids. In addition, by contracting the orbicularis oris along with its levators and depressors in a particularly subtle and idiosyncratic manner, a person can express various emotions spontaneously, either deliberately or involuntarily.

Muscle fibers of the orbicularis oris interdigitate with most, if not all, of the upper lip levators and the lower lip depressors. Although there is a certain interdependence with all the perioral muscles, the orbicularis oris also can function independently as an antagonistic muscle and deliberately oppose the actions of the labial levators and the depressors. For example, one can move the orbicularis oris and the lips intentionally to open or shut the mouth as one does when eating or drinking, and to purse or pucker the lips as one does when sucking or blowing air, liquid or solids in or out of the mouth. In addition, the lips function as the sentinels of sensation, monitoring temperature, and moisture content and consistency of the solid or liquid that is about to enter or exit the mouth.[1]

These subtle but functional differences in the way the various perioral muscles operate play a significant role in how to devise a treatment plan with OnaBTX-A. One cannot just identify a levator or depressor in the lower face and weaken it as one does in the upper face with injections of OnaBTX-A without affecting adjacent muscle fibers of differently functioning muscles and possibly producing adverse sequelae. Some of these untoward effects can include lip asymmetry; sphincter incompetence affecting mastication or deglutition; a disturbance in sound production and word pronunciation, and the inability

to accurately convey nonverbal communication and emotions in a deliberate or in a spontaneous, involuntary manner. However, as our injection techniques improve and our understanding of how the muscles in the lower one-third of the face respond to OnaBTX-A, it is becoming increasingly obvious that the lower face and neck should be treated in unison as a defined all-encompassing cosmetic unit. The approach to treating the lower one-third of the face should be similar to that of the upper one-third of the face, that is, to treat the area all-inclusively as a functional unit and not as separate, independent muscles. In the upper face, there is one large levator, the frontalis, that interdigitates with and opposes the four depressors of the brow and periorbital area. In the lower face, there is the one large depressor, the platysma that interdigitates with the levators and depressors of the lower face and perioral area. The platysma can either intentionally oppose or subtly and spontaneously supplement the movements of these lower face muscles. Therefore, because of these functional differences and complex muscle interactions in the lower face, only the very experienced physician should attempt to reduce the various rhytides of the lower face or correct anatomic variations and asymmetries of this area with injections of OnaBTX-A. Otherwise, what was intended to be remedied might be exacerbated.

PERIORAL LIP LINES AND RHYTIDES

Introduction: Problem Assessment and Patient Selection

Just as the eyes are the center of focus for the upper face, enabling an individual to express deep felt emotions and personal sentiment, the mouth also is the center of focus for the lower face, enabling one to express oneself with varying degrees of attitude and emotional spontaneity. Full and rounded lips with a smooth and distinct projected border of the vermilion, delineating it from the rest of the cutaneous lip, is the hallmark of youth with all its pristine beauty. With time and sun exposure, the lips become thin, flaccid, elongated, and wrinkled, lacking substance, contour, and projection. What once reflected a person's vitality and sensuality now reveals the passing years of trials and tribulation, leaving one appearing weary and worn, evidenced by a wrinkled face with thin lips and perioral rhytides.

Both static and dynamic wrinkling can be found around the mouth appearing as vertical lip lines perpendicular to the vermilion border. It has been shown that static perioral wrinkles are caused not only by intrinsic aging and photodamage, but also are precipitated and enhanced by the smoking of tobacco.[2] Frequent and chronic cigarette smoking also can augment perioral dynamic wrinkles, probably because of the persistent lip puckering and pursing needed to hold a cigarette in the mouth while inhaling and exhaling tobacco smoke, hence the epithet "smoker's lines" (Figure 15.1a, b). Dynamic perioral wrinkles are found in those who are genetically predisposed and frequently pout and repetitively purse their lips, whether deliberately or involuntarily. This is seen more commonly in women in the way they habitually move (i.e., pucker or purse) their lips during routine daily activities of eating, drinking, and speaking (Figure 15.2a). Activities, such as cigarette smoking, sipping liquids from a straw, whistling, and playing certain musical wind instruments, provide a supplemental cause in the formation of dynamic perioral rhytides. Repeated purse-string-like movements of the orbicularis oris exaggerate and intensify the dynamic perioral lines daily. Men usually are not in the habit of pursing or puckering their lips as women (Figures 15.1a and 15.2b). Some believe that because men also are "blessed" with facial

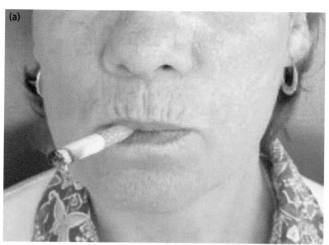
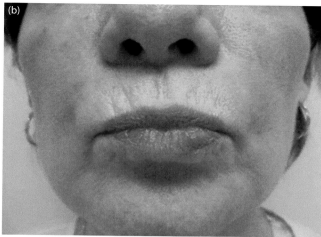

Figure 15.1 (a) Note the perioral wrinkles that are produced when this 56-year-old inhales on a cigarette. (b) Same patient puckering 1 month after treatment with OnaBTX-A. Note the absence of the intense perioral wrinkles in this smoker, and the fullness and eversion of the upper and lower vermilion (*pars marginalis*) after treatment.

and perioral beard hair, they unlike women, are spared from the fine infolding and wrinkling of facial and labial skin. However, Paes et al. performed a comparative study of the lips of fresh cadavers of both men and women. They meticulously performed full thickness anatomical dissections of the lips and then made histologic glass slide preparations of full thickness sagittal sections of the same lips and examined them microscopically. They then compared in a blinded fashion the lips of both women and men looking for gender specific differences in perioral skin. They found that women had significantly more and deeper perioral wrinkles than men possibly because of other more important reasons than just because of the lack of a beard.[3] The histologic examination of the full-thickness specimens of the perioral skin of men displayed a considerably higher number of sebaceous and sweat glands as well as a higher ratio of blood vessels to connective tissue in the labial dermis than that of women. Amazingly, the amount of hair follicles did not significantly differ between men and women, although the average number of sebaceous glands per hair follicle was greater in men. They concluded that because women's labial skin contains a significantly smaller number of appendages than men, women might be more susceptible to the development of perioral wrinkles. Incidently, Paes et al. also found the orbicularis oris, which surrounds

the lips, is anchored 1.5 times closer to the dermis in women than in men. This could conceivabley cause a stronger inward traction and pull on the skin of women's lips as they speak, eat, drink, and express themselves, thereby creating deeper perioral wrinkles on a constant and routine basis.[3] Although men are less afflicted than women with perioral wrinkling, they are not specifically bothered by them when and if they do occur. However, women are particularly frustrated by "lipstick bleeding," especially when lipstick channels up and down these rhytides blurring the outline of the vermilion (Figure 15.3).

There are many other causes for these perioral vertical lines besides repetitive puckering of the orbicularis oris. When they are produced by chronological aging and environmental exposure, these types of wrinkles are more static in nature. Static wrinkles can result from either identifiable causes, like aging and sun exposure, or unknown causes like genetics, gender differences, intrinsic soft tissue characteristics, and anatomic idiosyncrasies like the shape of the mouth and how it moves while functioning on a daily basis. Much of the static wrinkling of the perioral area can be reduced by invasive surgical procedures such as ablative skin resurfacing, (e.g., fractionated or nonfractionated laser resurfacing, mechanical dermabrasion, or chemical peeling) and possibly by other different types

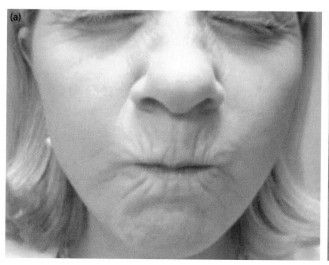
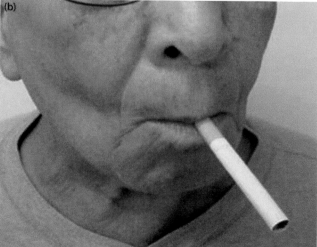

Figure 15.2 (a) Note the perioral wrinkles in this 57-year-old woman expressing her displeasure and exasperation by pursing her lips. She refused perioral OnaBTX-A treatments because she sang in a professional choir. (b) Note the lack of perioral wrinkles produced when this 77-year-old inhales on a cigarette.

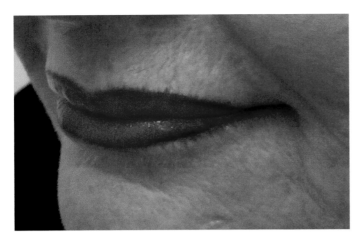

Figure 15.3 Blunting of the vermilion border in this 74-year-old is offset by lipstick. Note lines of lipstick tracking up and down the perioral rhytides.

of interventional surgical procedures, like rhytidectomy, subcision, excisions, implants and injections of synthetic soft tissue fillers or autologous fat.

It is extremely important to distinguish the dynamic wrinkles of the lips from those that are static. Static wrinkles usually are not substantially affected by injections of BoNTs. Static wrinkles can be easily distinguished from dynamic wrinkles by asking a person to purse their lips. If there are rhytides present in the lips prior to pursing them and there is minimal change or intensification of these wrinkles with movement, then their perioral rhytides are primarily static and generally not reducible by OnaBTX-A (Figure 15.4). Static wrinkles are more commonly found in someone over the age of 60–65 years or in a younger person who has acquired extensive solar elastosis of their exposed skin. If, on the other hand, the wrinkles accentuate and deepen with lip movement and puckering no matter how young or old a person is, then these are dynamic wrinkles and can be diminished with injections of OnaBTX-A (Figures 15.5a–d and 15.6a–d).

Functional Anatomy of Perioral Lip Lines and Rhytides (see Appendix 1)
The upper lip extends from the base of the nose to as far lateral as the nasolabial folds down to the free edge of the vermilion. The lower lip extends from the free edge of the vermilion down to the labiomental

sulcus. The shape of the mouth and the position of the lips are controlled by a complex three-dimensional arrangement of interlacing and decussating bundles of different mimetic muscles.[1] In the upper lip these include various levators, retractors, and evertors (i.e., levator labii superioris alaeque nasi, levator labii superioris, zygomaticus major and zygomaticus minor, levator anguli oris, and risorius). In the lower lip they include various depressors, retractors, and evertors (i.e., depressor labii inferioris, depressor anguli oris, mentalis, and platysma). Both the upper and the lower lips are interlaced with muscle fibers of the multilamellar, compound sphincter, the orbicularis oris, and those of the accessory muscle of mastication, the buccinator.[4]

The function of the orbicularis oris is to close the mouth by approximating the lips if and when they are opened by the buccal levators and depressors. By contracting the deep fibers and the superficial oblique ones, the orbicularis oris can apply the lips closely to the alveolar arches. The superficial interdigitating muscle fibers of the orbicularis oris, on the other hand, shape the lips in different configurations and either bring the lips together against the teeth or protrude the lips and the corners of the mouth forward to produce the maneuvers of pursing or puckering the lips for certain functions such as whistling or kissing. Because of its mouth-closing function, the orbicularis oris can be considered, in part, an antagonist to the lip levators and depressors.

The orbicularis oris was once assumed to be a series of complete ellipses of striated muscle that acted in unison as a sphincter around the oral cavity. However, the orbicularis oris is not just a simple sphincter like the orbicularis oculi. Instead the orbicularis oris is comprised of multiple lamellae of deep and superficial muscle fibers traversing in different directions around the orifice of the mouth that originate and emanate from the modiolus just lateral to the oral commissures.[1,5] The orbicularis oris is now understood to consist of four independent quadrants (right, left, upper, and lower) of striated muscle, each quadrant containing a larger *pars peripheralis* and a smaller *pars marginalis* (i.e., eight segments in total). These four right and four left anatomic parts (upper and lower right and left partes peripherals and upper and lower right and left partes marginales) are juxtaposed to each other, respectively, and roughly correspond to the exterior anatomic delineations of the free or unattached portion of the lips (Figure 15.7a). The smaller, but thicker *pars marginalis* corresponds to the vermilion of the lip and the larger, but thinner *pars peripheralis* corresponds to the remainder of the free unattached portion of the cutaneous lip. Consequently, the orbicularis oris is perceived as being composed of eight segments, each resembling a

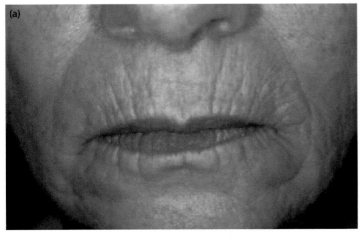
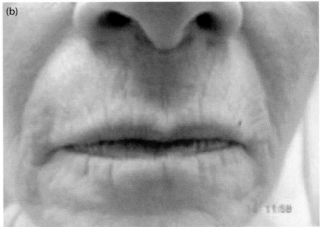

Figure 15.4 (a) A 72-year-old patient with deep perioral rhytides and moderate solar elastosis of the face and lips at rest. Her perioral rhytides barely intensified with puckering. (b) Note the persistence of the perioral rhytides 1 month after a treatment of OnaBTX-A injections, because the bulk of her wrinkles were age-related and static in nature. Note also the eversion and fullness of the upper lip at rest after treatment.

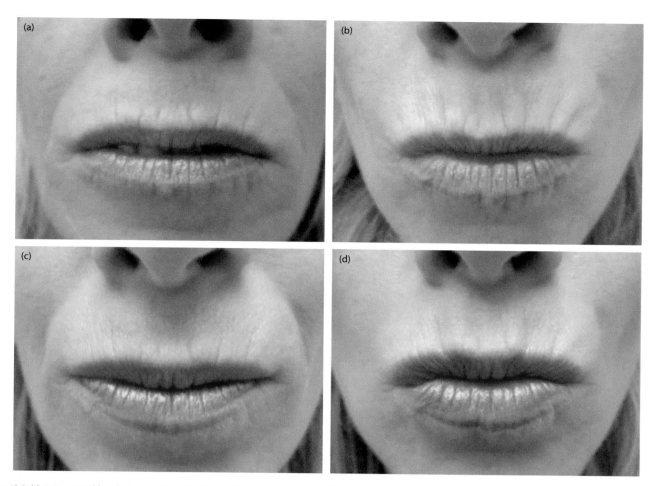

Figure 15.5 (a) A 53-year-old with deep perioral rhytides and severe solar elastosis of the face and lips is shown at rest and (b) with puckering before a treatment with OnaBTX-A. Note the rhytides intensify with puckering. (c) Same patient at rest and (d) puckering 3 weeks after her first treatment with OnaBTX-A. Note the rhytides at this early post-treatment time have only partially effaced. Note also the fullness and eversion of the vermilion after OnaBTX-A.

fan, whose apex begins at the modiolus, consisting of superficial and deep slips of muscle, one set on top of the other in different planes (Figure 15.7c).

The upper and lower lip muscle fibers of the *pars marginalis* are arcuate in form extending from the two corners of the mouth and blending with each other as they encircle the oral cavity parallel to the shape of the vermilion of the lip (Figure 15.7c). *Pars marginalis* forms a continuous band of muscle fibers across the lip, curling upward at the anterior aspect of the muscle, in the shape of a hook, forming the white roll seen along the interface between the *pars marginalis* and the *pars peripheralis*[6,7] (Figure 15.8c,d). This interface of the two muscle segments, also known as the vermilion border, is the only place where the *pars marginalis* and *pars peripheralis* meet and attach to the undersurface of the dermis. Since the muscle fibers of the *pars marginalis* of the orbicularis oris are thicker and bulkier, and occupy a more anterior frontal location of the lips than the *pars peripheralis*, they are responsible for the curled outward and upward curved "hook"-like projection and shape of the lip vermilion. This overall outline of a hook or curl of the lip has also been described by different authors as a "J" or hockey stick shape on sagittal sectioning of the lips, which becomes more pronounced as one contracts the lips when closing the mouth[8] (Figure 15.8b). In some individulas depending on their race and ethnicity this marginal "hook" is more marked in rounded and fuller lips, and less well defined in flatter, thin lips. It is also greater in length in the lower lip than in the upper lip[8] (Figure 15.8b). The *pars marginalis* of the orbicularis oris

functions more like a sphincter, opening and closing the mouth and lips.[5] The *pars peripheralis* has more of a dilatory function, widening and stretching the mouth and protruding the lips as one frequently must do at the dentist.[1,5] As the muscle fibers of the orbicularis oris enter their respective superior and inferior labial tissue, they aggregate into cylindrical bundles of muscle fascicles oriented parallel to the vermilion. The muscle fibers of the direct labial retractors procede to their areas of submucosal attachment in the *pars peripheralis* and *pars marginalis* by passing in between and beneath these cylindrical bundles of orbicularis oris.[4]

In the upper lip *pars peripheralis*, muscle fibers of the orbicularis oris insert into the incisive fossa of the maxilla, the nasolabial sulcus, the nasal ala, nasal spine, and caudal septum. In the lower lip *pars peripheralis*, fibers of the orbicularis oris insert onto the mandible at the mentolabial sulcus. Minor fascicles of the orbicularis oris also terminate in the connective tissue of the lips, into the dermis and submucosa as they traverse through all the quadrants of the free lips.[4]

In the upper lip, most muscle fibers of the orbicularis oris continue toward the midline, crossing over it at least 5 mm into the opposite side of the lip (Figure 15.7c). Consequently, these interlacing and crisscrossing muscle fibers just lateral to the midline in the center of the upper lip play a significant role in forming the lateral ridges of the philtrum as they insert into the dermis. The central depression or concavity called the philtrum is flanked on either side by these philtral ridges or escarpments, also called philtral columns. They begin at the base of the nose and continue down the upper lip and end at

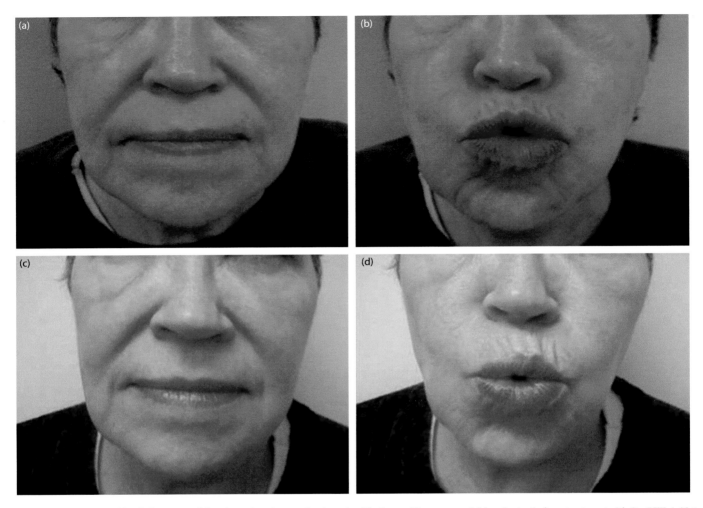

Figure 15.6 (a) A 66-year-old with deep perioral rhytides and moderate solar elastosis of the face and lips at rest and (b) puckering before a treatment with OnaBTX-A. Note that rhytides intensify with puckering. (c) Same patient at rest and (d) puckering 2 weeks after a treatment with OnaBTX-A. Note the fullness of the vermilion at rest and with puckering, and the reduction of rhytides with puckering.

the highest peaks of the vermilion border. The philtral depression, on the other hand, continues more inferiorly into the depth of the "V" shaped indentation in the center of the upper lip. The overall outline of the vermilion in the center of the upper lip is likened to *Cupid's bow*. The philtral depression is attributed to a sparseness of soft tissue and a lack of dermal insertions of decussating muscle fibers. It functions as a reservoir of extra distensible skin, facilitating a person's ability to open the mouth as wide as possible. The overall pattern of the philtrum can vary, depending on the overall size and shape of the face[6,9–11] (Figures 15.7c and 15.8e, f). Similarly, in the lower lip these crisscrossing muscle fibers interlace with their contralateral slips of muscle just a few millimeters beyond the midline and then attach to the dermis within and below the vermilion zone. This helps form the mental crease, an inverted "U" shaped depression, also known as the mentolabial sulcus.[4] This external lower border of the lower lip also corresponds to the inferior margin of the gingivolabial sulcus inside the mouth.[1] Similar muscle crisscrossing and overlap beyond the midline of the lip vermilion also occurs in the *pars marginalis*. It is the dense capillary network within the *pars marginalis* that gives it its vermilion color. The *pars marginalis* of the orbicularis oris is unique to humans and only found in the lips of hominids. Lips are crucial in the production of sound and necessary for the enunciation of speech.[12]

Direct labial retractors are those levators and depressors that enter directly into the tissue of the lips without passing through and

interlacing with the muscles of the modiolus (Figure 15.7b). For the most part, when these muscles contract, they exert a vertical pull at right angles on the buccal aperture. That is, they either elevate or evert in part or entirely the upper lip and they depress or evert in part or entirely the lower lip (Figure 15.8a). The position of the direct upper lip retractors is from medial to lateral: the lateral labial portion of the levator labii superioris alaeque nasi, levator labii superioris, and zygomaticus minor. In the lower lip, they are the depressor labii inferioris and platysma, pars labialis (Figure 15.8a). The pars labialis of the platysma is located in the same plane as the depressor anguli oris and depressor labii inferioris, and interdigitates its fibers with theirs, occupying any vacant space between them (Figure 15.9). In both the upper and lower lips, the direct labial retractors interlace their fibers into a continuous sheet of muscle superficial and deep to the intrinsic fibers of the *pars peripheralis* and *pars marginalis* of the orbicularis oris as they travel through the substance of the free lip and sequentially attach to the undersurface of the dermis and mucous membrane. The orbicularis oris interdigitates superficially and deeply with all the direct retractors as well as with the modiolar muscles of both the upper and lower lips. Movements of the direct retractors can be modified deliberately or spontaneously by the superseding activity of the modiolar muscles and the orbicularis oris to produce the fine and delicate labial movements required to whistle, enunciate different sounds, express certain emotions, and communicate nonverbally.[4]

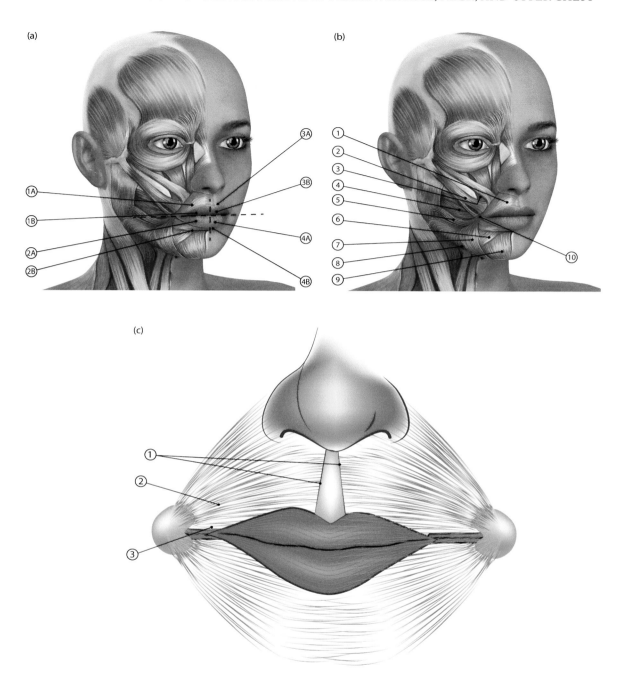

Figure 15.7 (a) The four quadrants (marked by dashed lines) and eight segments (black dots) of the orbicularis oris: 1A, *pars peripheralis* superioris; 1B, *pars marginalis* superioris; 2A, *pars marginalis* inferioris; 2B, *pars peripheralis* inferioris; 3A, *pars peripheralis* superioris; 3B, *pars marginalis* superioris; 4A, *pars marginalis* inferioris, 4B, *pars peripheralis* inferioris. (b) The modiolus is a small kidney-shaped nodule approximately 2 cm just lateral to the oral commissures (cheilion) where the orbicularis oris and indirect labial retractors converge and decussate with each other and then diverge, forming a dense, compact, but mobile, fibromuscular and tendinous mass of connective tissue. 1, orbicularis oris; 2, zygomaticus major; 3, levator anguli oris; 4, buccinator; 5, risorius; 6, depressor labii inferioris; 7, depressor anguli oris; 8, platysma (pars mandibularis); 9, mentalis; 10, modiolus. (c) In the upper lip, most muscle fibers of the orbicularis oris continue toward the midline, crossing over it at least 5 mm into the opposite side of the lip. 1, philtral columns; 2, orbicularis oris, *pars peripheralis*; 3, orbicularis oris, *pars marginalis* and vermilion.

The modiolus (Latin for *hub*) is a small button-shaped nodule approximately 2 cm just lateral to the oral commissures (cheilion) where the orbicularis oris and indirect labial retractors converge toward this centralized anatomic location. Their muscle fibers decussate with each other and then diverge from it, while forming a dense, compact, but mobile, fibromuscular and tendinous mass of connective tissue[13] (Figure 15.7). A well-developed modiolus can be palpated and often appears as a dimple when contracted.[14] It renders the lower face tonic, functioning as the main aesthetic landmark and natural aesthetic unit of the inferior third of the face.[15] The modiolus also is intimately connected with the nasolabial fold because the orbicularis oris and some of the levator muscles of the upper lip pass through the modiolus to participate in the formation of the nasolabial fold directly or indirectly.[16] A long convex nasolabial fold appears in individuals with a weak trophic modiolus, whereas a short concave nasolabial fold appears in persons with a large trophic modiolus.[13] In addition, the superficial fascia (superficial musculoaponeurotic system or SMAS) of the face at times can continue medial to the

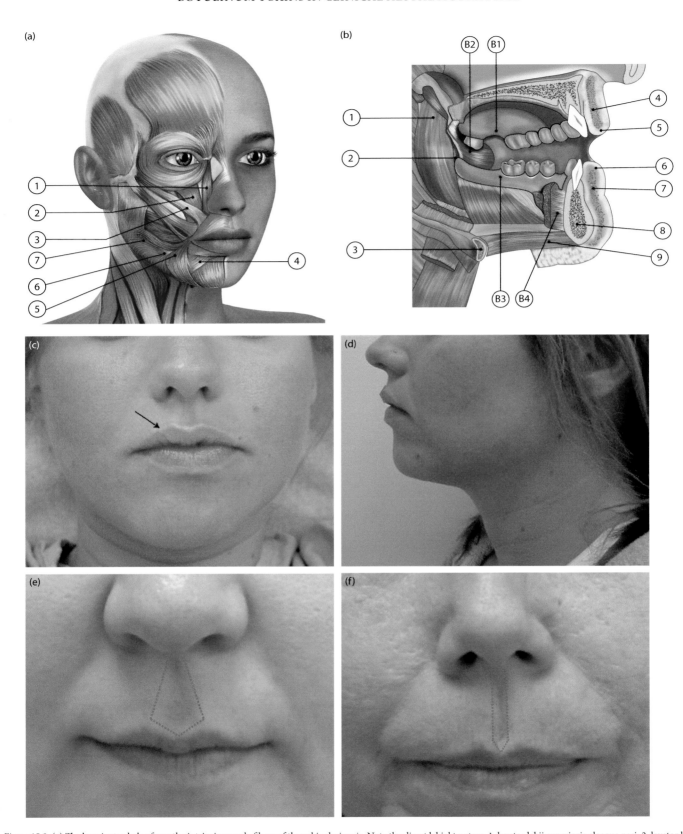

Figure 15.8 (a) The buccinator helps form the intrinsic muscle fibers of the orbicularis oris. Note the direct labial tractors: 1, levator labii superioris alaeque nasi; 2, levator labii superioris; 3, zygomaticus minor; 4, depressor labii inferioris; 5, depressor anguli oris; 6, platysma pars mandibularis; 7, platysma pars modiolaris. (b) The muscle fibers of the *pars marginalis* of the orbicularis oris are thicker and are responsible for the curved, curled, and upward "hook" like shape of the lip vermilion. 1, medial pterygoid; 2, pterygo-mandibular raphe; 3, hyoid bone; 4, orbicularis oris; 5, hook of upper lip; 6, lower lip protrusion; 7, orbicularis oris; 8, mandible; 9, mylohyoid; B1, buccinator band originating from the maxilla; B2, buccinator band extending from the pterygomandibular raphe; B3, B4, buccinator bands extending from the mandible. The white roll (arrow) can be seen along the interface between the *pars marginalis* and the *pars peripheralis* in (c) front and (d) side views of this 32-year-old patient. The anterior muscle fibers of the pars magi-nalis curl upward in the outline of a "hook," forming the white roll (arrow). It is the only area on the lips where the *pars marginalis* and *pars peripheralis* meet and attach to the undersurface of the dermis and identified as the vermilion border. (e) Divergent and (f) parallel shaped upper lip columellas, seen in 60% and 40% of the population respectively.

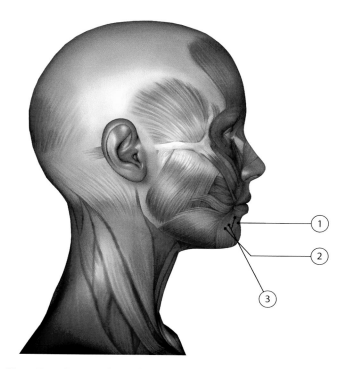

Figure 15.9 1, Depressor labii inferioris; 2, depressor anguli oris; 3, platysma, *pars labialis* occupying any vacant space between muscles 1 and 2.

nasolabial fold and also converges at the modiolus.[15,17] The facial artery courses along the lateral side of the modiolus to terminate into the angular artery after the superior labial artery branches off from it, while supplying the blood to the modiolus and the perioral region. This artery conveniently delineates the anterior limit of the buccal fat pad located at the lateral edge of modiolus which are both anatomically in the same plane. Conversely, the buccal fat pad is posterior to the facial vein and separated from the vein by the facial-vein canal. The fat present there is the fat within the buccal space. A large trophic modiolus with a large quantity of converging muscular fibers consequently can maintain the buccal fat pad in its original position and prevent it from descending and protruding with age.[13,15] Likewise, a well-controlled modiolus plays an important role of integrating the activities of the lips, the oral fissure and vestibule, cheeks, and jaws by the muscles that comprise it. There can be up to nine muscles which interlace and decussate within the modiolus, including: the zygomaticus major, platysma pars modiolaris, levator anguli oris, mentalis (sometimes), depressor labii inferioris (rarely), depressor anguli oris, risorius, and the main functional sphincteric effectors, the orbicularis oris and buccinator.[17] The muscles lie in different planes, their modiolar stems often form spirals, and most of them divide into two, three, or four bundles, each of them interlacing and attaching in diversely distinctive ways. Because of the high degree of three-dimensional functional complexity and individual patient anatomical and racial diversity, verification of modiolar functional anatomy and its location as a fixed, specific anatomical focal point cannot always be confirmed. In general, the modiolus has the overall configuration of a blunt kidney-shaped cone (Figure 15.7). Its base (basis moduli) is adjacent and adherent to the buccal mucosa. In Caucasians and Africans, it is generally located approximately 2 cm lateral to the center of the oral commissure and measures about 2 cm above and below an imaginary horizontal line that passes through the center of the oral commissure (cheilion). From mucosa to dermis, its vertical thickness is approximately 1 cm. In Asians, the modiolus is found less than 1.5 cm lateral and approximately 1.0 cm below the

horizontal line bisecting the cheilion.[18] The cone-shaped modiolus is extended by two rounded edges or cornua, which gives it its kidney shape and which extends into the lateral tissue of the free lip margin, above and below the angle of the mouth (Figure 15.7).

A set of suitably trophic modioli are required for the common three-dimensional mimetic muscular movements performed either bilaterally and symmetrically or unilaterally and asymmetrically. It is the modiolus that enables one to integrate common routine movements of the cheeks, lips, jaws, oral aperture, and vestibule. The modioli are responsible for monitoring changes in oral vestibular contents and controlling the pressure within the oral cavity. The modioli facilitate the innumerable precise variations in fine motor movements involved in speech and word formation, as well as the generation of abrasive harsh sounds and the modulation of harmonious musical tones and delicate soft whispers. They also bolster various deliberate activities such as biting, screaming, shouting, crying, chewing, drinking, spitting, sucking, swallowing, and whistling. All the permutations of facial expression, ranging from mere hints of satisfaction, elation, or purposeful determination to exaggerated distortions of sadness, pain, and discontent, be they symmetrical or asymmetrical, are enabled by the intricately synergistic and precise displacements of the modiolus.[17] These complicated modiolar movements are partly made possible because of the three muscular levels or strata of modiolar muscle insertions: the buccinator, levator anguli oris, and zygomaticus major.

Many of the movements of the modiolus seem to involve most, if not all, of its associated nine muscles (see above), whose actions are predicated on the amount of separation between the upper and lower teeth (i.e., the gape of the mouth). As the interlabial and interdental distances approach their maximum separation of about 4 cm, the modiolus occupies the interdental space, moves anteriorly 1 cm closer to the oral commissure, and becomes immobile. With the mouth wide open, the nasolabial sulci elongate, becoming straighter and more vertical, and the inferior labiomandibular sulci (marionette lines) are less deep and curved. With the lips in contact with each other and the teeth in tight approximation, the modiolus can move only a few millimeters in all directions. The mobility of the modiolus is maximized when the upper and lower teeth are separated by 2–3 mm, similar to its position when speaking. The muscular modiolar activities are enhanced by the partial separation of the jaws, integrating buccal functional movements with the direct labial retractors (levators of the upper lip and depressors of the lower lip) (Figure 15.8b). All of the delicate but intricate movements of the lips and mouth can be either intentionally or involuntarily set into motion from moment to moment by subtle and expeditious contractions of the diversely complex mimetic muscles of the perioral area.

A considerable number of the modiolar stem fibers are directly reinforced by different muscle fibers originating from the buccinator, an accessory muscle of mastication, which also reinforces the stratified complex of deeper intrinsic muscle fibers of the orbicularis oris. The buccinator in reality is not a typical mimetic muscle of the face. It is a deep, thin, quadrilateral muscle that spans the void between the maxilla and mandible and forms the deep muscular boundaries of the cheek (Figure 15.8b). Its posterior origins are from the outer surfaces of the alveolar processes of both the maxilla and mandible at the junction of the mandibular body and ramus, just posteromedial to the last molar and at the pterygomandibular raphe and ligament (Figure 15.10). This raphe stretches from the medial pterygoid process to the inner surface of the mandible, and represents the line of juncture between the buccinator and the superior constrictor of the pharynx (Figures 15.8b and 15.10). The buccinator is composed of four fibrous bands of muscle: a superior band originating from the maxilla, a central band extending from the pterygomandibular raphe, and two inferior bands of muscles extending from the mandible. The superior

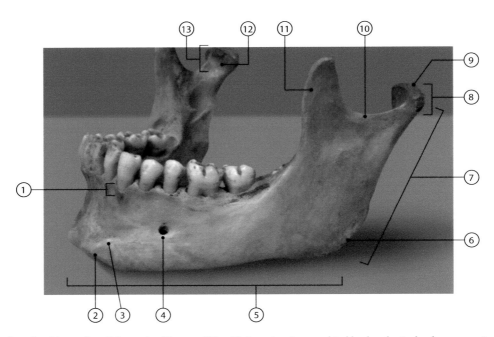

Figure 15.10 The anterior lateral and internal medial aspects of the mandible with its various topographical landmarks: 1, alveolar process; 2, mental protruberance; 3, mental tubercle; 4, mental foramen; 5, body; 6, angle; 7, ramus; 8, mandibular condyle; 9, head; 10, mandibular notch; 11, coronoid process; 12, neck; 13, mandibular condyle. (Adapted from Brennan PA, Mahadevan V, Evans BT, *Clinical Head and Neck Anatomy for Surgeons*, CRC Press: Boca Raton, FL, 2016, with permission.)

muscle band spreads anteriorly from behind the third maxillary molar to occupy the submucosa of the cheek and lips, as well as to converge into the modiolus. Also at the modiolus the central pterygomandibular fibers of the buccinator intersect and decussate with the orbicularis oris. The two inferior mandibular bands of the buccinator fibers from below cross to the upper part of the orbicularis oris, and those from above cross to the lower part of the orbicularis oris, crisscrossing each other as they continue on to their insertions in the upper and lower lips. However, the highest (maxillary) and lowest (mandibular) fibers of the buccinator continue forward to enter their corresponding upper and lower lips in a purse string fashion without decussating with the orbicularis oris (Figure 15.8b). As the buccinator courses through the cheek and modiolus, substantial numbers of its fibers are diverted internally to attach to the buccal submucosa.[4]

The buccinator's function is to keep the cheek against the gums and teeth during mastication. It also keeps food in between the teeth and prevents it from becoming lodged in the sulcus between the teeth and cheek. It also assists the tongue in directing and maintaining food between the teeth while chewing. As the mouth closes, the teeth glide over the buccolabial mucosa, which must be continuously and progressively retracted away from the occlusal surfaces of the teeth, otherwise a person would constantly inadvertently bite down on the inner surface of the buccal mucosa.

Contraction of the buccinator also prevents the cheeks from becoming overly distended by positive pressure when air, liquid, or solids fill the oral cavity. The buccinator assists in gradually expelling from in between the lips accumulated liquid, solids, or air within the oral cavity, as when spitting, blowing up a balloon, or playing a musical wind instrument (buccinator is Latin for trumpet player)[4] (Figure 15.8b).

Superficial to those deep intrinsic muscle fibers of the buccinator and orbicularis oris is another stratum of muscle fibers formed on either side of the mouth by the levator anguli oris and the depressor anguli oris. The fibers of both the levator and depressor crisscross each other at the corners of the mouth and continue away from each other. The muscle fibers of the levator anguli oris continue inferiorly into the lower lip and insert into the skin near the midline of the lower lip. The muscle fibers of the depressor anguli oris follow the same pattern into

the upper lip, inserting into the skin at the midline. Reinforcing these superficial transverse fibers of the upper and lower lips are interdigitating oblique muscle fibers from the levator labii superioris, the zygomaticus major, and the depressor labii inferioris. In addition, there are the intrinsic orbicularis oris muscle fibers of the lips, which run in an oblique direction and pass from the undersurface of the skin through the thickness of the lip and into the mucous membrane. Finally, there are additional slips of muscle fibers of the orbicularis oris which attach to the alveolar process of the maxilla, the nasolabial sulcus, and the nasal ala and septum superiorly and the alveolar process of the mandible inferiorly, anchoring the orbicularis oris in place as high as the nose and nasolabial folds, and as low as the mentolabial sulcus.

Dilution When Treating Perioral Lip Lines and Rhytides (see Appendix 3)

Injections of OnaBTX-A into the lips and the orbicularis oris must be done *intradermally* and with *minimal* dosing.[19] Because there may be

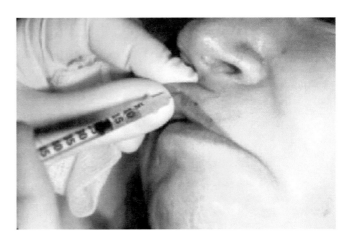

Figure 15.11 Injections of OnaBTX-A into the orbicularis oris at the junction between the upper *pars marginalis* and *pars peripheralis* in this 59-year-old patient were very painful.

a multitude of vertical lines across the lips, concentrated OnaBTX-A will not spread readily across the expansive surface of the superficial fibers of the orbicularis oris. To have the OnaBTX-A spread evenly, one can reconstitute a 100 U vial of OnaBTX-A with anywhere from 2 to 4 mL of normal saline. In this way, when injected intradermally, dilute, large volumes of OnaBTX-A can spread across the surface of the superficial fibers of the orbicularis oris even when only 1 or 2 U of OnaBTX-A are injected into each quadrant of the *pars peripheralis* of the upper and lower lips. Applying OnaBTX-A intradermally and in low doses will avoid any compromise in the sphincteric and synergistic functions of the deeper muscle fibers of both the orbicularis oris and the labial retractors and evertors.[20,21] However, there are those veteran expert injectors that are still using the same 100-unit vial of OnaBTX-A that was reconstituted with 1 mL of normal saline to treat perioral lip lines and rhytides.

Dosing: How to Correct the Problem (see Appendix 4), (What to Do and What Not to Do) When Treating Perioral Lip Lines and Rhytides

Because of the complex nature of the orbicularis oris and the way it functions, injections of OnaBTX-A in the perioral area should be performed only by an experienced physician injector. Each patient should be evaluated and treated individually and standard injection points should not necessarily be adhered to in this area or any other area of the face. OnaBTX-A should be injected into an area of maximal muscle contraction, indicated by the deepest vertical rhytides.

This is particularly important in the lips where the vertical lip lines may not be exactly symmetrical and do not always appear at the same depth or location in every patient. Perioral rhytides are dependent on the particular strength of the various superficial fibers of the orbicularis oris at that location (i.e., in that quadrant), which can vary from one patient to the next.

Place properly selected patients in the upright sitting or semireclined position and inject 1–2 U of OnaBTX-A into each *pars peripheralis* of the upper and lower lips *intradermally* and no deeper than the dermosubcutaneous junction. At this level, the superficial fibers of the orbicularis oris can be found. The appearance of fluid-filled wheals confirms the injections are performed at the proper depth. Injections can be placed into the border between the *pars peripheralis* and *pars marginalis*, which is the only location where the muscle fibers of both *partes* meet and insert into the dermis, the so-called "hockey stick" point of the vermilion border[1] (Figure 15.8b). This technique can be more painful than when OnaBTX-A is injected into the *pars peripheralis* 2 and no more than 4 mm away from the vermilion border of the upper and lower lips (Figure 15.12).

A further refinement of the injection technique is to stand behind the patient (Figure 15.13a,b). Reach around the patient's head with the nondominant hand and grasp the lip between the thumb and index finger, moderately squeezing the lip to distract the patient. The slight discomfort experienced by the patient when the lip is compressed between the fingers will help distract the patient from feeling the full impact of the pain experienced when the lips are pierced by the needle and the

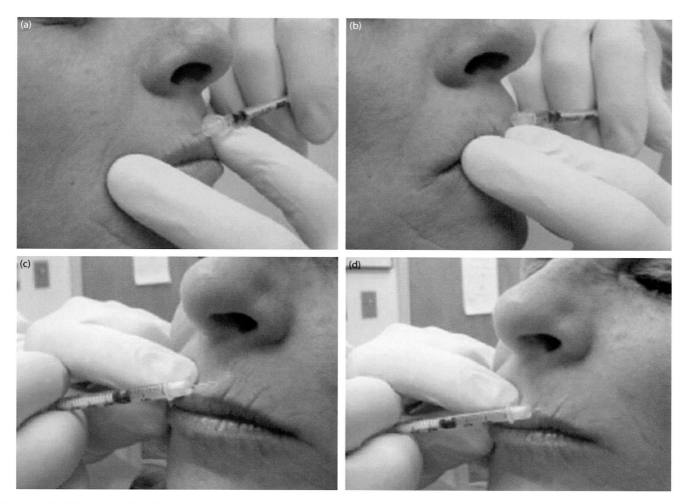

Figure 15.12 (a–d) Injections of OnaBTX-A placed 2–4 mm above the vermilion border into the center of the *pars peripheralis* of the orbicularis oris were less painful for this 53-year-old patient. (Same patient as in Figure 15.5.)

OnaBTX-A fluid is injected. Approaching the lip from behind on the opposite side of the head and from above the upper lip, pierce the skin of the cutaneous lip with a 30- or 31-gauge needle at less than a 45-degree angle, 2–4 mm above the vermilion border. Advance the needle tip downward to just underneath the lip's "white roll" of the vermilion border, that is, the "hockey stick" point. While simultaneously squeezing the lip a little harder with the thumb and index finger of the non-dominant hand, inject intradermally only 1 or 2 units of OnaBTX-A. Injections must be intradermal to affect only the superficial fibers of the orbicularis oris and to avoid deeper fibers of the upper lip retractors and inadvertent complications. The more superficial the injection, the more painful the injection, no matter what product is injected or where on the lip it is placed. Repeat this "squeeze and inject" maneuver all around the lips. However, when injecting the lower lip, return from behind the patient and stand facing the patient. Grasp the lower lip between the thumb and index finger with the nondominant hand. Approach the

patient from below the lower lip. Pierce the cutaneous lip with a 30- or 31-gauge needle at less than a 45-degree angle, 2–4 mm below the vermilion border. Advance the needle tip upward to just underneath the "white roll" border of the vermilion and cutaneous lip. Squeeze a little harder and inject 1 or 2 units of OnaBTX-A (Figure 15.13c,d). It is recommended that, at the initial treatment session, both quadrants of the *pars peripheralis* of the upper and lower lips be treated with no more than 2 U of OnaBTX-A. Inject each quadrant *intradermally* and *symmetrically* into 1–3 points per quadrant, depending on the severity of the wrinkling. The upper lip should not be injected with more than 10 U of OnaBTX-A at any given treatment session. OnaBTX-A should not be injected directly into the center of the philtrum, to avoid flattening of the philtral columns. If the lower lip does not possess the same type of deep rhytides as the upper lip, the lower lip still needs to be treated, but with only minimal amounts of OnaBTX-A, that is, no more than 2 units in each quadrant for a total of 4 U in the entire lower lip,

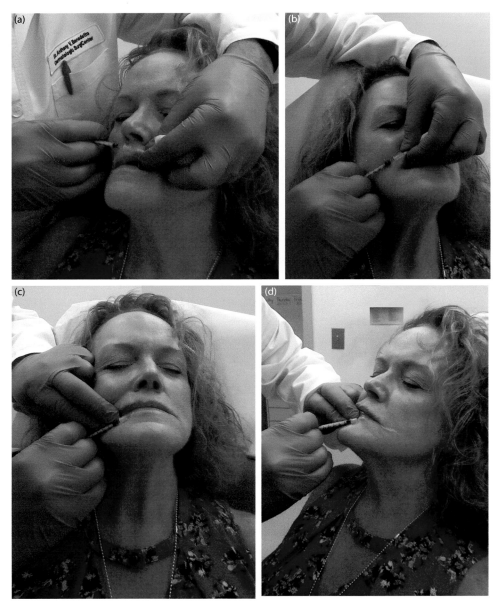

Figure 15.13 (a,b) Injection technique of the upper lip. Note the position of the fingers, compressing the lip between the index finger and thumb of the non-dominant hand. The approach is from behind the patient. The needle is inserted into the cutaneous lip 2–4 mm above the vermilion and then advanced under the vermillion raising a wheal with the injection. (c,d) Returning to the front of the patient, the injection technique is the same.

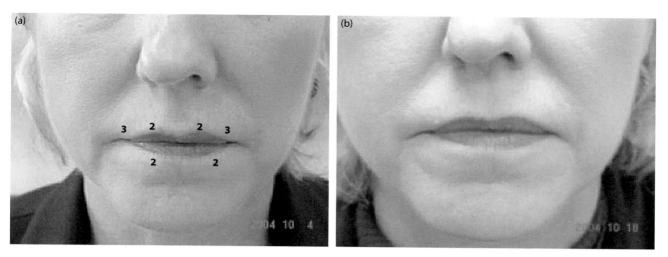

Figure 15.14 A 47-year-old patient at rest (a) before and (b) 2 weeks after her third OnaBTX-A treatment of perioral vertical rhytides. Note the subtle fullness of the vermilion and eversion of its border.

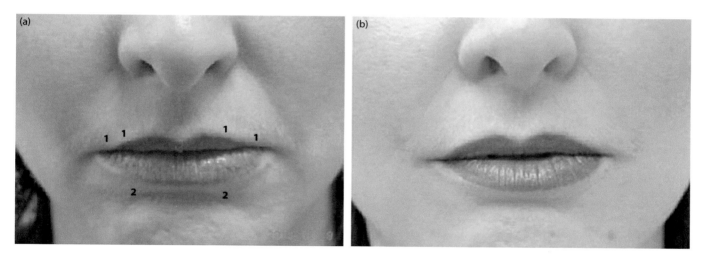

Figure 15.15 A 47-year-old patient at rest (a) before and (b) 2 weeks after her fourth OnaBTX-A treatment of perioral vertical rhytides. Note the subtle fullness of the vermilion and eversion of its border.

especially at the initial treatment session. It is advisable always to treat the lips symmetrically. By injecting the upper and lower lips in the four quadrants of the *pars peripheralis* at the same time, the orbicularis oris will weaken in a relatively proportionately symmetrical manner. This will allow the perioral muscles to adapt more easily to the subsequent changes in perioral muscle strength and proprioception, thereby maintaining the necessary and normal perioral functional competence of the overall sphincteric action of the lips.[21] The dose in each quadrant can vary depending on the number and depth of rhytides present. However, since only the superficial fibers of the orbicularis oris should be treated, then only 1–2 U of OnaBTX-A in 2 sites per quadrant, injected *intradermally*, will suffice to produce the desired effect of diminishing the perioral wrinkling while maintaining symmetrical movements and proper function of the lips.[20–22] In patients who have had treatments of OnaBTX-A repeated over many years and, therefore, are well known to the physician injector, slightly higher doses, but not more than 3 U of OnaBTX-A at each injection site on occasion, can be placed into each lip quadrant (Figures 15.14 and 15.15).

There was a report of some physicians using different patterns to inject the lips with OnaBTX-A that include as many as 10 or 11 injection sites between the upper and lower lips, usually at the points of maximal muscle contraction (Figure 15.16)[23] However, this large

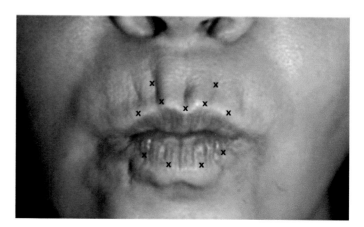

Figure 15.16 Illustrates previously suggested 11-point injection pattern to reduce vertical lip wrinkles, which should only be utilized in extreme cases of excessively deep rhytides. It usually is not advisable to inject any BoNT in the center of the upper lip, because doing so might flatten the philtral trough. (See further Reference Smychyshyn N, Sengelmann R. Botulinum toxin a treatment of perioral rhytides. *Dermatol Surg* 2003; 29: 490–5.)

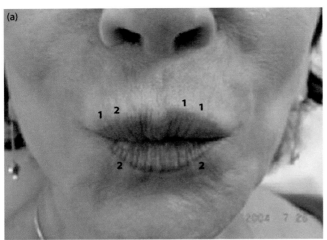
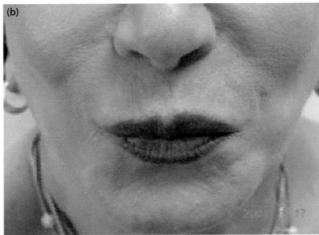

Figure 15.17 A 56-year-old shown puckering (a) before and (b) 3 weeks after a treatment of OnaBTX-A of the perioral rhytides.

amount of OnaBTX-A and these many injection points are not appropriate for most patients. In a dose ranging study where two different fixed doses (7.5 and 12 units) of OnaBTX-A were used to treat the upper and lower lips at the same time in 60 female subjects, the patients receiving the higher dose (12 units) seemed to develop adverse events more readily than those who received the lower dose (7.5 units).[24] This is the reason why it is imperative that the patient returns 2–3 weeks after a treatment session with BoNT so that the physician can evaluate the patient for any asymmetry or aberration in lip function.[21,22]

For those patients who also have their lips injected with soft tissue fillers, it has been found that injections of OnaBTX-A may prolong the effects of the fillers, since the constant muscle contraction and stress on the filler material by normal, routine lip movement is reduced by the effects of the OnaBTX-A.[21,22,25] Generally, when fillers are injected in the lips and other areas of the face during the same session OnaBTX-A treatments are given, OnaBTX-A should be injected first and before the fillers. This theoretically will allow the targeted muscles to become saturated with the OnaBTX-A first before having another product injected within the same area. If a

filler is injected first, however, some of the OnaBTX-A potentially can be injected into the filler and not into the targeted muscle, which can either dilute or disperse the OnaBTX-A and potentially diminish its effect and impact on the final outcome of either or both treatments. When other types of cosmetic procedures are performed during the same treatment session in which OnaBTX-A needs to be injected, for example, laser or other energy-based treatments or even a surgical procedure, they should all be completed before treating the patient with OnaBTX-A. The rationale for this is that most of the time during these types of procedures the patient is required to be mobile and either supine, prone, or in different recumbent positions. These particularly peculiar movements immediately following injections of OnaBTX-A potentially can be detrimental to the efficacy of the OnaBTX-A treatment, and potentially negatively affect the final results.

The total dose for OnaBTX-A injected into the upper lip should not exceed 10 U,[24] and that for the lower lip should never exceed 6 U, unless the physician knows the patient very well and has treated the patient successfully without complications in the past with high doses of OnaBTX-A (Figures 15.17 through 15.19).

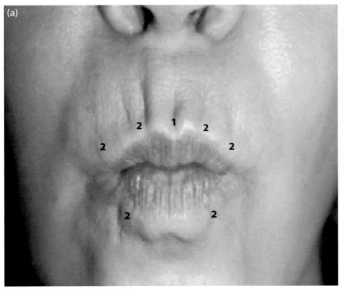
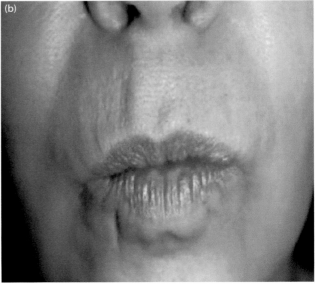

Figure 15.18 (a) A 59-year-old patient accentuating her dynamic perioral rhytides by puckering. She has had at least 4 OnaBTX-A treatments in the past. (b) Same patient puckering 5 weeks after an OnaBTX-A treatment. Note the subtle fullness of the lips and the eversion of the vermilion border.

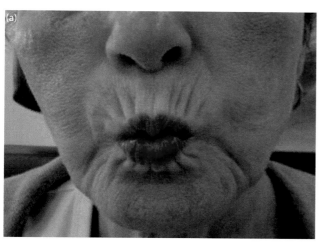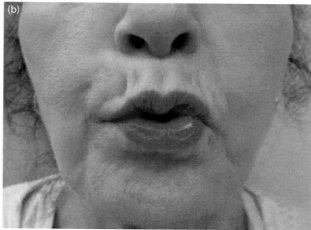

Figure 15.19 A 68-year-old patient is seen puckering (a) before and (b) 3 weeks after a treatment of OnaBTX-A. The patient experienced some difficulty puckering following the injections.

Outcomes (Results) When Treating Perioral Lip Lines and Rhytides (see Appendix 5)

Of all the areas of the face that are treated for wrinkling, the perioral area is the least predictable and responsive no matter what invasive or noninvasive modality is used, including injections of OnaBTX-A. Even so, the perioral area is high on the treatment list when patients request cosmetic rejuvenation of the face.

When OnaBTX-A injections of the lips are effective as intended, a pleasing effacement of the depth of the vertical lip lines occurs, which can dramatically improve the overall physical appearance and emotional outlook of the patient. In addition to relaxing the superficial fibers of the orbicularis oris and diminishing the wrinkles on the cutaneous surface of the lip, there also can be a slight widening of the philtrum and a noticeable eversion of the vermilion, producing an attractive "pseudo" augmentation of the lips (Figures 15.14, 15.15, and 15.18).[20,21,23,24] Many feel that this pseudoaugmentation and eversion of the lips are best produced when OnaBTX-A is injected directly into the white roll of the vermilion border (Figure 15.11). However, usually this technique can be very painful for the patient. Similar lip fullness and eversion also can be realized when OnaBTX-A is injected in a less painful way a few millimeters above and below the vermilion border in the upper and lower lips, respectively, as described above (Figure 15.12).[20]

Only dynamic perioral wrinkles can be attenuated by OnaBTX-A, not the static rhytides that result from photodamage and age (Figure 15.4). For correction of static wrinkles and solar elastosis, various soft tissue fillers, laser and energy-based treatments, and different resurfacing procedures with adjunctive treatments of OnaBTX-A when appropriate will give the best results.[21,25,26] Because only low doses should be used to efface perioral rhytides, the usual duration of effect from injections of OnaBTX-A is sometimes just a little more than 2 and generally no longer than 4 months.[24]

Complications (Adverse Sequelae) When Treating Perioral Lip Lines and Rhytides (see Appendix 6)

The perioral area is probably the most difficult location on the face to treat with injections of OnaBTX-A without frequent occurrence of adverse sequelae. This is because, unlike the sphincteric action of the orbicularis oculi, which has only one opposing levator muscle (i.e., the frontalis) and a few co-depressor muscles (i.e., the corrugator supercilii, procerus, orbicularis oculi, and depressor supercilii), the orbicularis oris is interlaced with muscle fibers from the different direct and indirect labial retractors and evertors of the upper

and lower lips, making it easy for injected OnaBTX-A to diffuse into any one or a group of adjacent interdigitating levators or depressors. Consequently, adverse sequelae or, annoying functional disturbances are bound to occur.

Using a range of higher doses ($\geq$8–10 U in the upper lip and $\geq$6–8 U in the lower lip) of OnaBTX-A will subject the patient to difficulties with lip puckering when attempting to whistle or kiss (Figure 15.19). A slightly asymmetric smile is relatively common in the general population (see sections "Gummy Smile," Chapter 14 and "Asymmetric Smile of the Lower Lip," Chapter 15). It also can be iatrogenically created or accentuated by unequal dosing and asymmetric placement of injections of OnaBTX-A in the lips. In the case of overdosing, many different adverse functional changes can occur which include but are not limited to the inability to form certain letters (e.g., M, F, B, P, V, W, O, and U), to articulate different sounds, and to pronounce certain words. Involuntary tongue, inner cheek, and lip biting and even paresthesia of the lips may result, along with flattening of the philtrum. There can be a disturbance in proprioception of the lips, which makes it difficult to apply lipstick, whistle, kiss, or brush the teeth. There also can be a concomitant inability to approximate the lips tightly enough to prevent air, fluid, or even food incontinence. Incontinence of fluid causes one to drool or actively dribble liquid out of the mouth while drinking from a glass or cup, or sipping from a straw, or eating from a spoon.[24,27–29] Incontinence of solids and food can be even more embarrassing, depending on one's social setting when it occurs. The inability to purse or pucker the lips can last beyond 2–4 weeks after a treatment of OnaBTX-A. Consequently, OnaBTX-A treatments of the lips should never be offered to certain types of people, for example, musicians and instrumentalists, or those who sing on a regular basis (e.g., in a choir at church or on stage) or professional vocalists. Other individuals who should avoid OnaBTX-A treatments of their lips are scuba divers and snorkelers; public speakers, especially television and radio announcers; and dog sitters and animal trainers who need to whistle and make subtle vocal sounds to enforce a learned response.

In the Cohen et al. dose ranging study, most of the untoward sequelae seemed to be dose-dependent, which included weakness and numbness of the lips, trouble eating and an inability to kiss, lip dryness, lip fullness, lip swelling, and decreased mobility of the lips and mouth. A few of those lip movement and functional difficulties (dryness of the lips, influenza-like syndrome, bruising of the left upper lip, and decreased mobility of the mouth) continued for more than 20 weeks beyond the termination of the study in 15%

of those patients who were treated with the higher 12-unit dose of OnaBTX-A.[27]

Therefore, one should not be tempted to inject progressively higher doses of OnaBTX-A into the lips similar to the way one can increase the dose injected in the periorbital area. Doing so will definitely lead to any number of the adverse sequelae as identified above. It is important to understand that there is only a very narrow margin for the successful treatment of the orbicularis oris with OnaBTX-A. If 2 U of OnaBTX-A per quadrant is injected into a patient's lips effectively and without untoward sequelae, then as little as an additional 1 or 2 U of OnaBTX-A in the upper or lower lip in that same individual may result in some or all of the adverse side effects previously detailed. Those most intolerable adverse effects are an asymmetric smile and lack of sphincter control, causing food and liquid incontinence, and difficulty with sound production and speech articulation. So, the temptation to inject even 1 U more in an upper or a lower lip to improve the results or extend the duration of an OnaBTX-A treatment must be overcome, unless visible ineffectiveness of a particular dose of a previous OnaBTX-A treatment already has been experienced by the patient. Then either additional units at the 2- to 3-week follow-up visit can be given, or a gradual increase in dose (by no more than 1 U of OnaBTX-A) and number of injection sites (one site at a time) can be attempted with each subsequent OnaBTX-A treatment session (Figure 15.20). When OnaBTX-A is ineffectively injected, or there is some loss of product while injecting, preventing a full complement of OnaBTX-A to reach the targeted muscle fibers, then an uneven outcome can result (Figure 15.20). Avoid injecting OnaBTX-A too close to the corners of the mouth. This can result in incompetent commissures, eclabion, an asymmetric smile, aberration in speech, drooling and dribbling, and even incontinence of solid food.

Of all the areas on the face to inject OnaBTX-A, the lips are the most painful. The more superficial (i.e., intradermal) the injection, the more painful it will be. Icing and the prolonged application of a topical anesthetic with occlusion may alleviate some of the pain that accompanies such superficial injections in the lips. Forewarning the patient of the potential side effects and the particular painfulness of the treatment does not seem to dissuade those who are determined to rid themselves of these unsightly lipstick-trailing rhytides. In contradistinction, superficial injections in the perioral area do not elicit ecchymoses with the same ease and frequency that superficial injections in the periorbital area do.

Figures 15.21 through 15.26 are additional examples of different patients treated with OnaBTX-A for perioral rhytides.

Treatment Implications When Injecting Perioral Lip Lines and Rhytides

1. Only dynamic wrinkles in the lips are reducible by OnaBTX-A treatments. A thorough and accurate assessment of the patient is the key to a successful outcome.
2. Treating hyperkinetic superficial fibers of the orbicularis oris with OnaBTX-A will relax surface rhytides, evert the vermilion, and create the appearance of fullness in the lips.
3. Inject low doses of high-volume OnaBTX-A *intradermally* in the lips, and see the patient 2–3 weeks after each treatment. It is absolutely imperative to employ a meticulous *intradermal* injection technique when injecting lips with OnaBTX-A, because the frequency, intensity, and duration of adverse sequelae is technique dependent.
4. Treat the lips with symmetrically placed injections of OnaBTX-A in all four quadrants of the *pars peripheralis*. Each individual injection site can be dosed differently with the tip of the needle advanced to just beneath the vermilion border.
5. Inject the lower lip conservatively and with a slightly lower dose of OnaBTX-A than the upper lip to avoid aberrations of normal labial function. Injecting OnaBTX-A into the base of the philtrum may flatten its contour.
6. Avoid injecting OnaBTX-A close to the corners of the mouth for risk of creating incompetent commissures, eclabion, an asymmetric smile, drooling, and even dribbling.
7. The pretreatment application of ice or a topical anaesthetic with occlusion may reduce the particular pain experienced when lips are injected.

ASYMMETRIC SMILE OF THE LOWER LIP
Introduction: Problem Assessment and Patient Selection
Many men and women are naturally born with an asymmetric smile (see Asymmetries, p. 127; Gummy smile, p. 220 and Figures 15.27 through 15.29). This also can be a manifestation of a family trait (Figure 15.30). For many who display this type of smile this is a source of considerable embarrassment, especially when they are in

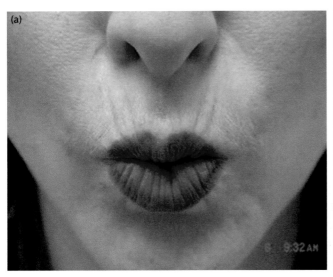
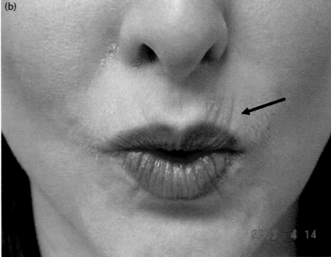

Figure 15.20 A 43-year-old patient puckering (a) before and (b) 3 weeks after her first OnaBTX-A treatment for perioral vertical rhytides. Note the persistence of wrinkles in the right upper quadrant (arrow) due to inadequate treatment on that side.

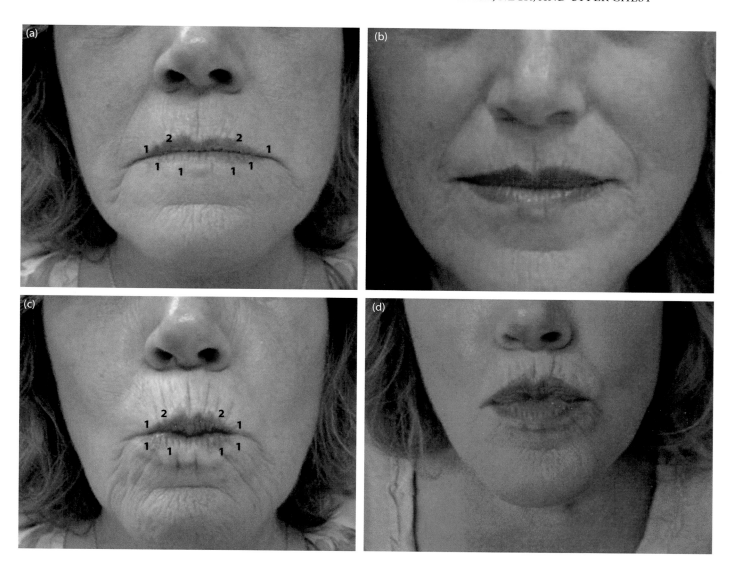

Figure 15.21 (a) A 53-year-old patient with deep perioral rhytides and severe solar elastosis of the face and lips at rest before and (b) 2 weeks after treatment with OnaBTX-A. Note the subtle fullness of the lips and the eversion of the vermilion border. (c) Same patient puckering before and (d) 2 weeks after treatment with OnaBTX-A. Many of the persistent wrinkles are of the static type, caused by photoaging. Note the subtle fullness of the lips and the eversion of the vermilion border.

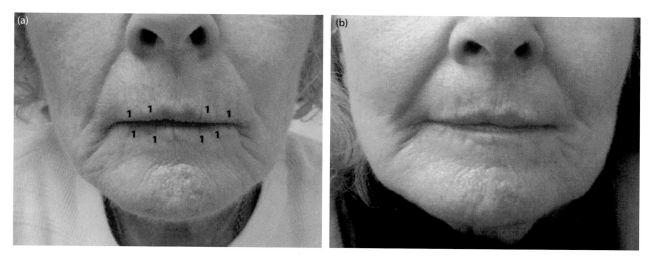

Figure 15.22 A 66-year-old patient is shown at rest with perioral rhytides (a) before and (b) 1 month after a treatment with OnaBTX-A in the upper and lower lips and a hyaluronic acid filler in the marionette lines, prementum, and prejowl areas.

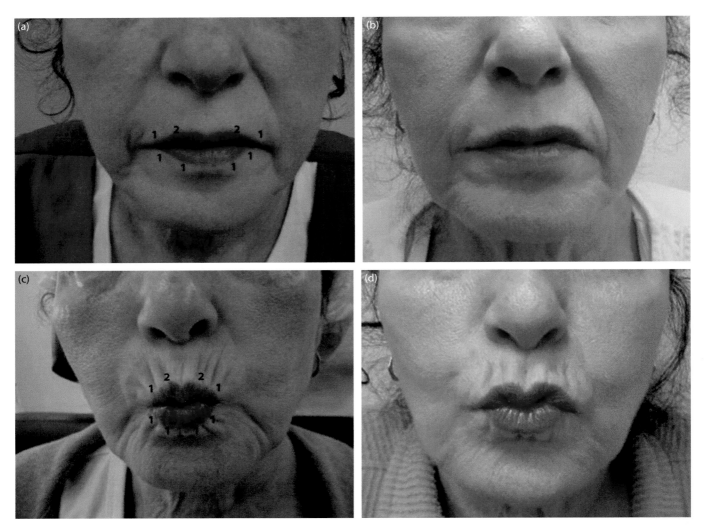

Figure 15.23 (a) A 68-year-old patient is shown at rest with perioral rhytides before and (b) 2 weeks after a treatment with OnaBTX-A. Note the subtle fullness of the lips and the eversion of the vermilion border. (c) Same patient puckering before and (d) 2 weeks after treatment with OnaBTX-A.

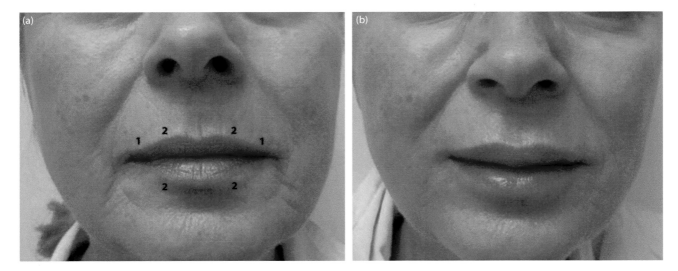

Figure 15.24 A 57-year-old patient is shown at rest with perioral rhytides (a) before and (b) 2 months after a treatment with OnaBTX-A of the upper and lower lips and a hyaluronic acid filler in the marionette lines, prementum, and prejowl areas.

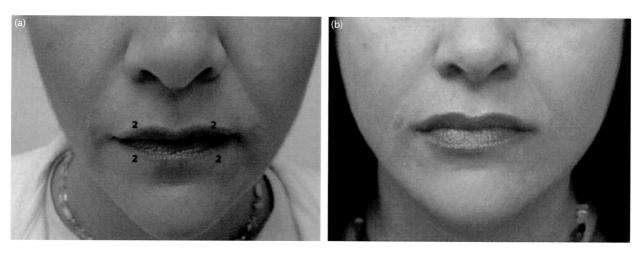

Figure 15.25 A 44-year-old patient is shown at rest with perioral rhytides (a) before and (b) 2 weeks after a treatment with OnaBTX-A. Note the subtle fullness of the lips and the eversion of the vermilion border.

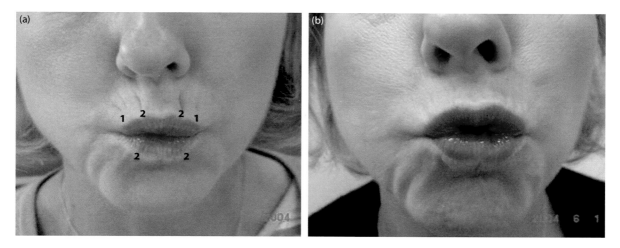

Figure 15.26 A 47-year-old patient is shown puckering with perioral rhytides (a) before and (b) 3 weeks after a treatment with OnaBTX-A. The mentalis and platysma were not treated; note the dimpling of the mentum and the perimental furrows.

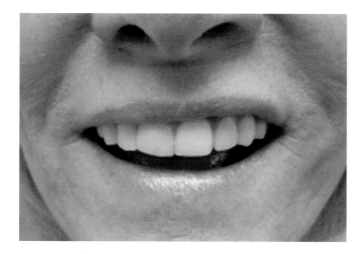

Figure 15.27 In this 55-year-old female, an asymmetric smile is caused by hyperkinetic lateral levators of the left upper *pars peripheralis* of the lips.

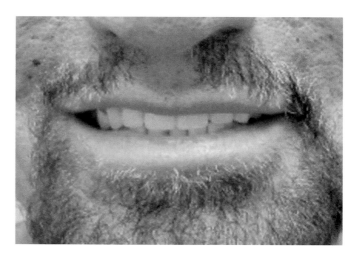

Figure 15.28 In this 62-year-old male, an asymmetric smile is caused by hyperkinetic central levators of the right upper *pars peripheralis* of the lips.

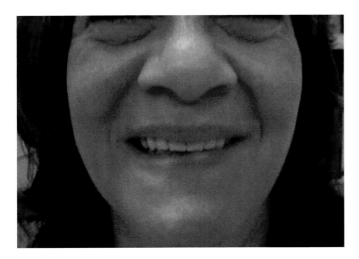

Figure 15.29 In this 61-year-old female, an asymmetric smile is caused by a hyperkinetic depressor labii inferioris in the right lower *pars peripheralis.*

a socially interactive situation. Just like those with a gummy smile (see pp. 220–230) they are reticent to freely grin in public, and seek different ways to conceal the gape of their mouths in the presence of others when laughing or smiling. Those who have a prominent position in society or in the workplace are especially self-conscious of their obviously "crooked smile." Many prefer not to smile when being photographed, and will avoid family and social events where photographs are being taken.

Functional Anatomy of a Lower Lip Asymmetric Smile (see Appendix 2)

No matter what type of smile one has (zygomatic, canine, or full denture), if it is asymmetrical or "crooked" it is always a source of anxiety and self-consciousness for the bearer, whether male or female[30–33] (see Figure 15.70 for types of smiles). Asymmetric smiles can occur because of segmentally weakened or hyperfunctioning muscles on either side of the upper or lower lips. If the asymmetry appears in the upper lip, one or more of the many upper lip levators or a segmental portion of the orbicularis oris may be involved unilaterally or bilaterally (see "Gummy Smile" earlier in this chapter). If the asymmetry appears in the lower lip, it is usually caused by a unilateral malfunctioning of a lower lip depressor that is usually weaker or stronger than its contralateral paired muscle with or without the segmental involvement of the orbicularis oris. Lower lip asymmetries are more easily corrected because unlike the intricate network of the upper lip levators, the problem commonly stems from a hyperkinetic depressor labii inferioris or occasionally a depressor anguli oris and rarely both.[33] Isolated quadrants or portions of the muscle fibers of the lower orbicularis oris theoretically also can be involved.

The depressor labii inferioris is a quadrilateral muscle that originates inferior to the mental foramen at the oblique line of the lower lateral surface of the body of the mandible between the symphysis menti and the mental foramen. As one of the direct labial retractors, its fibers travel upward and medially overlying the mental foramen to insert directly into the skin and mucosa of the lower lip, decussating with fibers of its paired muscle from the contralateral side along with some muscle fibers of the lower orbicularis oris. Inferiorly and laterally, it is continuous with the platysma (pars labialis) (Figure 15.31). At its origin, the depressor labii inferioris is approximately 3 cm wide, and superimposed laterally by muscle fibers of the depressor anguli oris for about 1–2 cm. It then narrows to approximately 2 cm wide before it inserts into the superior aspect of the lower lip.

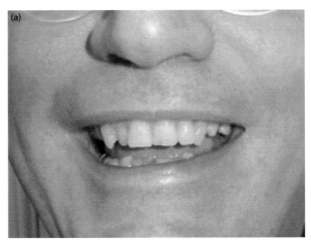

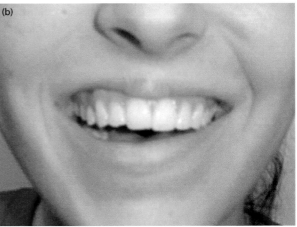

Figure 15.30 (a) A father (55 years old) and (b) his daughter (20 years old) demonstrate the same type of idiosyncratic, asymmetric smile caused by a hyperkinetic right depressor labii inferioris. The daughter also has an asymmetric smile of the right upper *pars peripheralis* with deep nasolabial grooves and folds.

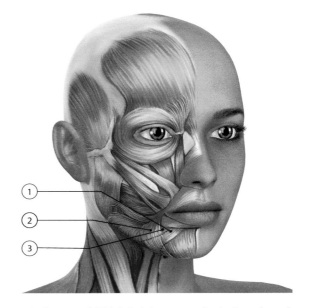

Figure 15.31 Depressor labii inferioris is a square, deeply situated muscle on the chin and it depresses the lateral aspect of the lower lip downward while gently everting the vermilion. It is one of the direct labial retractors inserting directly into the skin and mucosa while other fibers interdigitate with some of the lower fibers of the orbicularis oris and platysma (pars labialis). 1, depressor labii inferioris; 2, depressor anguli oris; 3, platysma–pars labialis passed underneath depressor anguli oris.

The function of the depressor labii inferioris is to pull the lower lip downward and laterally slightly everting the vermilion when a person is chewing, drinking, smiling, laughing, or speaking. Otherwise, one would bite or chew their lower lip while performing these functions. It should contract symmetrically and in unison with its paired counterpart on the opposite side of the chin. This is not always the case in some individuals. The depressor labii inferioris is one of the muscles used when expressing sorrow, irony, melancholy, and doubt.

Dilution When Treating a Lower Lip Asymmetric Smile (see Appendix 3)

Because of the extensive interlacing of muscle fibers in the perioral area, the success of treating a particular muscle in the lower face is predicated on not having OnaBTX-A diffuse beyond the area of injection and the targeted muscle. Consequently, minimal amounts of low-volume, highly concentrated OnaBTX-A should be used when injecting a perioral muscle. Therefore, experienced physicians will reconstitute a 100 U vial of OnaBTX-A with only 1 mL of normal saline.

Dosing: How to Correct the Problem (see Appendix 4) (What to Do and What Not to Do) When Treating a Lower Lip Asymmetric Smile

Ordinarily, a unilateral hyperkinetic muscle of the face, whether idiosyncratic or secondarily induced, can be weakened with injections of OnaBTX-A to correct an asymmetry (Figure 15.32). Depending on the type, location, and strength of the muscles creating the asymmetry, it is advisable for the physician injector to identify the offending muscle correctly and determine the dose of OnaBTX-A necessary for the correction of the asymmetry at the time of treatment. Each patient's problem should be evaluated individually and a suitable solution deduced from the presenting asymmetry of the patient's idiosyncratic anatomy. When treating muscles in the lower face, very low doses of OnaBTX-A are all that are necessary to produce a desired, long-lasting effect. Dramatic results can be obtained usually with less than 4 or 5 U of OnaBTX-A.

Prior to injection the patient should be in the sitting or semi-reclined position while forcibly contracting the muscle(s) to be treated. Commonly it is the depressor labii inferioris that is hyperkinetic and creating an asymmetric smile. As the patient smiles energetically, the location of the hyperkinetic muscle is easily visualized (Figure 15.32a,c). The needle should pass perpendicular to the skin's surface and enter directly into the thickest part of the muscle belly. This injection point should be inferior to the mental crease which are the lower limits of the orbicularis oris. Generally, 2–4 U of OnaBTX-A will weaken the hyperfunctional depressor labii inferioris sufficiently enough to realign an asymmetric smile (Figures 15.32 and 15.33).[33,34] Slow, deliberate injections will prevent pain and distant spread of OnaBTX-A, averting adverse sequelae.

Outcomes (Results) When Treating a Lower Lip Asymmetric Smile (see Appendix 4)

When the problem has been correctly assessed, and the proper *conservative* dose of OnaBTX-A determined, weakening the hyperkinetic muscle on the side of the face producing the asymmetry with injections of OnaBTX-A will correct the asymmetry (Figures 15.32 and 15.33). The effect of a single treatment can last beyond 5–6 months.[33] It is best to treat an asymmetry with a lower dose of OnaBTX-A which can be increased by a touch-up treatment 2–3 weeks later when the patient returns for his or her obligatory post-treatment evaluation. Correcting a problem conservatively, albeit possibly insufficiently, allows both the patient and the physician to assess clearly the appropriateness of the corrective action.[34] Subsequently, additional units of OnaBTX-A can then be injected with confidence to adequately treat the problem to the satisfaction

of patient and physician. In the lower face, the muscles are small, intermingled with indistinct borders, and do not always function in the same way in every patient.[35] The shape and contour of the mouth and whether it is symmetrical or asymmetrical will depend on how the perioral muscles function in a particular individual. When there is an obvious asymmetry, 1 or 2 U of OnaBTX-A can go a long way in modifying how perioral muscles contract and interact with each other.

In a study by Benedetto,[33] four females and one male were treated for lower lip asymmetry. Four were caused by a hyperkinetic right depressor labii inferioris, one by a left one. Four of the patients were aware of their asymmetry which was present since birth or early childhood. One was not aware of having an asymmetric smile. OnaBTX-A was used to correct the asymmetric smile of all the patients, with only 1–3 units. The smiles became level and symmetrical within one week of the treatments, which lasted anywhere from 6 to 7.5 months with the first treatment session and even longer with subsequent treatments, even when a lower dose was used. Such simple outpatient myorelaxation of the depressor labii inferioris when indicated for the properly selected patients has made invasive surgical resectioning of the depressor labii inferioris, a procedure of the past, unwarranted and virtually unnecessary.[34]

Complications (Adverse Sequelae) When Treating a Lower Lip Asymmetric Smile (see Appendix 6)

An erroneous assessment and fallacious conclusion to a problem in the lower face can produce incomplete and even untoward results, which can become an intolerable annoyance and even a functional problem to the patient. Therefore, a thorough knowledge of the anatomy and function of the muscles of the face in the particular area to be treated is absolutely necessary when one is attempting to treat a patient with OnaBTX-A. This is especially important when the problem is not a recognized, commonly occurring complaint with well-established and approved techniques of treatment as it is with glabellar and lateral canthal frown lines. Idiosyncratic or iatrogenic asymmetries need to be corrected on a case-by-case basis and expert understanding of functional anatomy is paramount. Overzealous treatment, especially in the lower face, of any problem can only lead to inadvertent adverse sequelae. In the case of an asymmetric smile, one or two extra units of OnaBTX-A can create the same complications of an adynamic smile and incompetent buccal sphincter, causing difficulty with eating, drinking, swallowing, and speech articulation.

Figures 15.34 through 15.36 are additional examples of different patients treated with OnaBTX-A for an asymmetric smile.

Treatment Implications when Injecting an Asymmetric Smile

1. Know the functional anatomy of the muscles to be treated.
2. Inject low-volume, minimal doses of OnaBTX-A directly into the belly of the hyperkinetic muscles in question.
3. First treatments should be conservative with low doses of OnaBTX-A to confirm the appropriateness of the treatment.
4. All first-time and subsequently treated patients must be re-evaluated 2–3 weeks after an OnaBTX-A treatment to assess their results and to monitor the patients' satisfaction with the outcome.
5. Assess and treat every patient individually. No two patients or their individual problems are alike and therefore cannot be treated in the same manner.
6. Reevaluate each patient's problem before every treatment because the dosage of subsequent injections may change depending on how the treated muscles respond and reanimate over time.
7. Treatment results are long lasting, and their duration can remain even longer with each subsequent treatment.

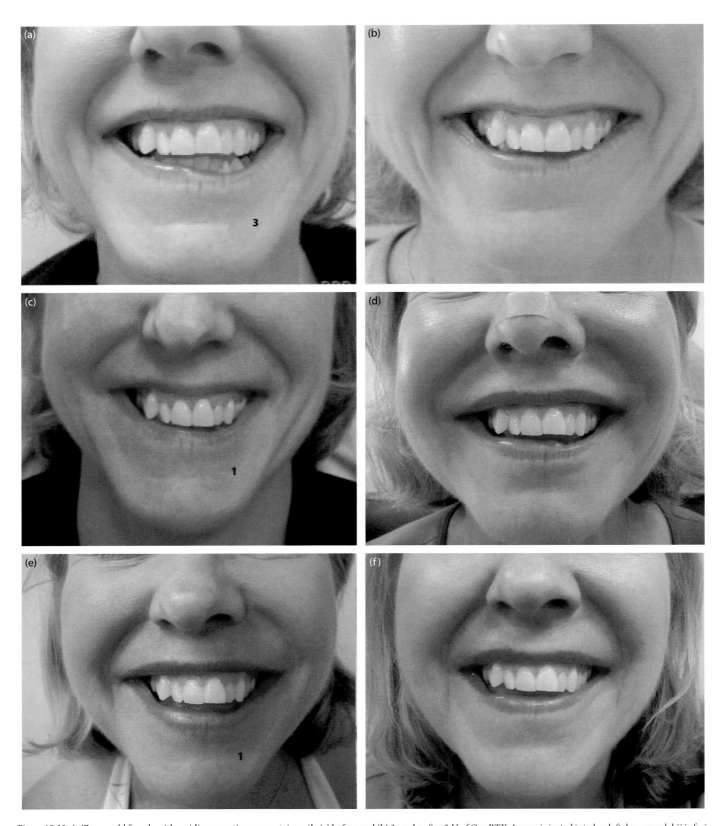

Figure 15.32 A 47-year-old female with an idiosyncratic asymmetric smile (a) before and (b) 3 weeks after 3 U of OnaBTX-A were injected into her left depressor labii inferioris. (c) Same patient seen 3 months after the first treatment of her left depressor labii inferioris. An additional 1 U of OnaBTX-A was injected at this time. (d) Same patient seen again 4 months after her second touch-up treatment. (e) Same patient seen with lasting results 8 months after her second treatment. An additional 1 U of OnaBTX-A was injected to maintain these results. (f) Patient seen again 7 months after her third treatment.

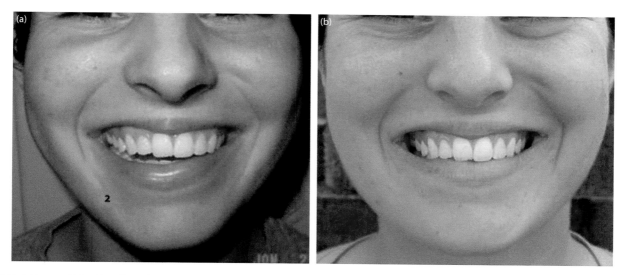

Figure 15.33 A 22-year-old female with an idiosyncratic asymmetric smile (a) before and (b) 4 months after 2 U of OnaBTX-A were injected into her right depressor labii inferioris for the second time. Note the absence of dental show of the lower teeth.

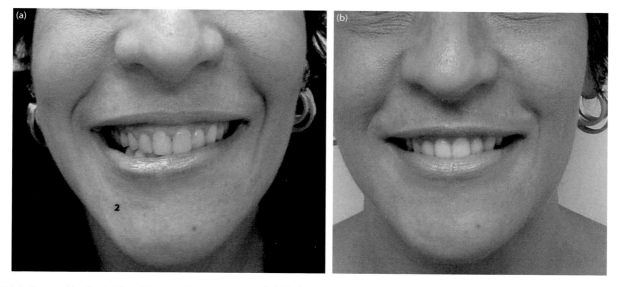

Figure 15.34 A 55-year-old patient with an idiosyncratic asymmetric smile (a) before and (b) 3 weeks after 2 U of OnaBTX-A were injected into her right depressor labii inferioris. Note the eversion of the vermilion border.

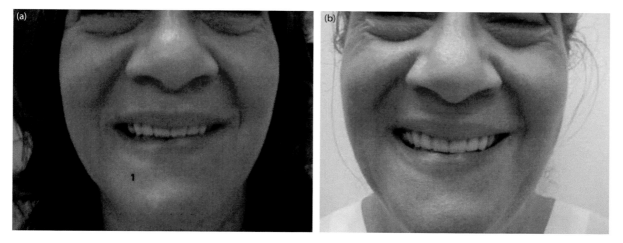

Figure 15.35 A 61-year-old patent with an idiosyncratic asymmetric smile (a) before and (b) 5 months after 1 U of OnaBTX-A was injected into her right depressor labii inferioris.

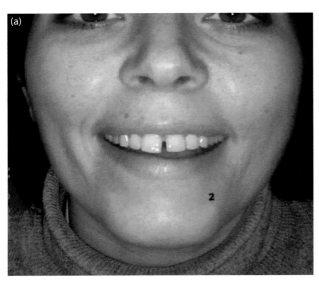
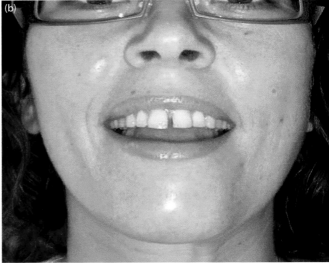

Figure 15.36 A patient with an idiosyncratic asymmetric smile (a) before and (b) 2 months after 2 U of OnaBTX-A were injected into her left depressor labii inferioris.

MELOMENTAL FOLDS

Introduction

Patients whose corners of the mouth chronically project downward commonly also will possess pronounced melomental folds. These superfluous folds of skin are created by deep furrows emanating away and downward from the oral commissures. They also are identified as a labiomandibular crease, "drool grooves," or "marionette lines." Their diverse appearance varies according to a person's individual muscular variations and the thickness of the subcutaneous fat.[36] Usually becoming more obvious in the fifth decade of life, melomental folds seem to appear more readily in smokers and when smiling or opening the mouth laterally. These telltale signs of aging involuntarily impart to others the negative expressions of sadness, tiredness, disapproval, unpleasantness, and melancholia, and even an angry demeanor, emphasizing negative impressions produced by an inverted smile.[35,36] When these "marionette lines" extend downward along the lateral sides of the mentum they reinforce the downward turn of the corners of the mouth creating an inverted smile or "Chinese moustache" and evoke the outward appearance of someone who is old and senile, no matter how young they might be chronologically (Figure 15.37). Marionette lines can be a source of frustration and embarrassment during daily social interactions, or for those who maintain a prominent position in the workplace. Until recently, the only way to efface these lines was either by invasive surgical procedures such as rhytidectomies, threading, lifting, subcision, and skin resurfacing, or injections of soft tissue fillers which can produce results that are remedial but temporary. Injections of OnaBTX-A can be given to supplement these procedures enhancing and even prolonging their results, bringing the treatments of melomental folds a little closer to a more satisfactory outcome.[37–39]

Functional Anatomy of Melomental Folds (see Appendix 2)

Formation of an inverted smile because of the downward projection of the corners of the mouth is produced by the hyperkinetic activity of the depressor anguli oris pulling down on the oral commissures (Figure 15.38).[40–42] The depressor anguli oris is a variably sized triangular muscle (also known as the triangularis) whose wide base originates on bone at the mental tubercle and along the external oblique

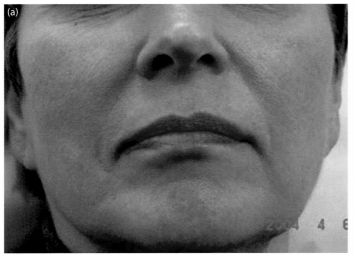
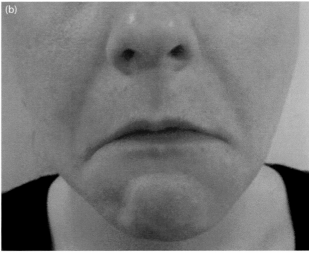

Figure 15.37 (a) This 52-year-old female at rest has marionette lines that extend down the lateral sides of the mentum creating an inverted smile because of a hyperkinetic depressor anguli oris. (b) This 37-year-old female grimacing displays a deep, inverted smile, also because of a hyperkinetic depressor anguli oris. Note the asymmetry in the depth and length of the marionette lines in both patients.

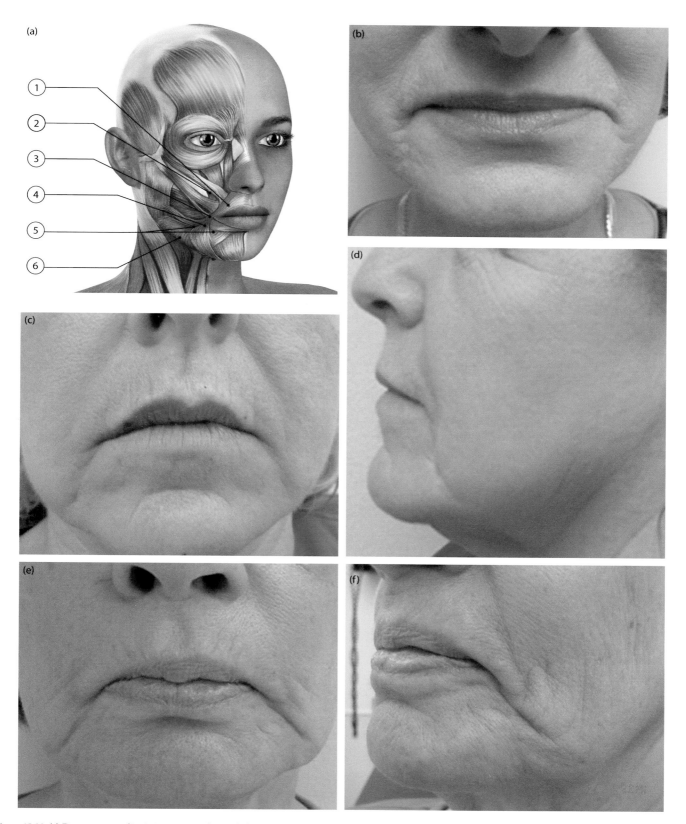

Figure 15.38 (a) Depressor anguli oris inserts into the modiolus before interdigitating with the risorius, platysma (*pars labialis*), levator anguli oris, and the orbicularis oris. It pulls the corners of the mouth downward. 1, orbicularis oris; 2, levator anguli oris; 3, modiolus; 4, depressor anguli oris; 5, platysma (pars labialis); 6, platysma (pars mandibularis). (b) An inverted smile with early formation of marionette lines. A hyperkinetic depressor anguli oris pulls the lateral oral commissures of the mouth downward, resulting in (c, d) early and (e, f) advanced melomental folds or "marionette" lines.

line of the body of the mandible below the canine premolar and first molar, lateral and superficial to the bony origin of the larger depressor labii inferioris, which it partially overlaps[40] (Figure 15.10). The muscle fibers of the depressor anguli oris narrow as they travel upward and converge onto the angle of the mouth, where some muscle fibers insert directly into the undersurface of the dermis while other fibers insert into the modiolus and then interdigitate with muscle fibers of the orbicularis oris, risorius, and levator anguli oris near the upper lip and the zygomaticus major and buccinator and platysma modiolaris at the oral commissures[18] (Figure 15.38). Its overall size can vary according to the shape of an individual's facial bony structure.[5] In addition, the lower posterior fibers of the depressor anguli oris interdigitate with those muscle fibers of the upper platysma (pars labialis) and cervical fascia that converge toward the lateral oral commissures. In some individuals, the depressor anguli oris will traverse the midline inferior to the mental tubercle and decussate with fibers of its paired muscle of the opposite side, creating the transversus menti or the "mental sling."[4]

Hur et al. investigated the topographical relationship of the depressor anguli oris to the mental foramen.[36] Although the position of the mental foramen can vary from individual to individual, depending on their idiosyncratic bone structure, it is generally found below the mandibular second premolar region. They also observed that most commonly the mental foramen was located under the middle third of the depressor anguli oris between the cheilion and the inferior border of the mandibule. In addition, the most common course of the buccal and marginal mandibular branches of the facial nerve was under the middle and lower thirds of the lateral border of the depressor anguli oris. In all cadaver specimens studied, the motor end plates were abundantly located in the lower portion of the depressor anguli oris inferior to the mental foramen, which they therefore concluded was the most effective site for injecting OnaBTX-A.[36]

The function of the depressor anguli oris is to depress the oral commissures slightly laterally and downward when opening the mouth. The depressor anguli oris is an antagonist to the levator anguli oris, risorius, and zygomaticus major, displacing the corners of the mouth downward and slightly laterally when it contracts in an expression of grief, sorrow, and sadness. The melomental sulcus, or marionette line, generally is located in the center and over the upper aspect of the depressor anguli oris[5,40] (Figure 15.38e, f). While in certain patients, the inferior aspect of the marionette line contributes to the formation of the prejowl or labiomandibular sulcus, fixed in place by the mandibular (retaining) ligament. Posterior to the depressor anguli oris and anterior to the jowl, the mandibular ligament adheres the dermis to the mandible.[5] On opening the mouth, the labiomental sulcus (mental crease) across the chin becomes more horizontal and deeper in its center.[4]

Dilution When Treating Melomental Folds (see Appendix 3)
When treating the depressor anguli oris and the perioral area, OnaBTX-A should not be allowed to diffuse beyond the targeted muscle fibers; otherwise, cosmetic aberrations such as an asymmetric smile, and functional disturbances such as drooling, dribbling, and even dysarthria are likely to follow. Therefore, the highest volume of diluent that should be used to reconstitute a 100 U vial of OnaBTX-A is 1 mL of normal saline. Any volume of diluent higher than 1 mL is sure to invite adverse sequelae.

Dosing: How to Correct Problem (see Appendix 4) (What to Do and What Not to Do) When Treating Melomental Folds
The downward angling of the "marionette lines" can be improved by injecting 3–6 U of OnaBTX-A intramuscularly in the center of the body of the mandible at a point that is most inferior to an imaginary vertical line that passes through the nasolabial sulcus (Figure 15.39b). This point should be approximately 8–10 mm lateral to the oral commissure

and 8–15 mm inferior to this point, depending on the idiosyncratic shape of the patient's face and anterior projection of the mandible. The appropriate injection point can be identified by palpating someone who is actively contracting the corners of the mouth downward (Figure 15.39c) while pronouncing the letter "E" in an exaggerated fashion (Figure 15.39d).[29,41] Having the patient smile intensely with the lower lip clenched upward and against the upper lip (i.e. a closed mouth smile) and then again enunciating the letter "E" also will help identify a hypertrophic depressor anguli oris. Another maneuver to assist in localizing the depressor anguli oris is to have the patient bite down, forcibly contracting the jaw muscles. This will contract and enlarge the belly of the masseter, which is a muscle very easily identified by palpation (Figure 15.40). In most individuals, the depressor anguli oris lies approximately 1 or 2 mm to 1 cm anterior to the masseter depending on the shape and projection of the jaw and mandible. After the patient clenches his or her teeth and the anterior border of the masseter is identified, have the patient exaggerate the pronunciation of the letter "E." The location of a hypertrophic depressor anguli oris should be easily palpated along the anterior border of the masseter and along the body of the mandible. At times, the depressor anguli oris can be detected more easily by palpating it intraorally along the inferior alveololabial sulcus as the patient actively contracts it (personal communication from Luitgard Wiest, MD). Yet another way to identify the appropriate injection point of the depressor anguli oris is to have the patient forcibly contract his or her platysma. Those patients who possess platysmal neck bands frequently will form a lateral neck band that is directly beneath the point where fibers of the platysma mandibularis and the depressor anguli oris decussate. Just cephalad to this lateral platysmal neck band on the superior aspect of the body of the mandible is the general vicinity where OnaBTX-A should be injected (Figure 15.39e,f).

Place the patient in the upright sitting or semireclined position. At the point where the contracted and thickened belly of the depressor anguli oris can be felt, insert the needle perpendicular to the skin surface over the body of the mandible about 3–5 mm above the inferior edge of the mandible. Advance the needle 3–4 mm deep into the skin until it passes through the subcutaneous tissue and barely into the muscle (approximately mid-depth) just superior to the bony origin of the muscle. Inject slowly 4–6 U of OnaBTX-A. Remember, a substantial amount of the lower medial aspect of the depressor anguli oris overlies the depressor labii inferioris (Figure 15.40a), so advancing the needle too deeply and anteriorly may unavoidably expose some of the posterior fibers of the depressor labii inferioris and possibly orbicularis oris to the injected OnaBTX-A. Also, if OnaBTX-A is injected too high and laterally from the depressor anguli oris, the zygomaticus major, risorius, and platysma can be affected.[18]

However, some authors prefer to inject lower dosages of only 2 units of OnaBTX-A into the depressor anguli oris at three separate locations.[1,5,40] The lower two injection points (I and II in Figure 15.40b) are applied deeply into the muscle until bone is contacted about 3–5 mm above the mandibular border in the same general vicinity of the muscle's lower bony origin, but much more deeply than what was discussed above. So, instead of one injection of 4–6 units of OnaBTX-A (Figure 15.39a), this technique recommends placing two injections of only 2 units of OnaBTX-A about 2–3 mm apart from each other, just anterior to the mandibular retaining ligament. Caution should be given not to inject OnaBTX-A too anteriorly toward the chin with this technique. Otherwise, the depressor labii inferioris will be unintentionally affected by these injections, producing speech difficulties and lip asymmetry at rest and in motion. The third injection point (III in Fig, 15.40b), when given, must be applied *superficially* in the midline of the upper aspect of the muscle before it inserts into the oral commissure, and always behind the marionette line, approximately 0.5 mm below and lateral to the commissure. A wheal should be elicited with this injection, otherwise the

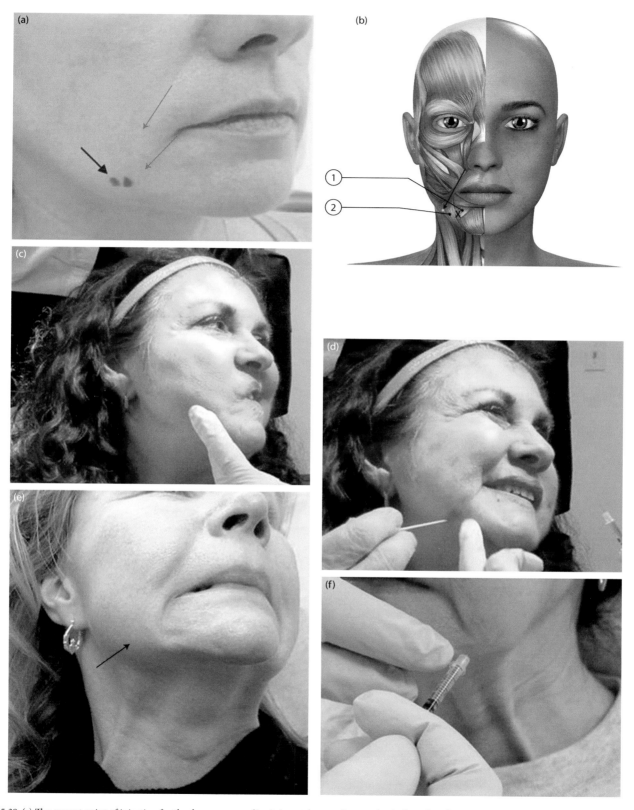

Figure 15.39 (a) The correct point of injection for the depressor anguli oris is not the anterior one that is directly inferior to the downward extension of the melomental crease (marking on the right), but slightly more posteriorly (marking on the left, *arrow*) at the most inferior point of an imaginary line that passes through the nasolabial sulcus; red arrows represent directional vectors of how to determine where to inject. (b) Placing the injection point too anteriorly (black X) injects the depressor labii inferioris. (1) The proper injection point is at the continuation of the nasolabial fold which extends to the mandibular border (dotted red line). This point is directly over the depressor anguli oris (2 and yellow dot). (c) The injection point can be identified by feeling the contraction of the depressor anguli oris as the patient actively contracts the corners of the mouth downward; (d) and pronounces the letter "E" in an exaggerated manner. (e) Note the lateral platysmal band, which points to where the depressor anguli oris can be injected with OnaBTX-A. (f) Injecting the depressor anguli oris at the most inferior point of the nasolabial sulcus in the center of the body of the mandible is approximately 1 cm lateral and 1 cm inferior to the corner of the mouth. Note how this usually corresponds to the uppermost aspect of the platysmal band.

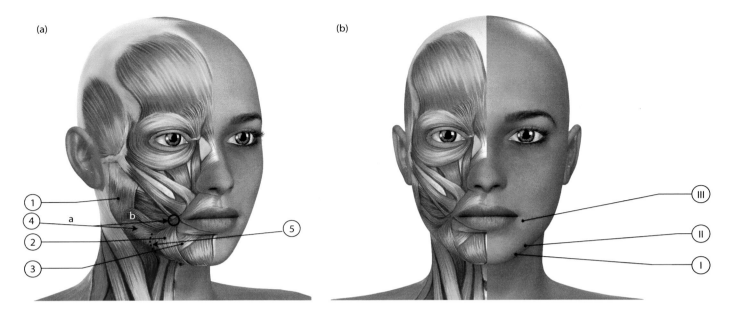

Figure 15.40 (a) The masseter can be easily palpated when patients clench their teeth. Note the position of the depressor anguli oris on the left. It normally is found laterally and superficially to the depressor labii inferioris and anteriorly to the masseter. 1, masseter; 2, depressor anguli oris; 3, depressor labii inferioris; 4a, platysma, pars mandibularis; 4b, modiolus; 5, mandibular retaining ligament (dotted black line). (b) This technique recommends placing two injections of only 2 units of OnaBTX-A about 2–3 mm apart from each other just anterior to the mandibular retaining ligament. These injection points, I and II, are applied deeply into the muscle until bone is contacted about 3–5 mm above the mandibular border in the same general vicinity of the muscle's lower bony origin. The third injection point, III, when given, must be applied superficially in the midline of the upper aspect of the muscle before it inserts into the oral commissure, and always behind the marionette line, approximately 0.5 mm below and lateral to the commissure.

injection will be given too deeply and the orbicularis oris will surely be affected, creating buccal incompetence and drooling at the very least.[40] This third, upper, superficial injection point to treat the depressor anguli oris has never been attempted by this author for fear of creating unnecessary untoward sequelae. Only one deep injection point with at least 4 units of low volume, concentrated OnaBTX-A at the mandibular border is the preferred technique and has always resulted in sufficient, naturally appearing results to satisfy patients without creating any additional adverse perioral functional changes.

In Asian patients, because of differences in the location of their modioli, from Caucasians and Africans, Choi et al. recommend injecting OnaBTX-A into a point that is less than 45 degrees lateral and less than 30 degrees medial to an imaginary vertical line that passes through the center of a palpable modiolus, which in reality is clinically similar in location to the injection technique described above for non-Asian patients.[18]

If the depressor anguli oris cannot be unequivocally identified and palpated, then it should not be treated. Inject precise amounts of OnaBTX-A accurately into the depressor anguli oris, since the orbicularis oris and depressor labii inferioris are immediately adjacent to it, and unsightly and dysfunctional perioral changes will be avoided. Otherwise, if either one of these two muscles are inadvertently weakened along with the depressor anguli oris, unintentional side effects will result. Care also should be taken not to inject into the marginal mandibular nerve and facial artery and vein that lie in this general vicinity in a bony groove just anterior to the masseter and posterior to the mandibular retention ligament. If the depressor anguli oris is palpated over this bony groove, lift the skin and muscle with the nondominant hand before injecting OnaBTX-A. With this technique, OnaBTX-A can be injected directly into the fibers of the depressor anguli oris, while avoiding injecting the neurovascular structures beneath the muscle in that area.[43] Since the depressor anguli oris is wider at its origin along the body of the mandible, it is advisable to inject it in this location and not near its insertion close to the corners of the mouth where it narrows and interdigitates with other perioral muscles (Figure 15.38). In fact, when there is an obvious platysmal band just inferior to where the depressor anguli oris is injected, an additional 2–3 U of OnaBTX-A also can be injected into the apex of that platysmal band approximately 2–3 cm inferior to the lower margin of the body of the mandible. This will ensure a complete relaxation of the depressor anguli oris and an uplifting of the oral commissures.

Outcomes (Results) When Treating Melomental Folds (see Appendix 5)

Injections of OnaBTX-A will relax the depressor anguli oris and permit the unopposed elevation of the corners of the mouth to occur by the upward pull of the levator anguli oris, the zygomaticus major, and risorius. When the corners of the mouth are relaxed and elevated by injections of OnaBTX-A, a person appears younger and naturally relaxed and pleasant (Figures 15.41 and 15.42a, b). Depending on the extent and depth of the marionette lines present, this area is best treated in combination with soft tissue fillers and some form of laser or energy-based treatments whether ablative or nonablative. OnaBTX-A then will usually prolong the beneficial effects of such rejuvenation procedures. The beneficial effects from injections of OnaBTX-A can last from 3 to 4 months and possibly even longer.[37]

Complications When Treating Melomental Folds (Adverse Sequelae) (see Appendix 6)

It is extremely important to exercise caution when injecting the depressor anguli oris too close to the mouth, since injections that are too *medial* can cause an ipsilateral weakness of the depressor labii inferioris, resulting in a flattening of the lower lip contour when the mouth attempts to form an "O," "U," or "W," in addition to an asymmetric smile (Figure 15.42d). Additional adverse sequelae when the depressor labii inferioris is inadvertently weakened include the inability to purse or pucker the lips symmetrically, seal the lips to contain solid food or fluid in the mouth or to drink from a glass, sip from a straw, or eat from a spoon (Figure 15.19b). To perform these maneuvers, a person

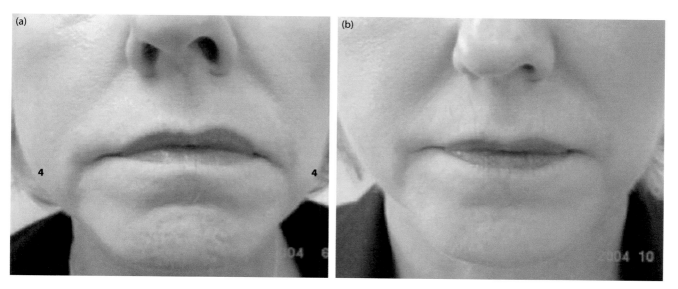

Figure 15.41 (a) This 47-year-old patient possesses a deep labiomental furrow and downward projecting corners of the mouth (a) before and (b) four months after a second treatment of 4 U of OnaBTX-A was injected into the depressor anguli oris bilaterally. Note the uplifted corners of the mouth and the patient's more pleasant appearance after a treatment of OnaBTX-A.

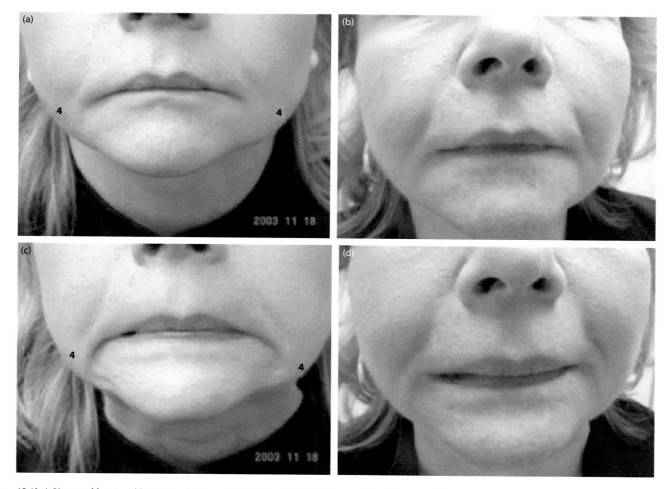

Figure 15.42 A 52-year-old patient (a) at rest and (b) 3 weeks after 4 U of OnaBTX-A were injected into each depressor anguli oris. (c) Same patient frowning before and (d) 3 weeks after that same treatment. Note the slightly asymmetric smile with forced frowning in (d), which lasted approximately 2-3 weeks after the initial OnaBTX-A treatment, and were of no concern to the patient. No other adverse sequelae were experienced by the patient.

with a weakened or adynamic depressor labii inferioris must manually depress the lower lip to open the mouth to eat, drink, and prevent biting the lower lip while chewing; so as not to dribble, drool, or lose any oral contents while masticating, the lower lip must be supported by light manual pressure throughout the entire processes of eating, drinking, and deglutition. Pronunciation of particular sounds can be hampered and the articulation of certain words will be difficult. When the depressor labii inferioris is profoundly affected, a disconcertingly adynamic smile is likely to occur, with only the upper lip moving. Overzealous injections with doses over 6–8 U of OnaBTX-A into the depressor anguli oris also will place patients at risk for developing the adverse sequelae as described above, even when the injection technique is flawless, if OnaBTX-A diffuses into the adjacent depressor labii inferioris. Even when the appropriate dose is precisely injected into the depressor anguli oris, vigorous massaging of the area after the injection can displace the OnaBTX-A into adjacent muscle fibers of the depressor labii inferioris or orbicularis oris and cause similar adverse effects as described above.

Injections that are too *high* and either adjacent to or above the mental crease can spread into the muscle fibers of the orbicularis oris and interfere with its sphincteric function, producing a localized area of inadequate sphincteric closure of the oral cavity (Figure 15.42d), difficulty with speech and suction maneuvers (e.g., kissing and drinking from a straw), and a segmental inability to pucker the lips, whistle, or perform similar functions (Figure 15.19b).[38,39]

Injections that are too *posterior* can affect the buccinator or the orbicularis oris or both and cause difficulty chewing and swallowing. Always remain below and far enough away from the mental crease and the orbicularis oris when treating the depressor anguli oris. Otherwise, OnaBTX-A can spread focally into the muscle fibers of the orbicularis oris and result in a localized area of eclabion, an asymmetric smile, drooling and even dribbling, and a change in speech and word pronunciation.

Injecting too *close* to the mental foramen could conceivably cause damage to the neurovascular plexus and mental nerve emerging from the mental foramen, resulting in the loss of sensation in the lips and chin. It may even result in lip biting, difficulty with speech, and diminished retention of saliva.[36] Therefore Hur et al. also concluded that injecting BTX-A into the lower third of the depressor anguli oris and below the mental foramen as described above has a lower risk of direct needle damage to the mental foramen neurovascular structures and a higher success rate in effectively and safely treating

unwanted melomental folds and the downward pull of the oral commissures compared to previously reported injection techniques.[36]

For the first-time patient, treatment in this area can produce similar but mild and transient sequelae that may be overwhelming to the uninformed and unprepared patient, so pretreatment warning of these potential side effects is mandatory (Figure 15.42).

Figures 15.43 through 15.46 are additional examples of different patients treated with OnaBTX-A to uplift the oral commissures.

Treatment Implications When Injecting Melomental Folds and Marionette Lines

1. Inject OnaBTX-A only when the depressor anguli oris can be unmistakenly identified and accurately palpated.
2. The depressor anguli oris usually can be identified at the inferior end of the nasolabial sulcus over the body of the mandible and anterior to the masseter.
3. A lateral platysmal band can identify the location where the depressor anguli oris and platysma pars mandibularis decussate along the inferior border of the mandible. It is at this point of maximal contraction of the depressor anguli oris that is the recommended site for an injection of OnaBTX-A.
4. Avoid injecting OnaBTX-A into the marginal mandibular nerve and facial artery and vein by lifting the skin and soft tissue before injecting.
5. Avoid injecting OnaBTX-A into the depressor labii inferioris and orbicularis oris by remaining at least 1 cm lateral and 1 to 1.5 cm inferior to the lateral oral commissure and in the center of or just above the body of the mandible.
6. OnaBTX-A should be injected intramuscularly just beneath the subcutaneous plane since the lower medial aspect of the depressor anguli oris is superficial to and overlies the posterior aspect of the depressor labii inferioris.
7. Always inject minimal doses of minimal volumes of highly concentrated OnaBTX-A in the perioral area.

CHIN PUCKERING AND A DEEP MENTAL CREASE
Introduction: Problem Assessment and Patient Selection
For some men and especially women, a hyperkinetic mentalis can produce involuntary localized dimpling (Figure 15.47) or an overall puckering of the chin, creating convolutions of deep ridges and furrows while they speak or convey a particular facial expression (Figure 15.48). For most individuals who consciously or involuntarily

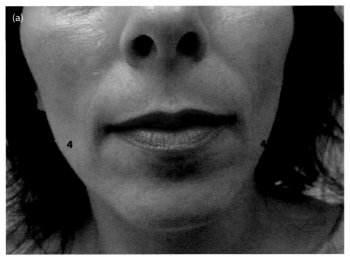
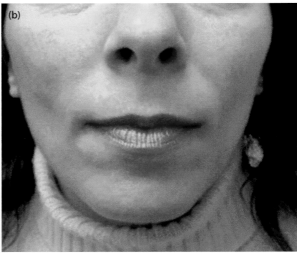

Figure 15.43 A 45-year-old patient (a) before and (b) 3 weeks after (b) 4 U of OnaBTX-A were injected into each depressor anguli oris. Note the slight uplifting of the corners of the mouth.

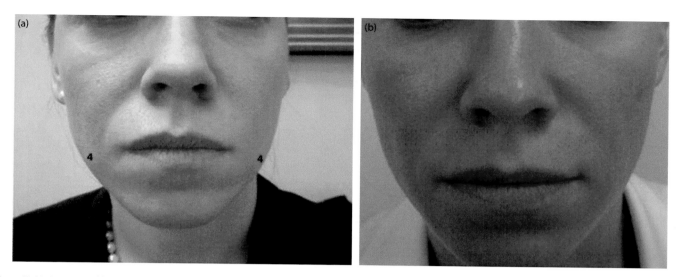

Figure 15.44 A 40-year-old patient (a) before and (b) 2 weeks after 4 U of OnaBTX-A were injected into each depressor anguli oris. Note the slight uplifting of the corners of the mouth.

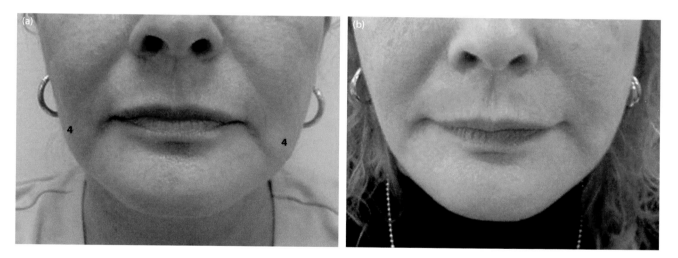

Figure 15.45 A 53-year-old patient (a) before and (b) 3 weeks after 4 U of OnaBTX-A were injected into each depressor anguli oris. Note the slight uplifting of the corners of the mouth.

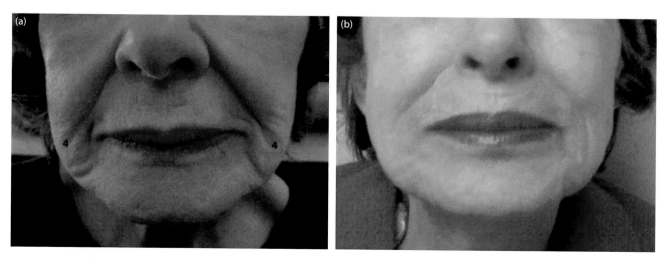

Figure 15.46 A 78-year-old patient (a) before and (b) after 4 U of OnaBTX-A were injected into each depressor anguli oris. Note the slight uplifting of the corners of the mouth. This patient also underwent ablative fractionated CO_2 resurfacing and injections of soft tissue fillers 2 weeks after the OnaBTX-A injections.

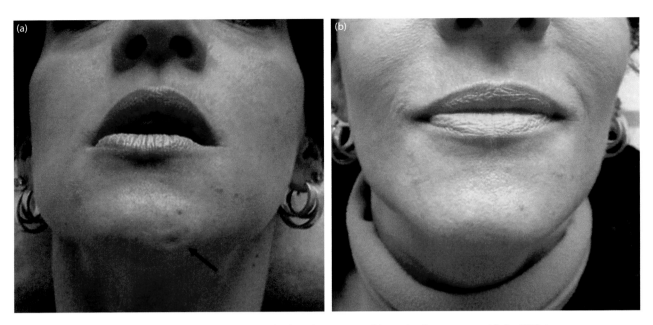

Figure 15.47 (a) This 49-year-old woman was unaware of her chin dimples (arrow) even at rest. (b) 3 weeks after treatment with OnaBTX-A.

crinkle their chin during animation or even while at rest, these changes generally go undetected by the person producing them unless disclosed by others. Once identified, chin puckering then can be verified by the patient personally, viewing these chin corrugations with a mirror while animating or speaking (Figure 15.49).

Any motion of the lower lip that causes the lip margin to evert as when pronouncing words that begin with the letter "F" or "V" will usually accentuate chin puckering (Figure 15.50). In other individuals, chin puckering can be a disquieting annoyance when it occurs postoperatively as a secondary synkinesis from an augmentation mentoplasty (Figure 15.51a).[43,44] Because not all of the bony attachments of the muscle fibers of the mentalis can reposition and reapproximate exactly as they were prior to the instillation of a chin implant, the contracting fibers of the mentalis then become anomalously reattached to the mentum, producing irregular crimping of the skin surface, either at rest or with each movement of the chin and mentalis (Figure 15.51a, c). This can be an unexpected and frustrating side effect for a surgical correction of an inadequately projecting chin.

In still another group of people, a hyperkinetic mentalis produces an accentuated, deep transverse (labio)mental crease between the lower lip and the prominence of the chin that amplifies the forward projection of the apex of the mentum (Figures 15.52 and 15.53). This is viewed as a sign of dotage or senility by the casual observer, because with age the tip of the chin can elevate and project forward, producing the so-called "wicked witch's chin." Men are not as frequently bothered by similar changes and even less often do they seek relief from them.

Functional Anatomy Chin Puckering and a Deep Mental Crease (see Appendix 2)

Dynamic wrinkling and corrugations of the surface of the chin or the deep infolding and indentation of a labiomental crease is produced by a hyperkinetic mentalis. The mentalis is a short, stout, conical, two-bellied muscle that originates below the depressor labii inferioris on the anterior aspect of the alveolar mandible on either side of the midline and symphysis menti, at the level of the incisive fossa and root of the lower lateral incisors and canines (Figure 15.54). It travels obliquely

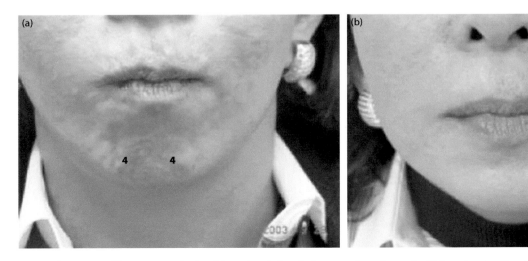

Figure 15.48 This 50-year-old was unaware that her chin puckered when she became animated or spoke. (a) Forced contraction of her mentalis produced multidirectional corrugations before OnaBTX-A, which disappeared (b) 2 weeks after 8 U of OnaBTX-A were injected in her mentalis.

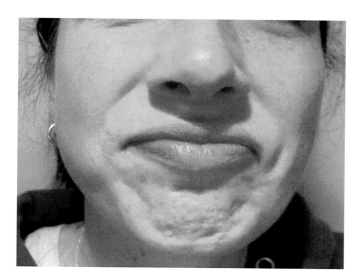

Figure 15.49 This 30-year-old was unaware of her chin corrugations until she was actively animating and puckering in front of a mirror. Note the localized dimpling of her chin.

downward, converging its two muscle bellies toward the midline in a V-shaped triangle to insert with multiple fibrous attachments into the skin of the apex of the chin on either side of the frenulum of the lower lip. Some of its other fibers interdigitate superiorly with fibers of the orbicularis oris and laterally with the fibers of the depressor labii inferioris, contributing to the formation of the mental crease. The mentalis elevates the skin at the base of the lower lip upward, helping to force the lower lip against the gums. The mentalis assists other reciprocating synergistic perioral muscles (e.g., depressor labii inferioris and orbicularis oris) to depress, protrude, and evert the lower lip during drinking, eating, and speaking. These synergistic functional movements also intensify the indentation of the labiomental crease. The mentalis also wrinkles the skin of the chin when it is contracted in pouting to produce an expression of doubt, displeasure, sadness, or disdain. With age comes the loss of dermal collagen, elasticity, and soft tissue support. Ageing also promotes the diminution and retrusion of the bony mentum and a reduction in subcutaneous fat. In conjunction with a hyperkinetic mentalis, all of these structural changes can facilitate the appearance of uncontrollable chin convolutions and dimpling. In most individuals, when frowning in displeasure or projecting an expression of sadness, doubt, or disdain, the depressor anguli oris contracts simultaneously with the mentalis, so the melomental ("marionette") lines also are accentuated. Therefore, for many patients, it is advisable

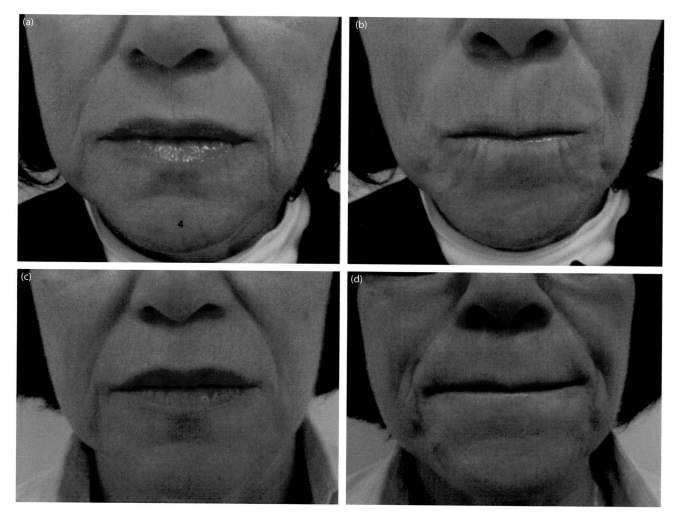

Figure 15.50 A 63-year-old woman (a) at rest before 4 U of OnaBTX-A were injected into her mentalis. (b) Note the crimping of the chin and deep mental crease at rest and while pronouncing words containing the letter "F." Same patient (c) at rest and (d) 3 weeks after the OnaBTX-A treatment. Note the reduction of chin crimping and effacement of the mental crease.

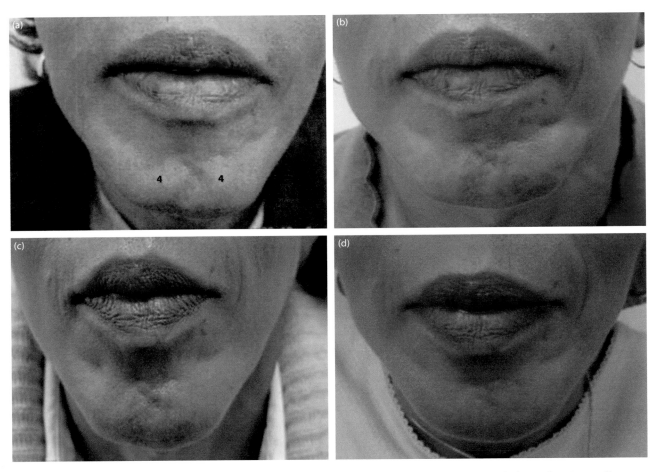

Figure 15.51 A 67-year-old (a) before and (b) 6 weeks after her third OnaBTX-A treatment with 8 U of OnaBTX-A into her mentalis for a synkinesis caused by an augmentation mentoplasty 2–3 years previously. Note the difference in the pattern of chin crimping before and after a treatment with OnaBTX-A. The same patient was plagued with the appearance of chin crimping both at rest and during animation seen here (c) before and (d) 3 weeks after her fourth treatment of OnaBTX-A.

to treat both the presence of marionette lines and chin dimpling at the same time during the same session.

Dilution When Treating Chin Puckering and a Deep Mental Crease (see Appendix 3)

When treating the mentalis, lateral diffusion of the OnaBTX-A runs the risk of weakening the depressor labii inferioris and producing sphincter and motor movement incompetence of the mouth, causing an inability to depress the lower lip when smiling, laughing, speaking, drinking, and eating. Therefore, accurately reconstituted, low volumes of concentrated OnaBTX-A must be precisely injected when treating the mentalis. The preferred way to accomplish this is to reconstitute a 100 U vial of OnaBTX-A with only 1 mL of normal saline.

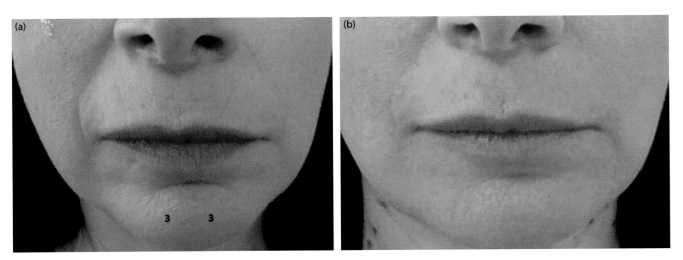

Figure 15.52 A 52-year-old patient seen (a) before and (b) 1 month after 6 U on OnaBTX-A were injected into the mentalis. Note the slight diminution of the mental crease.

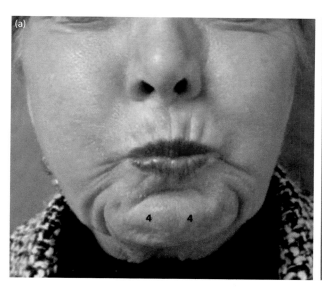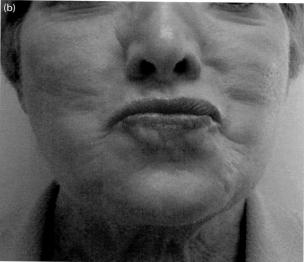

Figure 15.53 This 58-year-old patient seen (a) before and (b) 3 weeks after 8 U of OnaBTX-A were injected into the mentalis. Note the deep transverse labiomental crease prior to treatment and its diminution after treatment.

Dosing: How to Correct the Problem (see Appendix 4) (What to Do and What Not to Do) When Treating Chin Puckering and a Deep Mental Crease

Injections of the mentalis are best done with the patient in the upright sitting or semireclined position. A hyperactive mentalis can be relaxed by inserting the tip of the needle perpendicular to the surface of the skin and injecting 3–4 U of OnaBTX-A deeply into the muscle at one point about 5 mm on both sides of the midline into the apex of the protuberance of the mentum, approximately 1 cm above the tip of the chin. This two-point injection technique is especially appropriate if the patient has a vertical mental cleft or a widely shaped, square chin (Figures 15.51 through 15.53). If the patient has a narrow, rounded, or a more pointed chin, the insertion of the mentalis into the undersurface of the skin with its paired muscle belly of the contralateral side probably is more centrally located in a narrower, overlapping V-shape. For these patients, an alternative one-point injection technique is more appropriate (Figure 15.55). This is accomplished by injecting 4–6 U of OnaBTX-A deeply into one point only into the center of the mentum at the apex of the mental protuberance, approximately 1 cm above the tip of the chin (Figure 15.56).

It is imperative to avoid inadvertent diffusion of OnaBTX-A into any of the muscle fibers of the orbicularis oris, which can result in sphincter and motor movement irregularities. This can be accomplished by injecting OnaBTX-A significantly lower than the transverse mental crease and into the center of the apex of the mental protuberance. Light massage will relieve the pain of injection. Vigorous massage will displace the OnaBTX-A laterally or superiorly, particularly if the two-injection point technique is used, and cause the OnaBTX-A to spread into the fibers of the depressor labii inferioris or the orbicularis oris or both producing untoward sequelae.

Outcomes (Results) (see Appendix 5)

Relaxing the hyperkinetic muscle fibers of the mentalis can reduce or eliminate the involuntary convolutions and corrugations of the chin when one is at rest, speaking, or emotionally expressing oneself (Figures 15.53 and 15.56). A weakening of the mentalis also can drop the anterior projection of the skin of the chin slightly downward, attenuating an already deep transverse labiomental crease and possibly rotating the lower lip slightly upward (Figures 15.53 and 15.57). When the transverse labiomental crease is exceptionally deep and resistant to treatment with OnaBTX-A, elevating and effacing it with

soft tissue fillers is an advisable alternative. Deeply placed injections of soft tissue fillers across the anterior aspect of the mentum will recontour and rejuvenate the chin. Injections of OnaBTX-A into the mentalis will actively sustain and prolong the improvement.

For those patients who have a distorted convoluted chin because of a previous augmentation genioplasty with a chin implant, injections of OnaBTX-A can produce a softening and a relaxation of the chin. This is much appreciated by those who are vexed by these anxiety provoking wrinkles and convolutions of the mentum and for whom additional surgery is not an option (Figure 15.51). The addition of a soft tissue filler will augment and prolong the corrective effects produced by the injections of OnaBTX-A. The effects of the injections of OnaBTX-A of the mentalis can last anywhere from 4 to 6 months.

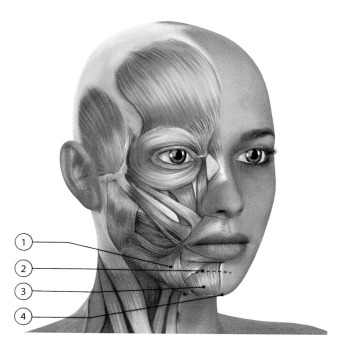

Figure 15.54 The mentalis elevates the lower lip, indents the mentolabial crease, and creates surface corrugations over the mentum: 1, depressor anguli oris; 2, mentolabial crease (dotted line); 3, mentalis; 4, mentum.

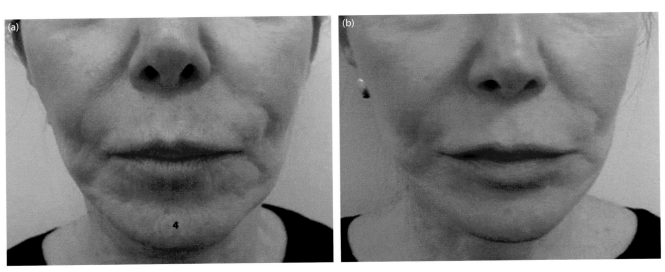

Figure 15.55 This 70-year-old woman accentuated chin puckering by pursing her lips (a) before and (b) 1 month after 4 U of OnaBTX-A were injected into a single site at the apex of the mentum.

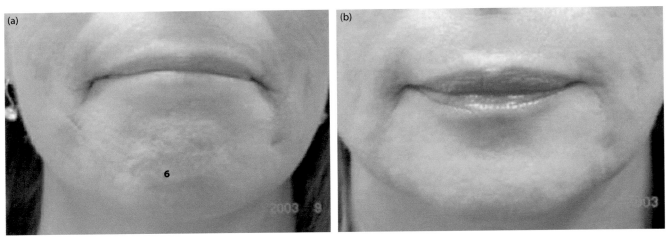

Figure 15.56 A 53-year-old, with chin puckering at rest that was exacerbated with animation, is seen (a) before and (b) 2 weeks after 6 U of OnaBTX-A were injected into a single site at the apex of the mentum. Note the narrowness of the apex of the mentum and the location of the single injection point.

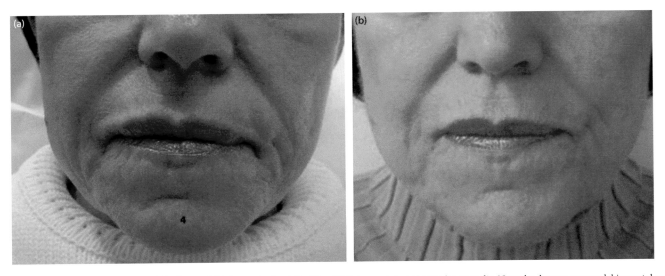

Figure 15.57 A 58-year-old patient seen (a) before and (b) 1 month after 4 U of OnaBTX-A were injected into the mentalis. Note the deep transverse labiomental crease prior to treatment and its slight diminution after treatment.

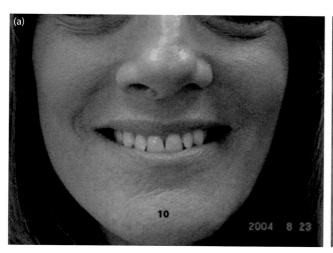
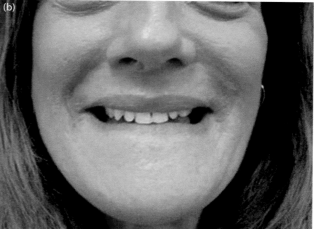

Figure 15.58 A 55-year-old patient smiling (a) before and (b) after 10 U of OnaBTX-A were injected into her mentalis. Note the inability of the mentalis to lower the center of the lower lip after her excessively high dose treatment, which also might have diffused into the depressor labii inferioris. The patient had to manually lower her lip to avoid biting it while eating and drinking. She had incontinence with liquids and difficulty with articulating certain sounds and words.

Complications When Treating Chin Puckering and a Deep Mental Crease (Adverse Sequelae) (see Appendix 6)

When dosing is excessive or if the injections of an appropriate amount of OnaBTX-A are placed too high on the lower lip, that is, above the transverse (labio)mental crease, the orbicularis oris, and even the depressor labii inferioris can certainly be weakened, particularly when using the two-point injection technique. Diffusion of OnaBTX-A into the depressor labii inferioris and orbicularis oris also can occur when the injections are too superficial or vigorous massaging is performed immediately after injection. If either the orbicularis oris or the depressor labii inferioris is inadvertently affected by OnaBTX-A, a relaxation of a tight oral sphincter, a reduction in lip competence, and a diminution in buccal motor movements will occur (Figure 15.58). This can cause a patient to form certain letters, such as P, B, W, F, O, and U, and articulate certain sounds and words with embarrassing difficulty. Also, an asymmetric smile can be produced because of an adynamic or synkinetic lower lip. An overzealous treatment of the mentalis with too high a dose of OnaBTX-A that virtually immobilizes the mentalis will cause an inability to evert and approximate the lower lip tightly against the teeth, or against a glass or cup,

producing a disconcerting predicament with incontinence of solid food when eating, dribbling from the lower lip when drinking, and drooling from the corners of the mouth when at rest (Figure 15.58). Excessive dosing also can inadvertently spread to fibers of the adjacent depressor labii inferioris, intensifying the total weakness of the lower lip, resulting also in a profound inability to depress the lower lip. When this occurs, the person affected is obligated to manually lower his or her lower lip to avoid biting it while eating, drinking, and even speaking. Proper enunciation of speech is temporarily and overwhelmingly impeded.

Figures 15.59 through 15.63 are additional examples of different patients treated with OnaBTX-A for chin puckering and a deep mental crease.

Treatment Implications When Injecting the Mentalis

1. Inject OnaBTX-A far below the transverse mental crease and at the apex of the mental protuberance.
2. Injections should be placed deeply, in one site centrally or in two sites separately on either side of the midline depending on the width of the chin.

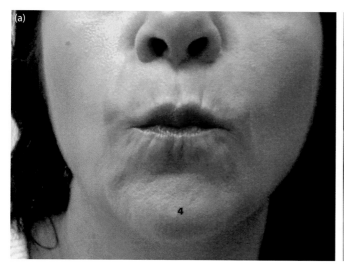
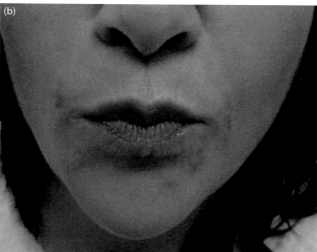

Figure 15.59 This 44-year-old with chin puckering and perioral rhytides is seen (a) before and (b) 3 weeks after 4 U of OnaBTX-A were injected into the mentalis. Note the softening of the lower face and fullness of the lip vermilion with additional OnaBTX-A injections of the perioral rhytides.

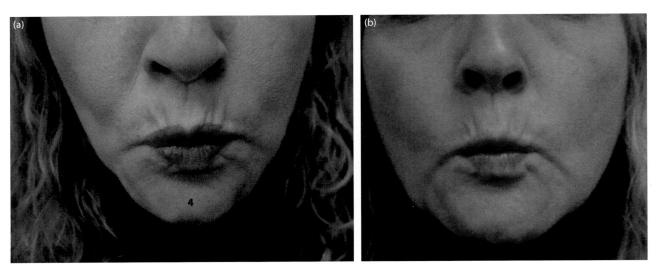

Figure 15.60 A 53-year-old with chin puckering is seen (a) before and (b) 2 months after 4 U of OnaBTX-A were injected into the mentalis. Note the transverse widening of the mentum. Perioral rhytides were also treated with OnaBTX-A.

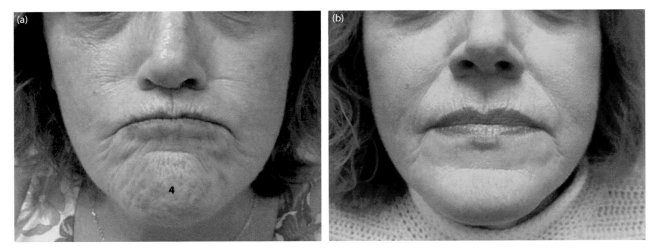

Figure 15.61 A 53-year-old with chin puckering is seen (a) before and (b) 6 weeks after 4 U of OnaBTX-A were injected into the mentalis. Note the softening of the lower face and a fullness of the lip vermilion with the additional treatment of her perioral rhytides with onaBTX-A.

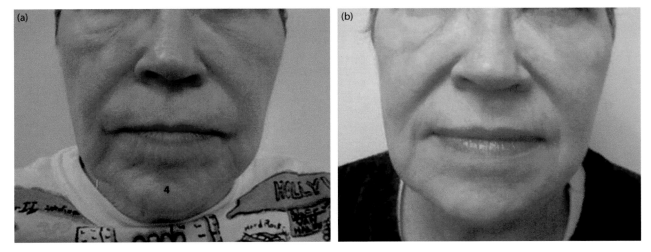

Figure 15.62 A 66-year-old is shown at rest with chin puckering and perioral rhytides (a) before and (b) 2 weeks after 4 U of OnaBTX-A were injected into the mentalis and additional OnaBTX-A was injected in the perioral rhytides. Note the excessive wrinkling of the lower lip and chin before treatment that softened after treatment.

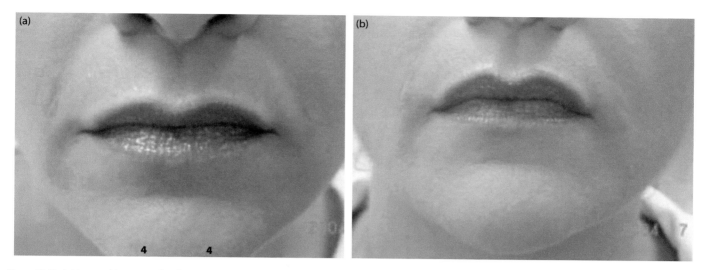

Figure 15.63 A 38-year-old at rest with a deep transverse mental crease (a) before and (b) 3 weeks after 8 U of OnaBTX-A were injected into the mentalis. Note the efface-ment of the mental crease and upward rotation of the lower lip vermilion.

3. High-volume injections or an improper heavy-handed tech-nique can cause the spread of OnaBTX-A into the depressor labii inferioris or the orbicularis oris or both, and result in an inability to move the lower lip inferiorly, causing sphincter incompetence of the buccal aperture.

4. Immobilizing the mentalis with a high dose of low-volume OnaBTX-A can prevent the lower lip from approximating tightly against the teeth or a drinking vessel, resulting in drib-bling while drinking and drooling while at rest. Inability to articulate words and sounds distinctly also can occur.

5. Injections of OnaBTX-A can correct postoperative chin puckering and distortions resulting from an augmentation mentoplasty.

6. The use of OnaBTX-A can prolong the enhancement produced by soft tissue filler injections of the perimental and perioral areas.

7. OnaBTX-A treatment of the lower face and perioral area should always include injecting the mentalis.

JAWLINE BLUNTING AND WRINKLING OF THE PERICOMMISSURAL AREA AND LOWER MANDIBULAR BORDER

Introduction: Problem Assessment and Patient Selection of Jawline Blunting and Wrinkling of the Upper Platysma

With age, the effects of gravity, genetics, and the environment cause our skin to slacken and become redundant as we lose dermal elastic-ity. There is a descent of soft tissue from the mid face toward the man-dibular border.[45] With time, the platysma can become hyperkinetic and the skin of the face and neck becomes lax and drapes randomly in the lower face, over the mandibular border, overhanging and blunting the cervicofacial angle (Figure 15.64a). Patients who can elevate their platysma, blunting their sharp mandibulocervical angle by pulling down hard on their platysma are ideal candidates for treatment with OnaBTX-A (Figure 15.64b).

In addition, there is a small subset of patients whose upper pla-tysma is very active and hyperkinetic creating various types of lower face wrinkling. For example, one type of hyperkinetic platysmal lower face wrinkling can be attributed to the long-term changes occurring

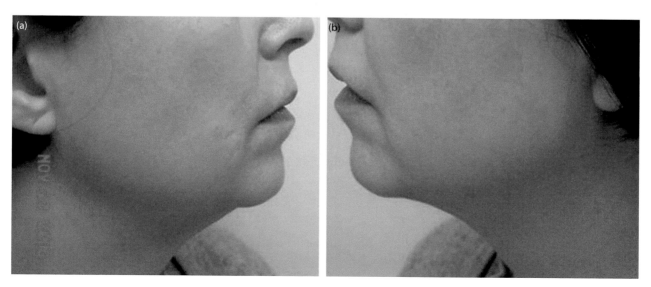

Figure 15.64 (a) This patient has a hyperkinetic platysma, creating a blunting of the cervicofacial angle. (b) Same patient tightening her platysma and further blunting the cervicofacial angle.

after a surgical rhytidectomy. These patients by grimacing can form different atypical wrinkles parallel to the mandibular border, which are produced by the compensatory contractions of the mandibular platysma (*pars mandibularis*) as it becomes hypertrophic and more active with time (Figure 15.65a, b).

Still another type of lower face wrinkling attributed to a hyperkinetic mandibular platysma are the naturally occurring pericommissural horizontal lines, which become visible with the slightest bit of buccal movement. These lines in particular will deepen with smiling or laughing and are an annoyance to those who possess them (Figure 15.66). Lower facial platysmal lines become more obtrusive when their bearer loses weight and the lower facial skin continues to become lax and inelastic with time and progressive photoaging.

Functional Anatomy of the Upper Platysma (see Appendix 2)

The platysma is composed of two separate paired broad, flat, thin sheets of muscle originating over the chest and shoulders, extending over the full length of the neck. It continues up the frontal and lateral aspects of the neck subcutaneously from the upper chest to the mandible, fusing and blending its paired muscle fibers just below the chin, and participating in the formation of the superficial musculoaponeurotic system (SMAS) in the lower, lateral and superior aspects of the face (Figure 15.67).[46–50] The platysma can vary considerably in thickness and extent; in general, women have a thinner platysma than men.[51] In some individuals, the platysma may even be absent.

The platysma ascends obliquely upward and inward in a superomedial direction from the upper anterior thorax and deltoid, and laterally from across the clavicle and acromion of the scapula and up the lateral neck. It continues up the anterior and lateral aspect of the neck and inserts into the chin anteriorly, while laterally, it inserts above the mandible into the anterior one third of the oblique line of the mandibular ramus (Figures 15.10 and 15.67). The more posterior fibers of the lateral platysma partially cover and interdigitate with fibers of the sternocleidomastoid, running posterior to it. Then some of these posterior platysmal fibers assume a more anterior course, while traversing over the lower border of the mandible, and pass superficially over the marginal mandibular branch of the facial nerve, artery, and vein and insert into the oral commissures. These posterior superior muscle fibers of the platysma move in a "lazy S" configuration as they travel from the chest, up the neck, over the mandible, onto the lower face and into the corners of the mouth (Figures 15.9 and 15.67).[52] The platysma can reach as high as the ear or zygoma because it then joins the layers of the temporalis fascia over the zygomatic arch near the origin of the zygomaticus major which it envelopes and can continue up to the margin of the *orbital* orbicularis oculi. This is because as the plastysma continues cephalad from the neck onto the face it is indistinguishable from and persists as the SMAS of the face.[48,49]

The upper portion of the platysma muscle, before it becomes an aponeurosis and part of the SMAS, is composed of three parts, the mandibular, labial, and modiolar parts, and functions as an accessory muscle

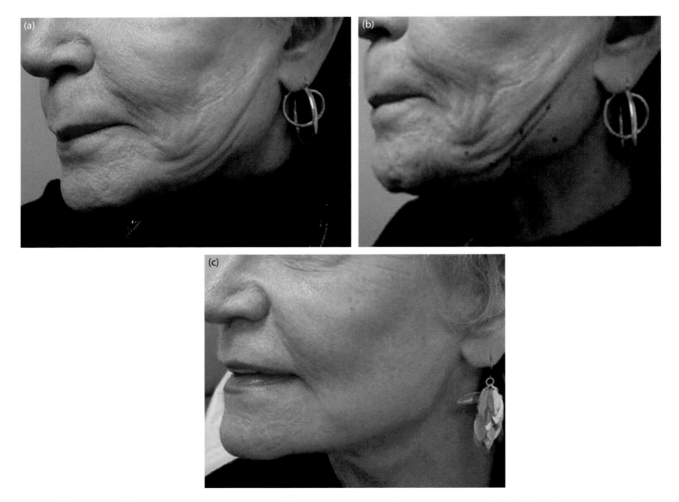

Figure 15.65 (a) This 68-year-old has a very active upper platysma which creates a set of perioral horizontal rhytides with the slightest buccal movement. Same patient is seen grimacing prior to (b) 20 U of OnaBTX-A that were injected 2–4 mm above and below the inferior border of the body of the mandible. (c) Same patient shown 1 month after treatment.

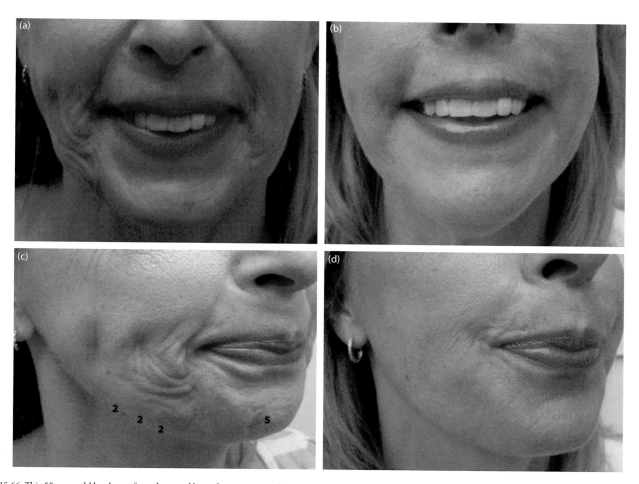

Figure 15.66 This 55-year-old has lower face platysmal lines due to aging and weight loss. Patient is seen before (a, c) and 3 weeks after (B, D) 6 U of OnaBTX-A were injected into the platysma pars mandibularis along the inferior border of the mandible. The mentalis was injected with 5 U of OnaBTX-A and a hyaluronic acid soft tissue filler was injected into the nasolabial folds during the same treatment session.

to the orbicularis oris complex[4] (Figures 15.7, 15.9, and 15.67). The upper fibers of the platysma identified as the platysma *pars mandibularis* insert onto the lower border of the mandible below the oblique line and into the skin and subcutaneous tissue of the lower part of the face (Figures 15.10 and 15.67). Posterior to this attachment, a substantial number of flattened muscle bundles separate and pass superomedially to interdigitate with muscle fibers of the lateral border of the depressor anguli oris (Figure 15.9). Other fibers of the platysma pars mandibularis travel deep to the depressor anguli oris and re-emerge medial to it.

Some of these medial platysmal fibers known as the platysma *pars labialis* continue within the tissue of the lateral half of the lower lip, as a direct labial retractor. The pars labialis occupies the interval space between the depressor anguli oris and depressor labii inferioris, and is in the same tissue plane as both of these muscles. The adjacent margins of all three muscles interdigitate with each other and have similar labial dermal attachments. They then also blend into some of the muscle fibers surrounding the buccal commissures (orbicularis oris and risorius) and the chin (mentalis) (Figures 15.67).

The platysma *pars modiolaris* is comprised of all the remaining muscle fibers of the upper platysma posterior to the platysma pars labialis other than a few fine fascicles that end directly into buccal dermis or submucosa. The pars modiolaris is posterolateral to the fibers of the depressor anguli oris. They pass superomedially, deep to the risorius and into the apical and subapical modiolar attachments[4] (Figure 15.7).

The platysma slightly depresses the mandible, partially opening the mouth during an expression of surprise. The platysma also is active

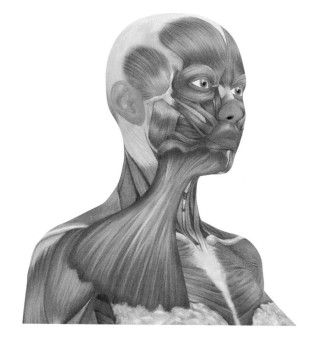

Figure 15.67 Anterolateral view of the extent of platysma (pars mandibularis, pars labialis, and pars modiolaris), from its origin in the chest and pattern of ascent, to insertion along the mandible. (Note that only the right side of platysma is shown here; the left side has a paired symmetrical extent.)

during sudden, rapid, and deep inspiration. The anterior portion and thickest fibers of the platysma can pull the lower lip and corners of the mouth downward and laterally, widening the buccal aperature at the corners of the mouth as in an expression of horror. Contracting the platysma can increase negative pressure in the superficial jugular veins of the neck, facilitating venous circulation. Electromyographic studies have demonstrated that the platysma is not actively contracting during laughing, opening the mouth, or moving the head.[40,46,47] However, deliberate maximum contraction of the platysma pulls the skin lying over the clavicles upward and wrinkles the skin of the neck in an oblique direction increasing the diameter of the neck, as one does when relieving the pressure of a tight collar. Platysmal cords and bands also may be unmasked with this maneuver in those so predisposed to develop them (see Vertical Bands below).

Dilution (see Appendix 3) When Treating Jawline Blunting and Wrinkling of the Upper Platysma

When treating the upper fibers of the platysma, it is safer and results will be more consistent if small volumes of OnaBTX-A are injected. This will avoid any unintended diffusion beyond the targeted thin muscle fibers of the platysma. Therefore, a 100 U vial of OnaBTX-A is best reconstituted with 1 mL of normal saline. If a more far-reaching technique simulating the "microbotox" technique is desired (Chapter 17 by Dr. Seo), then a 100 U vial of OnaBTX-A can be reconstituted with 2–5 U of normal saline. This more highly diluted OnaBTX-A should only be injected with the small volume, intradermal, microinjection technique.

Dosing: How to Correct the Problem (see Appendix 4) (What to Do and What Not to Do) When Treating Jawline Blunting and Wrinkling of the Upper Platysma

The platysma plays a predominant role in the overall contour of the mandibular border and the cervicofacial angle. It also is responsible for the horizontal wrinkles seen just below and adjacent to the modiolus and the oral commissure (Figure 15.66). To treat either the blunting of the jawline or the horizontal wrinkles lateral to the mentum and inferior to the oral commissure along the upper mandibular border, place the patient in a sitting or semireclined position. Because of the intricate way the upper platysma interdigitates with the muscles of the lower face above the mandible, those horizontal rhytides that become more prominent when the corners of the mouth

are compressed by the contraction of the modiolar area should be treated with injections of onaBTX-A only submandibularly and never over or above the body of the mandible. These horizontal lines along the upper border of the mandible frequently are caused mainly by the platysma mandibularis and platysma labialis, and occasionally reinforced by the platysma modiolaris. Place 2–3 U of OnaBTX-A in the upper neck, approximately 1.5–2.0 cm below the inferior margin of the mandible and directly beneath those horizontal wrinkles in 2–4 injection points 1.5–2.0 cm apart from each other (Figure 15.66). The injections should begin just lateral to the bony origin of the depressor labii inferioris and not any more anterior to this point. These injections usually should be performed at the same time the depressor anguli oris and mentalis are treated, since these muscles all interdigitate and function codependently with each other.

In addition, Levy found that he could delineate more sharply the mandibulocervical angle by injecting 2–3 U of OnaBTX-A at multiple sites along the upper cervical border of the platysma just adjacent and inferior to the mandibular border and over the entire lateral side of the neck in patients who did not need a lower face or cervical rhytidectomy. He called this injection technique the "Nefertiti" lift (Figure 15.68).[53,54] These injections should begin no higher than 1.5–2.0 cm beneath the mandibular border just underneath and lateral to the bony origin of the depressor labii inferioris. This places the first injection point directly beneath the bony origin of the depressor anguli oris. Continue the injections along the upper border and over the entire lateral side of the neck. However, the injections should not cross over the anterior border of the sternocleidomastoid (Figure 15.69). The total dose for each lateral side of the neck should not exceed more than 20–25 U of OnaBTX-A, that is, a total dose of 40–50 units of OnaBTX-A on both sides of the entire neck during any given treatment session. If there are prominent platysmal bands in the anterior and lateral neck, they also should be included in the treatment of this "Nefertiti lift" (Figure 15.68a,b) (see Vertical Bands below and Figure 15.69a,b).

The platysma with or without platysmal bands in the submandibular area of the lateral neck can be easily treated by grasping skin or the band with the thumb and index finger of the nondominant hand and injecting 2–3 U of OnaBTX-A between those fingers in a "T"-like pattern along the lateral side of the neck. Six to a maximum of 8 points of injection along one lateral side of the neck is sufficient to produce a Nefertit

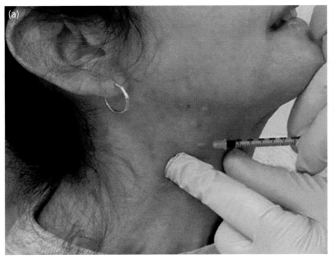
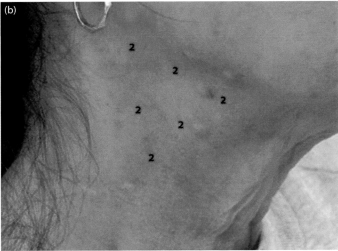

Figure 15.68 (a, b) Note the multiple injection points along the upper cervical border of the platysma, along the lateral aspect of the neck. Approximately 2 U of OnaBTX-A were injected at each point (wheal).

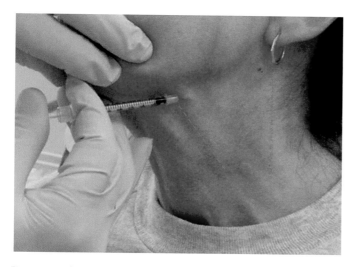

Figure 15.69 The injection points are posterior to the lateral border of the depressor anguli oris (dashed lines) and anterior to the belly of the sternocleidomastoid (red dashed lines).

lift. Eight to a maximum of 12 points of injection along one lateral side of the neck is sufficient to diminish prominent platysmal banding when they are present. (Figures 15.68, 15.69, and 15.79).

Outcomes (Results) When Treating Jawline Blunting and Wrinkling of the Upper Platysma (see Appendix 5)

Hyperkinetic platysma and inelastic, saggy skin cause blunting of the jaw line. Injections of OnaBTX-A along the inferior border of the mandible and down the lateral sides of the neck relax the upper lateral platysma and pars mandibularis, allowing the levators of the face to lift the skin of the lower face and upper neck. This in turn redefines the mandiblar border and sharpens the mandibulo-cervical angle closer to 90 degrees by redraping the skin over the jaw line for a tighter, more youthful, contoured appearance. This technique also elevates the corners of the mouth giving the overall visual effect of a "mini-lift" of the lower face and upper neck[53] (Figures 15.70, 15.71, and 15.74). Levy named this technique the "Nefertiti lift" to emphasize the final visual effect of an elegant, perfectly recontoured jawline similar to that of the famous bust of the Egyptian Queen Nefertiti (Figure 15.72).

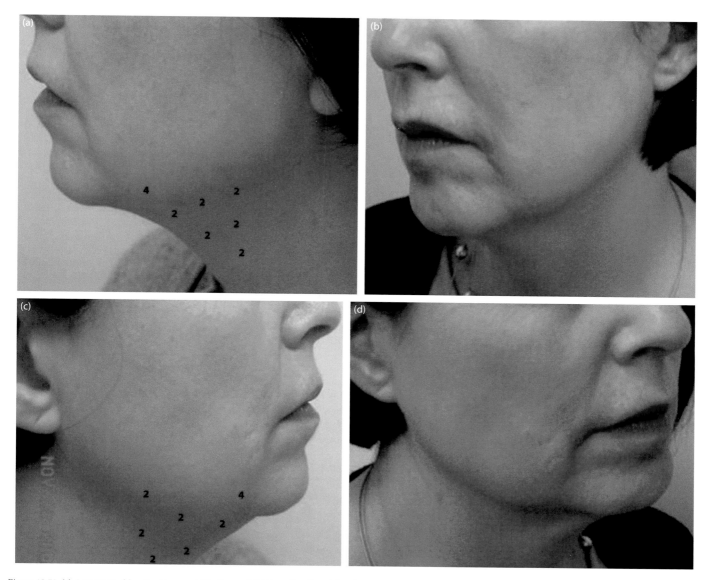

Figure 15.70 (a) A 59-year-old patient is seen (a) before and (b) 2 weeks after 12 U of OnaBTX-A were injected in her left plastysma, pars mandibularis and left depressor anguli oris. Same patient is seen (c) before and (d) 2 weeks after the identical treatment with OnaBTX-A was completed on the right.

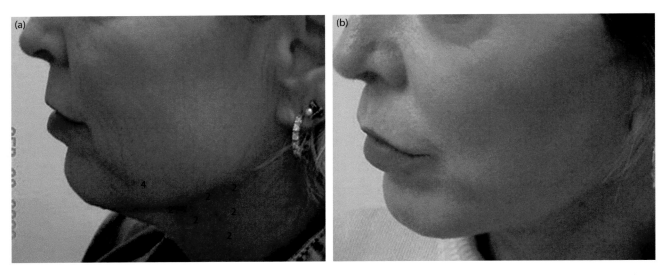

Figure 15.71 A 58-year-old patient is seen (a) before and (b) 2 weeks after 12 U of OnaBTX-A were injected in her left platysma, pars mandibularis and left depressor anguli oris.

For those horizontal platysmal wrinkles lateral to the mentum and inferior to the oral commissures, a treatment with 4–8 U of OnaBTX-A will diminish them, and the results can last 3–4 months (Figures 15.65 and 15.66). Levy, however, reports the effects of the "Nefertiti lift" to last even longer, an average of 6 months.[53]

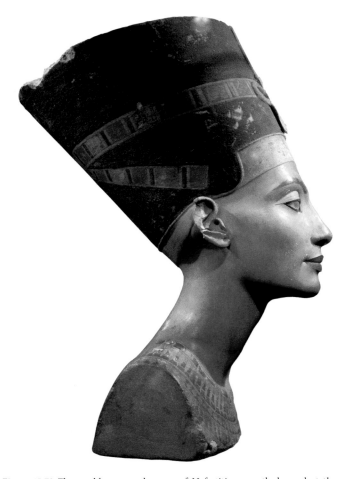

Figure 15.72 The world-renowned statue of Nefertiti, currently housed at the Neues Museum in Berlin, illustrates the ideal cervicofacial angle of 80°–95°.

Complications When Treating Jawline Blunting and Wrinkling of the Upper Platysma (Adverse Sequelae) (Appendix 6)

Injecting the platysma pars mandibularis is no easy task and should only be performed by the expert injector. If there is diffusion of OnaBTX-A beyond the immediate site where it is injected, the depressor labii inferioris, the orbicularis oris, and other segments of the platysma will be affected, which can adversely impact the final results (Figure 15.73). In addition, if OnaBTX-A is injected unevenly or if it is taken up by the different muscle fibers of the platysma that interdigitate with the lower lip depressors, then an asymmetry and a malfunctioning of the mouth and distortion of the lower face will be experienced by the patient (Figure 15.73). This can occur when performing the Nefertiti lift or when one attempts to eliminate the horizontal lines of the lateral mentum inferior to the oral commissures. Injections too close to the inferior border of the mandible and too far anteriorly, that is, directly under the origin of the depressor labii inferioris will cause lower lip fuctional disturbances, as was also seen in de Almeida's recent retrospective study[81] and first described in the previous edition of this text (Figure 15.73).[82] Other predictable adverse sequelae that can occur when injections of OnaBTX-A are not placed properly in the neck are an asymmetric smile, disruption of lip competence causing incontinence of food and liquids, dysarthria, disphonia, and dysphagia. When treating the platysma pars mandibularis along the inferior mandibular border posteriorly, OnaBTX-A should not inadvertently penetrate the sternocleidomastoid either by direct injection or unintentional spread. If this occurs, the patient will have difficulty with lateral and rotational movements of the neck, resulting in an instability of head positioning and difficulty raising it from a supine position.

When treating the lower face and the platysma, there is an exquisitely delicate balance of levators and depressors just like in the midface, that is, a narrow margin of dosing for successful and uneventful outcomes. Increasing a proven efficacious dose of OnaBTX-A by 1 or 2 U may cause adverse sequelae when a lower dose did not. Therefore, only a minimal amount of concentrated, low volume OnaBTX-A should be injected in the mid and lower face, if predictable and reproducible beneficial treatments without adverse side effects are expected. Most importantly, when treating the platysma in the lower face, keep the injections superficial (i.e., intradermal) and far away from the orbicularis oris and depressor labii inferioris.

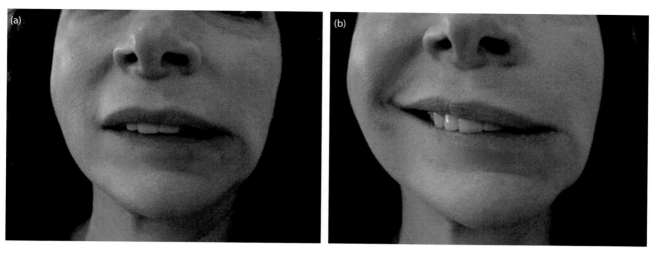

Figure 15.73 (a, b) This patient experienced asymmetry of the lower right *pars peripheralis* of the lips and distortion of the lower face after submandibular injections of OnaBTX-A diffused into the right depressor labii inferioris. Note the synkinesis of the levators in the upper lateral quadrant. The right submandibular injection was placed anterior to the posterior border of the depressor anguli oris and possibly too close to the lower edge of the mandible.

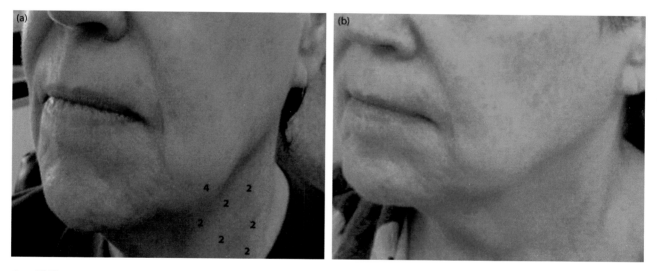

Figure 15.74 (a) This 66-year-old patient is seen before (a) and 3 weeks after (b) 12 U of OnaBTX-A were injected in her left platysma, pars mandibularis, and 4 U of OnaBTX-A were injected in her left depressor anguli oris.

Treatment Implications When Injecting the Jawline and Upper Platysma

1. Horizontal rhytides just lateral to the mentum and oral commissures can be diminished by intradermal injections of OnaBTX-A only along the undersurface of the mandible and never above it.
2. Hyperkinetic fibers of the upper platysma (pars mandibularis) can blunt the jawline.
3. Properly placed intradermal injections of OnaBTX-A along the underside of the mandible and down the lateral neck can sharpen the jawline and lift the skin of the lower face and upper neck.
4. Injections of the submandibular upper platysma with OnaBTX-A should be performed posterior to the origin of the depressor labii inferioris and 2–3 cm inferior to the lower border of the body of the mandible.
5. Avoid injecting the sternocleidomastoid by placing the injections of OnaBTX-A in the lateral neck in front of the anterior border of the muscle to prevent difficulty with neck movements and head positioning.

6. For optimal results, the lower face should be treated as one cosmetic unit with injections of OnaBTX-A placed intradermally in the superficial labial orbicularis oris, deeply into the mentalis, subcutaneously and intramuscularly into the depressor anguli oris, and intradermally in the upper platysma.
7. Avoid injecting the depressor labii inferioris and the deep fibers of the orbicularis oris with OnaBTX-A to prevent oral sphincter incompetence and a disruption in buccal function.

HORIZONTAL LINES AND VERTICAL BANDS OF THE NECK

Introduction: Problem Assessment and Patient Selection

Frequently, the neck can be a more accurate gauge of a person's chronologic age than the overall appearance of his or her face. This is especially true in those individuals who have spent a lot of time outdoors and who have taken advantage of various cosmetic procedures available to rejuvenate their faces. The neck as well as the perioral region have remained the bane of aesthetic rejuvenation for most age-conscious individuals seeking relief from the ravages of time and the innumerable hours spent outdoors, whether for work or pleasure. None of the available invasive surgical procedures (i.e., cervicoplasties

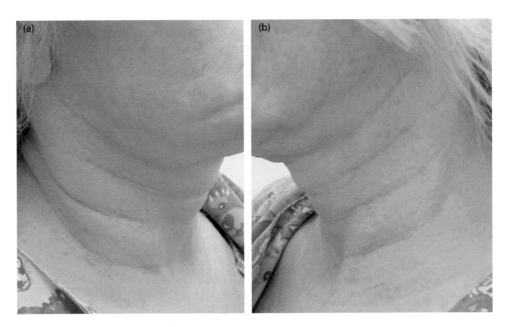

Figure 15.75 (a, b) This 55-year-old began to notice deep horizontal wrinkles of the anterior neck at age 40.

or rhytidectomies) have ever eliminated satisfactorily and safely horizontal necklace lines or vertical platysmal bands for any substantial length of time.[53] Since the 1990s, more innovative and aggressive approaches to neck rejuvenation have been introduced, albeit not as invasive as a surgical intervention. These include minimally invasive suture-based suspensory thread-lifting techniques and superficial skin surface altering procedures, for example, chemical peeling or ablative and nonablative fractionated laser resurfacing. A multitude of transepidermal and subdermal approaches to facial and neck rejuvenation have become popular, including sequential treatments with nonablative laser and light devices, for example, pulsed dye laser and polychromatic intense pulsed light, radiofrequency (RF) and high-intensity focused ultrasound (HIFU). The routine use of energy-based treatments in combination with BoNT, soft tissue fillers and implants, and daily topical treatments with cosmeceuticals is probably the only way to effectively maintain a harmoniously youthful appearance of the neck with the rest of the face.[55] (See Carruthers, Chapter 7.)

With age, the skin of the neck progressively loses its elasticity, becoming increasingly lax and redundant. There also is a diminution of soft tissue support, causing the skin of the neck to be susceptible to frequent and continuous horizontal creasing in some individuals. These idiosyncratic movements of the neck can lead to persistent transverse wrinkles that are perpendicular to the normal vertical contractions of

the platysma. These horizontal lines traverse the anterolateral aspect of the neck between the anterior borders of the right and left sternocleidomastoid, which start just below the submandibular border and continue downward toward the clavicles like multiple parallel rings around the neck, also referred to as "necklace lines" (Figure 15.75).

A hyperkinetic anterior platysma also produces the detested platysmal neck bands, whether a person is actually at rest or intentionally tightening their neck muscles. Upon animation with different neck movements, vertical bands and cords may become prominent at an early age (in the fourth or fifth decade) in predisposed individuals or eventually in the sixth or seventh decade for many others (Figures 15.76 and 15.77). Neck bands are caused by the platysma and not by the skin of the neck, whether the skin is inelastic or lax.[5] When an individual's platysma is hyperkinetic, anterior neck bands will be noticeable even when that person is at rest. Intentionally contracting the platysma will intensify these bands significantly.

When the platysma becomes less elastic with age, it separates anteriorly and can be appreciated clinically as two or more divergent bands or folds of skin that extend from the lower margin of the mandible to the medial aspect of the clavicles. These anterior neck bands often tighten and become more visible, especially when the patients turn the head from side to side as they speak or gesticulate (Figure 15.76).[56] Vertical bands and cords develop as the result of a hyperactive platysma attempting to support the ptotic structural

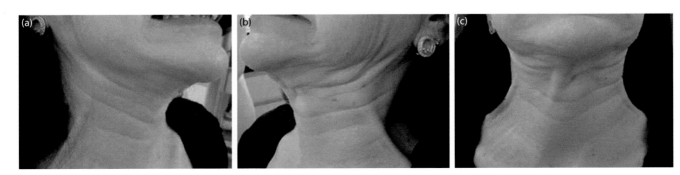

Figure 15.76 (a, b, c). This 52-year-old began to notice deep horizontal wrinkles of the anterior neck at age 38. Note the platysmal neck bands when she forcibly contracts her platysma.

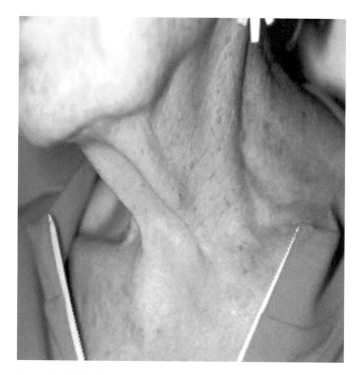

Figure 15.77 Note the pendulous "turkey neck deformity" in this 73-year-old woman.

changes so characteristic of a senescent neck. The anterior edges of the fibers eventually lose muscle tone, separate over time, and protrude anteriorly, creating the cords and bands that are sometimes referred to as the "turkey neck" deformity[52] (Figure 15.77). For some carefully selected individuals who still possess a reasonable amount of cutaneous elasticity, but who develop prominent platysmal neck bands because of idiosyncratic platysmal hyperactivity, injections of OnaBTX-A have become a viable treatment option to reduce the prominence of those platysmal neck bands. For others demonstrating a similar integrity of cutaneous elasticity, but who either are unable for medical reasons or are unwilling for other personal reasons, to undergo the burden of the postoperative morbidity of an invasive surgical procedure such as a cervicoplasty or rhytidectomy, injections of OnaBTX-A have become a frequently requested and reliable solution to their problem.

Functional Anatomy of Horizontal Lines and Vertical Bands of the Neck (see Appendix 2)

The platysma is composed of two separate paired broad, flat, thin sheets of muscle originating from the superficial fascia of the upper part of the thorax over the pectoralis major and deltoid, extending over the full length of the neck. In certain patients, the platysma can originate lower than the second, and as far down as the fourth to the sixth intercostal space (Figure 15.67). It continues running up the frontal and lateral aspects of the neck subcutaneously from the upper chest to the mandible, fusing and blending its paired muscle fibers just below the chin, and participating in the formation of the SMAS in the lower, lateral and superior aspects of the face (Figure 15.67).[46–49] The platysma can vary considerably in thickness and extent; in general, women have a thinner platysma than men.[51] In some individuals, the platysma may even be absent.

The platysma ascends obliquely upward and inward in a superomedial direction from the upper anterior thorax and deltoid, and laterally from across the clavicle and acromion of the scapula and up the

lateral neck. It continues up the anterior and lateral aspect of the neck and inserts into the chin anteriorly, while laterally, it inserts above the mandible into the anterior one third of the oblique line of the mandibular ramus. The more posterior fibers of the lateral platysma partially cover and interdigitate with fibers of the sternocleidomastoid, running posterior to it. Then some of these posterior platysmal fibers assume a more anterior course, while traversing over the lower border of the mandible, and pass superficially over the marginal mandibular branch of the facial nerve, artery, and vein and insert into the oral commissures (Figures 15.9 and 15.67).

The medial, anterior fibers of the platysma in the neck are the most variable. Both sheets of the anterior fibers of the platysma on either side of the neck converge at the level of the thyroid cartilage and form an inverted "V," decussating at various levels in the submental area or directly under the chin at or near the symphysis menti of the mandible. Consequently, the submental area can be either totally covered or even devoid of muscle fibers of the platysma.[49,52,57,58] Some authors like to emphasize the different anatomic variations of the platysma based on the pattern of decussation of its interlacing fibers as they approach the submental region (Figure 15.78b).[48,49,52,57,59–61] One can appreciate from many of the existing anatomical studies in the literature why some individuals develop platysmal neck bands and cords, while others do not. Most of these reports are of cadaver dissections, and they differ according to race, sex, and age of the cadavers, depending on the country in which the study took place. One of the first and frequently referred to studies of cadaver dissection was that of Cardoso de Castro. In 1980, he characterized the various configurations of the anterior, medial muscle fibers of the platysma based on his dissection of 50 cadavers, in which he observed three patterns of platysmal decussation.[57] The most common variant was seen in approximately 75% of the cadavers. Identified as type I, the fibers of the platysma showed convergence and decussation with its counterpart from the opposite side of the neck 1–2 cm below the chin. Another 15% of the cadavers (type II) showed muscle fibers which decussated at the level of the thyroid cartilage and became a unified sheet of muscle from thereon up and over the entire submental region. Only type III, or 10% of the cadavers, demonstrated two separate straps of platysma which ran parallel to each other up the neck, attaching to the undersurface of the chin and mandible and into the skin without decussating its fibers (Figure 15.78b).[46,57,60–63]

Pogrel et al. in their later study categorized four similar but different patterns of anterior platysma decussation.[58] Approximately 40% of their cadavers had platysma fibers from the level of the thyroid cartilage converging in the center of the neck just beneath the chin, but they did not decussate. They formed what they called a "V-shaped dehiscence." Another 35% of their specimens, converged lower in the center of the neck; however, these muscle fibers criss-crossed over the midline, decussating with each other, also in a "V-shaped dehiscence." These two groups of "V-shaped dehiscence" (75%) seem to correspond to Cardoso de Castro's group I cadavers. Another 15% of the cadavers in the Pogrel et al. study showed total interdigitation of platysmal fibers in the midline throughout the submental region. In this group, no area in the submental region was free of muscle and there were no free borders of dehisced platysma fibers. Their submental area was completely covered in a sheet of muscle forming a submental sling or what they considered a platysmal "diaphragm." These were the patients who were least likely to form platysmal bands, even with advancing age. In the final 10% of their cadavers, Pogrel et al. found the right and left platysma were the farthest apart from each other, but eventually merged and interdigitated with each other closest to the chin in a "U-shaped dehiscence" rather than in a "V-shaped dehiscence." They felt that this configuration of the submental area was the freest of muscle and had the greatest potential for a "turkey

(a)

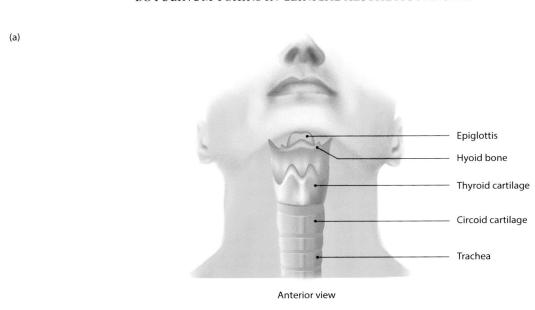

Epiglottis

Hyoid bone

Thyroid cartilage

Circoid cartilage

Trachea

Anterior view

(b)

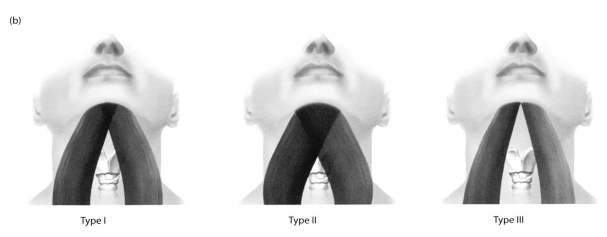

Type I   Type II   Type III

Figure 15.78 (a) Anatomical landmarks of the anterior neck. (b) Three types of decussating platysma. (From Brennan PA, Mahadevan V, Evans BT, *Clinical Head and Neck Anatomy for Surgeons*, CRC Press: Boca, 2016, with permission.)

neck" deformity.[58] These results are similar to what Cardoso de Castro found in 10% of his cadavers where both sides of the platysma approached the menton without prior decussation.

The simplest explanation why some people develop platysmal bands and chords and others do not is that, according to Vistnes et al.[52] and Hoefflin,[49] there are just two basic decussating configurations of the platysma in the anterior neck. Vistnes et al. found in approximately 60% of their cadavers that the free medial borders of the paired platysma formed an inverted "V" around the prominence of the thyroid cartilage, with its apex at the hyoid bone (Figure 15.78a). At the level of the hyoid bone, the muscle fibers decussated across the midline, forming a sling from the hyoid bone to the tip of the chin (menton)[52] (Figure 15.78b). Hoefflin further simplified the classification of the platysma as either decussating two-thirds of the time, or not at all.[49]

There are two distinctly separate depots of fat in the submental region of the neck that must be taken into consideration when planning rejuvenation procedures for the aging neck. The more superficial one of the two is the submental or submandibular fat pad, which lies directly anterior to the platysma in the subcutaneous plane. The other, the subplatysmal fat pad, lies more deeply in the neck, residing behind and posterior to the platysma. Herniation and protrusion of the subplatysmal fat pad in the aging neck are predicated on the type of anatomic variant and amount of platysmal central dehiscence present in an individual and whether there is a significantly wide enough separation of the two muscle sheets inferior to the mentum. In those individuals with excessive amounts of submental fat in the subplatysmal layer, the loss of platysmal muscle tone permits the subplatysmal fat pad to herniate through the free borders of the platysma and establish a central fullness of submental fat in between vertical columns of neck bands, blunting a youthful 110-degree cervico-mental angle and creating the so-called turkey neck deformity[50,52] (Figure 15.77).

The submandibular salivary glands are secondary salivary glands which measure approximately 3×5 cm and are located one-third of the way between the chin and mastoid process and are found in the lateral floor of the mouth, positioned under the border of the mandibule.[55] With time, the gland becomes enlarged and ptotic and can herniate through a weakened or attenuated platysma. This creates a small bulge at the sides of the neck, characteristic of someone of advanced age. Injections of OnaBTX-A can contribute to this deformity by decreasing the support of the platysma and superficial cervical fascia. However, direct injections of OnaBTX-A into the body of the submandibular glands are somewhat successful in reducing the size of enlarged and ptotic submandibular glands and minimizing their appearance for prolonged periods of time.[55] Such BoNT-A treatments usually are performed more frequently in the East[64] (see Chapter 17 by Kyle Seo).

Dilution When Treating Horizontal Lines and Vertical Bands of the Neck (see Appendix 3)

Because the platysma is a large sheet of muscle that drapes over the anterolateral aspect of the neck, injections of large volumes of dilute OnaBTX-A may be more expedient when the entire neck needs to be treated. Therefore, reconstituting a 100 U vial of OnaBTX-A with 2–4 mL of normal saline is more practical than reconstituting it with a smaller volume when injecting the platysma.

Dosing: How to Correct the Problem (see Appendix 4) (What to Do and What Not to Do) When Treating Horizontal Lines and Vertical Bands of the Neck

To eliminate most of the dynamic horizontal lines of the neck, inject approximately 2–3 U of OnaBTX-A above and below the entire anterior and lateral extent of the main horizontal line at points 2–3 cm apart into the deep dermis, rather than the subcutaneous plane (approximately 2–3 mm deep), using dilute volumes of OnaBTX-A. Elevated wheals will confirm that the injections were placed correctly. Repeat this technique above and below the other horizontal lines along the anterior and lateral aspects of the neck. Injections are performed with the patient sitting upright or in a semireclined position and forcibly contracting their platysma by clenching their teeth (Figure 15.76). Depending on the size of the patient's neck, no more than 25–35 U of OnaBTX-A should be given at any given treatment session for this indication.[65]

In the properly selected patient, OnaBTX-A also can be used to reduce the appearance of vertical bands and cords of the neck.[37–39,41–43,56,66] In those patients with extensive cutaneous laxity and flaccid platysmal cords, injections of OnaBTX-A can actually cause the patient to appear worse, and therefore should not be attempted (Figure 15.77).

Again, with the patient sitting upright or in a semireclined position and contracting their platysma, grasp the platysmal band between the thumb and index finger of the nondominant hand (Figure 15.79). Inject 2–3 U of OnaBTX-A intradermally, or just subcutaneously (2–3 mm deep) into each injection site along the vertical extent of the band. Start the injections approximately 2 cm below the inferior border of the mandible centrally in the submental area, 1–2 mm lateral to the origin of the depressor labii inferioris or posterior to the mandibular retaining ligament. This technique avoids the spread of OnaBTX-A into the lower fibers of the depressor labii inferioris and may prevent unexpected visible distortions of the chin and functional disturbances of the lower lips. Repeat each injection at intervals of 1.5–2 cm from each other, descending down the neck toward the upper border of the clavicle, stopping at the level of the thyroid cartilage.[5,60] Raising a visible wheal with each injection attests to the appropriately superficial placement of the injected OnaBTX-A (Figure 15.80). Keeping the injections as superficial as possible will avoid postinjection ecchymoses that result from puncturing superficial vasculature of the muscle. The application of ice to the area before and especially immediately after injecting OnaBTX-A as well as gentle massage helps to alleviate some of the pain that accompanies an intracutaneous injection. It also may help reduce the potential for bruising. Most patients require 3–5 injection points along the vertical length of a platysmal band to treat it adequately, and some may require even more, depending on the length of their neck. It is advisable to inject no more than 6–12 U of OnaBTX-A along the vertical extent of each platysmal band for a total of 30 to 50 U per treatment session when two or three neck bands are treated on both sides of the neck.[46] When more than two platysmal bands are present on each side

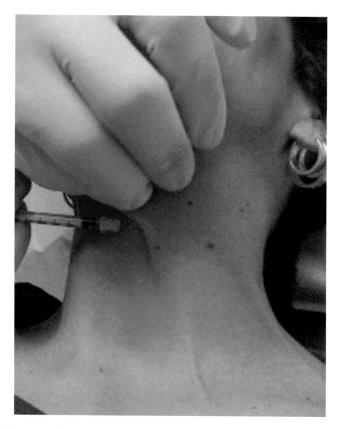

Figure 15.79 Contracting the platysma makes grasping the skin and band easy to inject OnaBTX-A into the lower dermis.

of the neck, the other platysmal bands should be treated at another treatment session, 2–4 weeks later, especially if more than 50 U of OnaBTX-A have already been injected. When the neck bands present as thick cords and a hypertrophic platysma can be palpated, an additional 1 or 2 units of OnaBTX-A can be applied at each injection point. Some authors have injected as much as 200 U per treatment session in the same patient, a practice that is not necessary in most cases.[62,63] There are others who use electromyographic guidance to accurately place a minimum amount of OnaBTX-A in a platysmal band when treating the neck. By utilizing electromyographic guidance, they can use less than a total of 20 U of OnaBTX-A in the neck of a patient in any given treatment session.[67]

Outcomes (Results) When Treating Horizontal Lines and Vertical Bands of the Neck (see Appendix 5)

Relaxation of a hypertrophic platysma with diminution of horizontal neck lines and vertical bands will occur 5–7 days after a treatment with OnaBTX-A. The effects can last anywhere from 3 to 5 or more months, depending on the precision of the injections, the strength of the platysma, and the frequency and intensity of the patient's neck movements. Usually patients who are too young for rhytidectomies or older patients who have had rhytidectomies and have minimal skin excess will have the best results when there is reasonably tight cutaneous elasticity and minimal ptosis of subplatysmal fat and soft tissue. It is advisable to have patients return 2–3 weeks after a treatment session with OnaBTX-A to assess their response to the treatment and their satisfaction with the overall results. Touch-up injections always can be done to correct any asymmetry or lack of a response along a particular neck band or cord.[65]

Treatment with OnaBTX-A has been beneficial in preparing a patient for submental liposuction because, by relaxing the neck bands,

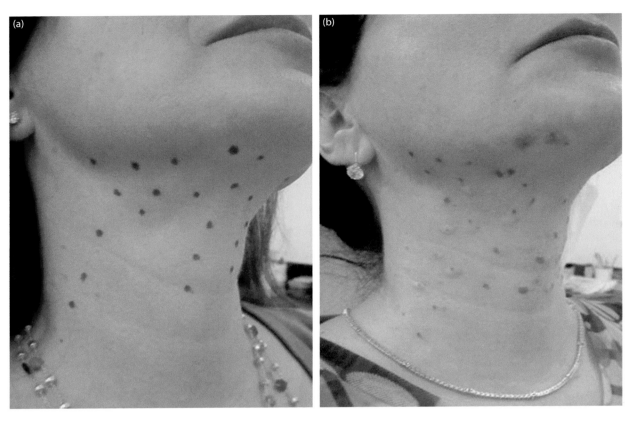

Figure 15.80 (a, b) Raising a wheal while injecting OnaBTX-A in the neck attests to the superficial placement of the product.

a more even draping of the anterior neck skin can be achieved in the postoperative period after liposuction. In those patients in whom liposuction surgery has unmasked vertical neck bands postoperatively, injections of OnaBTX-A will help conceal them again after surgery.[68] When there is a significant amount of fat herniation from in between the two lateral sheets of platysma in certain patients, along with submandibular fat occupying the submental area, deoxycholic acid injections or liposuction with or without a platysmaplasty and possibly a rhytidectomy, are the only treatments that will be corrective (Figure 15.81). Injections of OnaBTX-A in these patients are marginally helpful. On the other hand, when there is no herniation or protrusion of subplatysmal fat and the presence of submental fat is negligible, injections of OnaBTX-A will be effective in reducing the vertical neck bands and cords created by a hypertrophic platysma (Figure 15.82). In some authors' experience, the anatomic type or configuration of platysmal decussation (Figure 15.78b) does not necessarily prove to be predictive of whether a treatment of OnaBTX-A will be successful.[62] It is the length of the platysma, the extent of muscle flaccidity, and the degree of muscle hypertrophy that seem to be the predictive factors that mostly influence the success rate of a treatment of OnaBTX-A in the neck. In fact, flaccid neck bands that are heavy and loose can be made worse with injections of OnaBTX-A (Figure 15.77).

In patients who experience suboptimal results with residual banding and asymmetric draping of the anterior neck skin after

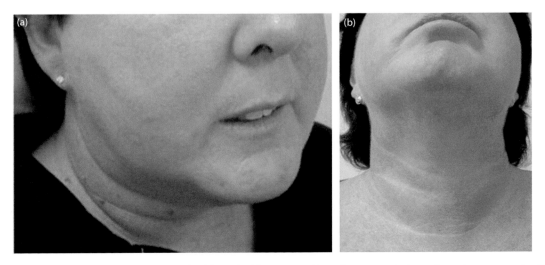

Figure 15.81 (a, b) The significant amount of fat in between bands of the neck of this 49-year-old may be more conducive to alternative treatment, i.e., liposuction.

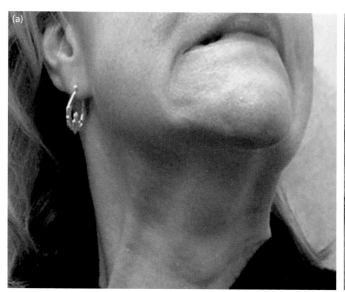 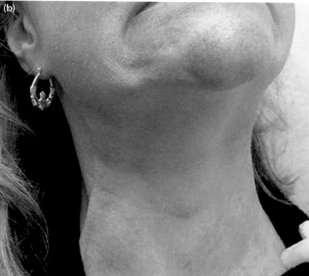

Figure 15.82 A 52-year-old patient is seen (a) before and (b) 3 weeks after treatment with OnaBTX-A.

rhytidectomy, injections of OnaBTX-A can help normalize these types of unwanted outcomes. The additional benefit of a slight elevation of the lower lip and buccal commissures and a tightening of lower cheek jowl has been known to occur.[62,63,67] This effect of lower face lifting takes place when OnaBTX-A diffuses from the fibers of the upper platysma pars mandibularis into the decussating fibers of the depressor anguli oris and the platysma (pars labialis), which are immediately subjacent to the mandible during injections of platysmal bands.[62,63,67] This allows for compensatory muscle contractions by the zygomaticus major, levator anguli oris, and risorius, contributing to a "mini-chemical face lift." This relaxation of the upper platysma (pars mandibularis), along with a secondary tightening of the cerviofacial angle[62,63,67] was recently described as the Nefertiti lift.[53]

Complications (Adverse Sequelae) When Treating Horizontal Lines and Vertical Bands of the Neck (see Appendix 6)

Treatment of horizontal rhytides and vertical bands in the neck with OnaBTX-A usually is very safe, and there is a very low incidence of untoward sequelae, provided the injections are place intradermally. When complications do occur, however, they usually are the result of improper technique and overzealous dosing.

Since the underlying nine muscles of deglutition, phonation, and neck flexion are also cholinergic in origin, overdosing with OnaBTX-A when treating the neck bands can result in xerostomia, dysphagia, dysphonia, dysarthria, and neck weakness.[62,69,70] The static wrinkles caused by solar elastosis and age usually are not affected by OnaBTX-A. Injections of more than 50 U of OnaBTX-A in the neck increases the risk for temporary hoarseness and difficulty with swallowing (dysphagia). Older patients are more at risk for such complications because they present with more wrinkling and banding of their necks and commonly require higher doses of OnaBTX-A to achieve satisfactory results. They also have a diminution in the soft tissue support of the neck, making it easier for the OnaBTX-A to diffuse to other deeper muscles of the neck, which will affect deglutition, speech, and the overall strength of the neck in keeping it upright, especially if the sternocleidomastoid is weakened. Similar complications can be produced in younger patients when OnaBTX-A is injected too deeply, because it can affect the deeper musculature of the neck.

In patients treated for cervical dystonia in whom over 200 U of OnaBTX-A commonly are injected into the strap muscles of the neck during one treatment session, dysphagia, hoarseness, dry mouth, and flu-like syndromes have been frequently observed.[62,63,70–72]

When OnaBTX-A is injected in the neck only to reduce platysmal banding and transverse rhytides, mild and transient neck discomfort can occur 2–5 days after treatment, with only a rare occurrence of neck weakness experienced with head elevation and flexion.[62] Only 1 patient out of 1500 in a multiple center treatment study experienced clinically significant dysphagia, which resolved spontaneously within 2 weeks. Profound dysphasia was reported in 1 patient when more than 75–100 U of OnaBTX-A were used to treat platysmal bands during one treatment session.[73] A nasogastric tube was temporarily required to feed the patient until she could swallow without assistance.

Commonly observed and expected side effects include transient edema and erythema, both of which usually resolve within 1–2 days. Postinjection ecchymoses may last a few days longer. Other less commonly occurring adverse sequelae can include muscle soreness or neck discomfort and mild headache. A few patients complain of either difficulty or, in extreme cases, an inability to lift the head from the supine position and then to keep it still, steady, and upright. When OnaBTX-A injections are placed less than 1–2 cm beneath the menton at the inferior margin of the mandible, centrally, fibers of the depressor labii inferioris can be weakened by spread of the product. This can cause a reduction in the strength of the lower lip and the integrity of perioral sphincteric balance (Figure 15.73). For many patients, the cost–benefit ratio is not significant enough to make this procedure a regularly sought-after treatment.

Figures 15.83 through 15.86 are additional examples of different patients treated with OnaBTX-A for horizontal lines and vertical bands of the neck.

Treatment Implications When Injecting the Neck

1. Superficial intradermal injections of OnaBTX-A can diminish horizontal wrinkles and vertical bands of the neck.
2. The platysma lies superficial to the muscles of deglutition and neck flexion while deep injections of large amounts of OnaBTX-A too low down the neck can weaken these muscles and cause varying degrees of dysphonia, dysphagia, and an inability to raise the head and keep it steady and upright. Injections should not go below the level of the thyroid cartilage.

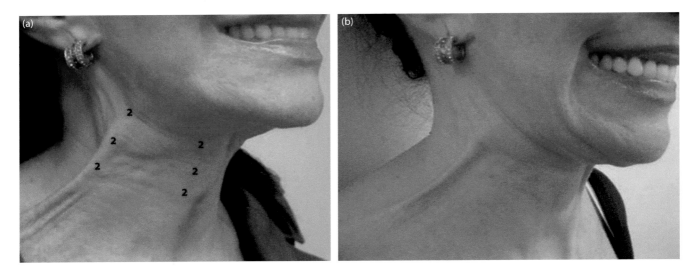

Figure 15.83 A 71-year-old patient is seen (a) before and (b) 3 weeks after treatment with OnaBTX-A.

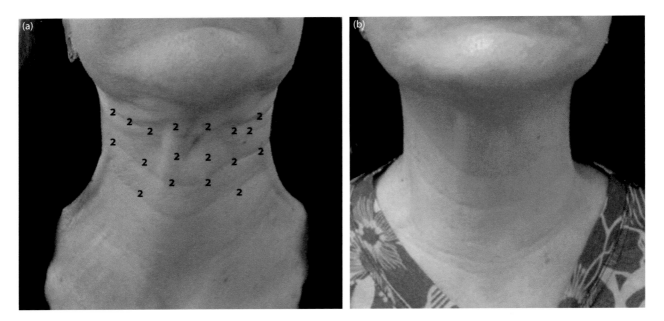

Figure 15.84 This 52-year-old patient (the same patient as in Figure 15.80) is seen (a) before and (b) 2 months after treatment with OnaBTX-A. Note the additional attenuation of the horizontal wrinkles.

3. Injecting the platysma pars mandibularis can affect the corners of the mouth, lower lip, chin, and inferior border of the mandible because of the interdigitation of platysmal fibers into the mimetic muscles of the lower face. Therefore, injections of onaBTX-A should start at least 1.5–2 cm below the mandibular border.

4. In older patients with lax, redundant skin and attenuated platysma fibers that are separated and form flaccid neck bands and cords, so-called "turkey neck deformity", injections of OnaBTX-A may enhance rather than diminish the appearance of those neck bands.

5. Injections of OnaBTX-A cannot correct the herniation of subplatysmal fat or reduce the fullness of excessive amounts of submental or submandibular fat.

6. Injections of OnaBTX-A should be applied at least 1.5–2.0 cm inferior to the mandibular origin of the depressor labii inferioris to prevent distortions of the skin of the chin and dysfunction of the lower lip.

7. Horizontal neck lines do not always completely efface with injections of OnaBTX-A, especially in an older person with lipodystrophy, and excessively lax and severely photodamaged skin.

UPPER CHEST AND DECOLLETE WRINKLING
Introduction: Problem Assessment and Patient Selection

When the fashion of women's clothing becomes more revealing, the décolleté takes on an entirely new significance, revealing the tell-tale skin surface changes caused by the innumerable number of hours one has spent in the sun, either at leisure or for work. Inelastic, sagging facial and neck skin that has been rejuvenated to a more youthful appearance by myorelaxation redraping and resurfacing techniques and with soft tissue fillers and implants will be marred by the appearance of the crepe paper-like wrinkling of the "V" of the upper chest. On the upper chest, both static and dynamic wrinkling can coexist. When they do, the person exhibiting them

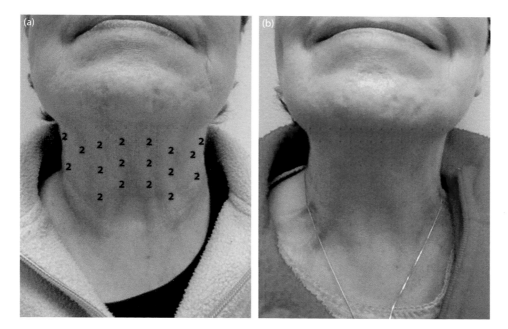

Figure 15.85 This 66-year-old patient is seen (a) before and (b) 2 weeks after treatment with OnaBTX-A. Note the dimpling of the mentalis, because it was mentalis was not treated in this patient.

appears deceptively older than their stated age, spoiling the youthful impression that is portrayed by a supple and wrinkle-free face and neck. Recently, superficial and middepth wrinkles on the upper anterior chest wall have been successfully treated with OnaBTX-A.[19,74,78]

There also have been reports describing the use of OnaBTX-A to relax postsurgical myospasm of the fibers of the pectoralis complex after breast implantation surgery.[75,76] Subsequently, there appeared a report describing the use of injections of AboBTX-A to reduce wrinkles of the lower anterior neck and upper chest wall attributed to the excessive contractions of the platysma.[76]

Functional Anatomy of Upper Chest and Decollete Wrinkling (see Appendix 2)

The platysma is composed of two separate paired broad, flat, thin sheets of muscle originating from the superficial fascia of the upper part of the thorax over the pectoralis major and deltoid, extending over the full length of the neck. In certain patients, the platysma can originate lower than the second, and as far down as the fourth to the sixth intercostal space (Figure 15.67). The platysma can vary considerably in thickness and extent; in general, women have a thinner platysma than men.[51] However, in some women when a large, thick and extensive platysma is in constant, hyperkinetic contraction,

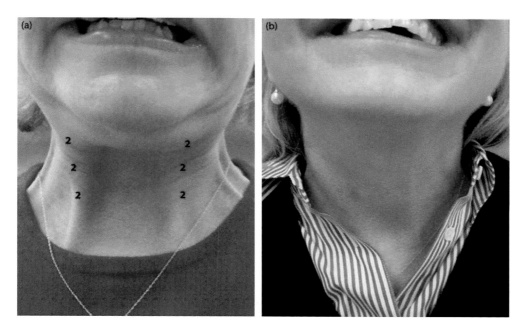

Figure 15.86 A 47-year-old patient (a) before and (b) 1 month after treatment of the platysmal bands with OnaBTX-A. The mentalis, depressor anguli oris, and perioral rhytides were also treated with OnaBTX-A.

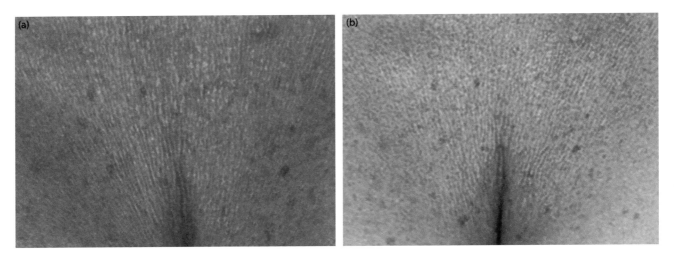

Figure 15.87 (a, b) Area of the central upper chest with extensive vertical and some horizontal wrinkling.

excessive horizontal and vertical wrinkling in the center of the chest, from mid to the lower décolleté can occur[75] (Figure 15.87). These changes are more commonly seen in individuals who have spent the better part of their daily activities and leisure time outdoors in low cut, revealing clothing.

Dilution When Treating Upper Chest and Decollete Wrinkling (see Appendix 3)

Because of the large surface area of the upper chest, a more extensive coverage of OnaBTX-A is necessary and widespread diffusion is encouraged. Therefore, a 100 U vial of OnaBTX-A can be reconstituted with 2–4 mL of normal saline.

Dosing: How to Correct the Problem (see Appendix 4), (What to Do and What Not to Do) When Treating Upper Chest and Decollete Wrinkling

The patient can be treated more comfortably in the semireclined rather than in the upright position. OnaBTX-A can be injected into each site on the anterior chest wall in several different treatment patterns. The key to a successful outcome is to have the OnaBTX-A diffuse throughout the entire anterior expanse of the upper chest wall.[75] Injections should be applied superficially into the deep dermis or at the dermosubcutaneous junction, particularly because the soft tissue

density of the chest is relatively thin. Intercostal muscle injection with OnaBTX-A must be avoided; otherwise, the patient may have severe difficulty with deep respirations. The pattern of injection depends on the particular shape of an individual's upper chest. Accordingly, the area to be treated is outlined as either an upside down isosceles or equilateral triangle, whose apex is at a point over the middle of the xiphoid process of the sternum and whose base is an imaginary line that connects two points placed over the middle of both clavicles (Figure 15.88).[74] This triangle corresponds to the points of interdigitation of the clavicular portion and the sternocostal portion of the platysma and pectoralis major. Approximately 2–4 U of OnaBTX-A are injected into the dermosubcutaneous plane at multiple sites that are roughly 1.5–2.0 cm apart from each other within the triangle. The total dose injected should range from 20 to 50 U (average is 35 U) of OnaBTX-A, depending on the overall strength of the platysma, the number and depth of the wrinkling, and the size and expanse of the anterior chest wall of the patient being treated. Some chests will require anywhere from 6 to 12 injection sites to be successfully treated.

Gentle massage and point pressure with ice to the area injected can prevent postinjection bleeding and ecchymoses. Severely photodamaged chest wall skin also needs to be treated by fractionated nonablative laser, light and energy-based devices that are readily available for such situations to assure the long-term success of BoNT-A treatments.

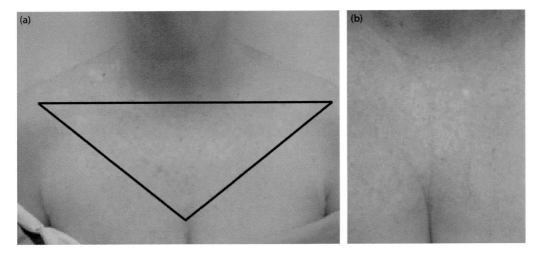

Figure 15.88 (a) An upside-down triangle represents the area where the OnaBTX-A can be injected to reduce wrinkling. (b) Note fine wrinkling on chest in close-up.

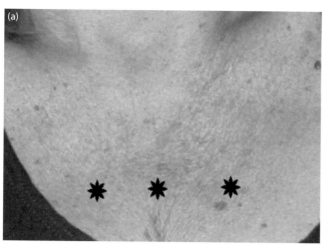 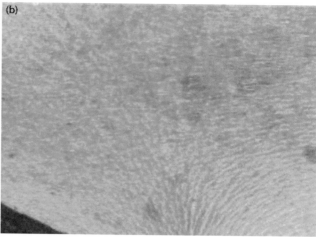

Figure 15.89 (a) Asterisks represent points where 5 U of OnaBTX-A were injected; (b) post-treatment. (Courtesy of Dr. Francisco Perez-Atamoros.)

Outcomes (Results) When Treating Upper Chest and Decollete Wrinkling (see Appendix 5)

A smoothening of the surface of the mid to lower décolleté usually occurs within 1–3 weeks after a treatment session of OnaBTX-A (Figures 15.89 through 15.91).

The diminution of chest wrinkling usually commences more slowly than when OnaBTX-A is injected in the face, and it may be effective for only 2–3 months (Figures 15.89 and 15.92). Widespread diffusion of the injected OnaBTX-A is necessary to achieve total coverage and complete reduction in the wrinkling of the skin surface of the upper chest wall. Therefore, injections in the upper chest wall are performed preferably with high volumes of low concentrations of OnaBTX-A.[38] For many patients with severely photodamaged skin of the upper chest wall, a combination of treatments with soft tissue fillers, laser, light and energy-based devices, and daily application of collagen enhancing cosmeceuticals along with regular OnaBTX-A injections is the only way to recapture a youthful decollete.

Complications (Adverse Sequelae) When Treating Upper Chest and Decollete Wrinkling (see Appendix 6)

The most common side effect reported when treating the decollete with OnaBTX-A is inadequate clinical results because of insufficient dosing. Additional adverse sequelae include a reduction in upper extremity muscle strength, especially on adduction and internal rotation as when performing a hugging motion. If OnaBTX-A is injected too deeply and at higher doses, exceeding 75–100 U per treatment session, unintended weakening of the intercostal musculature can occur, which may interfere with deep respiration. This absolutely needs to be avoided in both young patients who are physically active in sports and during routine daily activities, and in older patients who may already suffer from some sort of respiratory compromise.

The clinical results of pectoral platysma weakening can take up to 15 days or longer to occur, a much slower onset of effect compared to that which occurs after OnaBTX-A injections of facial muscles.[76,77] The more severely photodamaged the skin of the chest, the more readily bruising occurs with the injections of OnaBTX-A no matter how carefully the treatements are performed. The other frustrating adverse result is the quantity and the cost of so much OnaBTX-A that often produces so little appreciable changes. Therefore, for many, the cost–benefit ratio is not an incentive to have this procedure performed on a regular basis.[77]

Treatment Implications When Injecting the Upper Chest

1. Injections of high-volume, low concentration OnaBTX-A in the upper "V" of the anterior chest wall can suppress the fine surface wrinkling of the skin of the decollete.

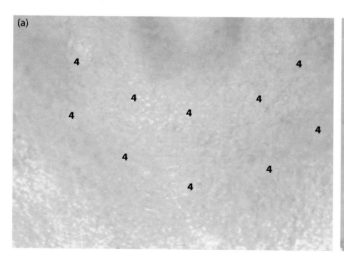 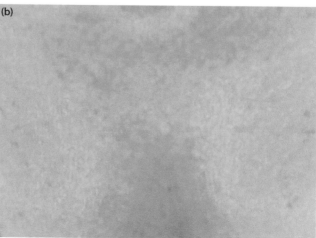

Figure 15.90 (a) Area of the central upper chest of a 56-year-old treated with OnaBTX-A before and (b) 5 weeks after treatment. (Courtesy of Dr. Francisco Perez-Atamoros.)

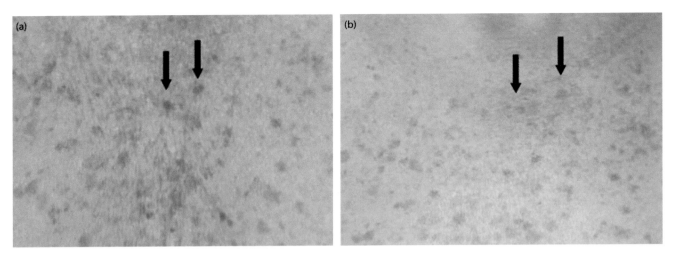

Figure 15.91 (a) Area of the central upper chest of a 49-year-old treated with OnaBTX-A before and (b) 6 weeks after 42 U of OnaBTX-A were injected. (Courtesy of Dr. Francisco Perez-Atamoros.)

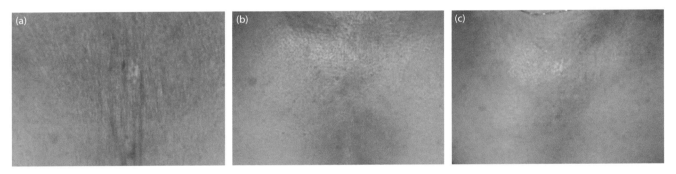

Figure 15.92 Area of the central upper chest which has been treated with OnaBTX-A: (a) before; (b) 2 weeks after; and (c) 4 weeks after.

2. Induction of effect after a treatment with OnaBTX-A in the upper chest wall takes longer and lasts for a shorter amount of time compared to OnaBTX-A injections in the face.

3. Overdosing OnaBTX-A can cause difficulty with deep inspiration or with adducting the upper extremities, as is done when one performs a hug.

4. Injections of OnaBTX-A must be performed intradermally to prevent weakening of the intercostal musculature and difficulty with deep inspiration.

5. For many individuals, the cost and questionable benefit of having the upper chest treated with OnaBTX-A to diminish fine wrinkling is not conducive to frequent and regular treatments.

6. Combination treatments with fillers, laser, light and energy-based devices along with OnaBTX-A is the only way patients with severely photodamaged skin of the upper chest will be able to realize a noticeable rejuvenation of the decollete.

7. Injecting severely photodamaged skin of the upper chest can cause easy bruising no matter how carefully and gently the injections are performed.

REFERENCES

1. Azib N, Charrier JB, de Saint Cyr BC et al. *Anatomy & Lip Enhancement*. Master Collection Volume 4. Paris, France: Expert 2 Expert SARL; 2013.

2. Freiman A, Bird G, Metelitsa AI et al. Cutaneous effects of smoking. *J Cutan Med Surg* 2004; 8(6): 415–23.

3. Paes EC, Teepen HJ, Koop WA, Kon M. Perioral wrinkles: Histologic differences between men and women. *Aesthet Surg J* 2009; 29(6): 467–72.

4. Standring S (ed). *Gray's Anatomy. The Anatomical Basis of Clinical Practice*, 41st ed. New York: Elsevier; 2016.

5. Lamilla GC, Ingallina FM, Poulain B, Trevidic P. *Anatomy and Botulinum Toxin Injections*. Master Collection Volume 1. Paris, France: Expert 2 Expert SARL; 2015.

6. Rogers CR, Meara JG, Mulliken JB. The philtrum in cleft lip: Review of anatomy and techniques for construction. *J Craniofac Surg* 2014; 25(1):9–13.

7. Mulliken JB, Pensler JM, Kozakewich HP. The anatomy of Cupid's bow in normal and clef lip. *Plast Reconstr Surg* 1993; 92: 395–403.

8. Vinkka-Puhakka H, Kean MR, Heap SW. Ultrasonic investigation of the circumoral musculature. *J Anat* 1989; 166: 121–33.

9. Latham RA, Deaton TG. The structural basis of the philtrum and the contour of the vermillion border: A study of the musculature of the upper lip. *J Anat* 1976; 121(1): 151–60.

10. Bo C, Ningbei Y. Reconstruction of upper lip muscle system by anatomy, magnetic resonance imaging, and serial histological sections. *J Craniofac Surg* 2014; 25: 48–54.

11. Baker SR. *Local Flaps in Facial Reconstruction*, 2nd ed. Philadelphia: Mosby; 2007.

12. Rogers CR, Mooney MP, Smith TD et al. Comparative microanatomy of the orbicularis oris muscle between chimpanzees and humans: Evolutionary divergence of lip function. *J Anat* 2009; 214: 36–44.

13. Zufferey JA. Importance of the modiolus in plastic surgery. *Plast Reconstr Surg* 2002; 110(1): 331–4.

14. Salasche SJ, Bernstein G, Senkarik M. *Surgical Anatomy of the Skin*. Connecticut: Appleton & Lange; 1998.

15. Yu SK, Lee MH, Kim HS et al. Histomorphologic approach for the modiolus with reference to reconstructive and aesthetic surgery. *J Craniofac Surg* 2013; 24: 1414–17.

16. Rubin LR, Mishriki Y, Lee G. Anatomy of the nasolabial fold: The keystone of the smiling mechanism. *Plast Reconstr Surg* 1989; 83: 1–10.

17. Al-Hoqail RA, Abdel Meguid EM. An anatomical and analytical study of the modiolus: Enlightening its relevance to plastic surgery. *Aesthet Plast Surg* 2009; 33: 147–52.

18. Choi YJ, Kim JS, Gil YC et al. Anatomical considerations regarding the location and boundary of the depressor anguli oris muscle with reference to botulinum toxin injection. *Plast Recontr Surg* 2014; 134: 917–21.

19. Atamoros FP. Botulinum toxin in the lower one third of the face. *Clinics in Dermatol: Botulinum Toxin in Clinical Medicine (Part 1)* 2003; 21: 505–12.

20. Fagien S. BOTOX® for the treatment of dynamic and hyperkinetic facial lines and furrows: Adjunctive use in facial aesthetic surgery. *Plast Reconstr Surg* 1999; 103: 701–13.

21. Carruthers JA, Glogau RG, Blizter A. Advances in facial rejuvenation: Botulinum toxin type A, hyaluronic acid dermal fillers and combination therapies – consensus recommendations. *Plast Reconstr Surg* 2008; 121(5 Suppl): 5s–30s.

22. Carruthers J, Fagien S, Matarasso SL et al. Consensus recommendations on the use of botulinum toxin type A in facial aesthetics. *Plast Reconstr Surg* 2004; 114(Suppl 6): 1s.

23. Smychyshyn N, Sengelmann R. Botulinum toxin a treatment of perioral rhytides. *Dermatol Surg* 2003; 29: 490–5.

24. Cohen JL, Dayan SH, Cox SE et al. OnabotulinumtoxinA dose-ranging study for hyperdynamic perioral lines. *Dermatol Surg* 2012; 38: 1497–1505.

25. Coleman KR, Carruthers J. Combination therapy with BOTOX and fillers: The new rejuvenation paradigm. *Dermatol Ther* 2006; 19(3): 177–88.

26. Carruthers J, Carruthers A, Moheit GD et al. Multicenter, randomized, parallel-group study of onabotulinumtoxinA and hyaluronic acid dermal fillers (24-mg/mL smooth, cohesive gel) alone and in combination for lower facial rejuvenation: Satisfaction and patient-reported outcomes. *Dermatol Surg* 2010; 36(Suppl 4): 2135–45.

27. Klein AW. Complications and adverse reactions with the use of botulinum toxin. *Seminars Cut Med Surg* 2001; 20: 109–20.

28. Alam M, Dover JS, Klein AW et al. Botulinum A exotoxin for hyperfunctional facial lines. Where not to inject. *Arch Dermatol* 2002; 138: 1180–5.

29. Mazzuco R. Perioral wrinkles. In Hexsel D, de Almeida ART, (eds). *Cosmetic Use of Botulinum Toxin*. Porto Allergre, Brazil: AGE Editora; 2002.

30. Rubin LR. The anatomy of a smile: Its importance in the treatment of facial paralysis. *Plast Reconstr Surg* 1974; 53: 384–7.

31. Rubin LR. The anatomy of the nasolabial fold: The keystone of the smiling mechanism. *Plast Reconstr Surg* 1999; 103: 687–91.

32. Mazzuco R, Hexsel D. Gummy smile and botulinum toxin: A new approach based on the gingival exposure area. *J Am Acad Dermatol* 2010; 63: 1042–51.

33. Benedetto AV. Asymmetric smiles corrected by botulinum toxin serotype A. *Dermatol Surg* 2007; 33(Suppl 1): s32–s36.

34. Lindsay RW, Edwards C, Smithson C et al. A systematic algorithm for the management of lower lip asymmetry. *Am J Otolaryngol* 2011; 32(1): 1–7.

35. Hur MS, Kim HJ, Lee KS. An anatomic study of the medial fibers of depressor anguli oris muscle passing deep to the depressor labii inferioris muscle. *J Craniofac Surg* 2014; 25: 214–6.

36. Hur MS, Hu KS, Cho JY et al. Topography and location of the depressor anguli oris muscle with a reference to the mental foramen. *Surg Radiol Anat* 2008; 30: 403–7.

37. Carruthers JD, Glogau RG, Blitzer A. Advances in facial rejuvenation: Botulinum toxin type A, hyaluronic acid dermal fillers, and combination therapies – consensus recommendations. *Plast Reconstr Surg* 2008; 121: 5s–36s.

38. Carruthers J, Carruthers A. Aesthetic botulinum A toxin in the mid and lower face and neck. *Dermatol Surg* 2003; 29: 468–76.

39. Carruthers J, Carruthers A. Botulinum toxin A in the mid and lower face and neck. *Dermatol Clin* 2004; 22: 151–8.

40. Trevidic P, Sykes J, Criollo-Lamilla G. Anatomy of the lower face and botulinum toxin injections. *Plast Reconstr Surg* 2015; 135(Suppl 5): 84s–91s.

41. Pessa JE et al. The anatomy of the labiomandibular fold. *Plast Reconstr Surg* 1998; 101(2): 482–6.

42. Blitzer A, Brin MF, Green PE et al. Botulinum toxin injection for the treatment of oromandibular dystonia. *Ann Otol Rhinol Laryngol* 1987; 98: 93–7.

43. Loos BM, Mass CS. Relevant anatomy for botulinum toxin in facial rejuvenation. *Facial Plast Surg Clin N Am* 2003; 11: 439–43.

44. Papel ID, Capone RB. Botulinum toxin A for mentalis muscle dysfunction. *Arch Facial Plast Surg* 2001; 3: 268–9.

45. Rohrich RJ, Pessa JE. The fat compartments of the face: Anatomy and clinical implications for cosmetic surgery. *Plast Reconstr Surg* 2007; 119(7): 2219–27.

46. Sposito MM. New indications for botulinum toxin type A in cosmetics: Mouth and neck. *Plast Reconstr Surg* 2002; 110(2): 601–11.

47. Carruthers A, Carruthers J. Clinical indications and injection technique for the cosmetic use of botulinum A exotoxin. *Dermatol Surg* 1998; 24: 1189–94.

48. Hoefflin SM. The platysma aponeurosis. *Plast Reconstr Surg* 1996; 97: 1080–8.

49. Hoefflin SM. Anatomy of the platysma and lip depressor muscles. A simplified mnemonic approach. *Dermatol Surg* 1998; 24: 1225–31.

50. Ellengbogen R, Karin JV. Visual criteria for success in restoring the youthful neck. *Plast Reconstr Surg* 1980; 66: 826–37.

51. Petrus GM, Lewis D, Maas CS. Anatomic considerations for treatment with botulinum toxin. *Facial Plast Surg Clin N Am* 2007; 15: 1–9.

52. Vistnes LM, Souther SG. The anatomical basis for common cosmetic anterior neck deformities. *Ann Plast Surg* 1979; 2: 381–8.

53. Levy PM. The "Nefertiti lift:" A new technique for specific re-contouring the jawline. *J Cos Las Ther* 2007; 9: 249–52.

54. Levy PM. Neurotoxins: Current concepts in cosmetic use on the face and neck–jawline contouring/platysma bands/necklace lines. *Plast Reconstr Surg* 2015; 136(Suppl 5):80s–83s.

55. Mulholland RS. Nonexcisional, minimally invasive rejuvenation of the neck. *Clin Plast Surg* 2014; 41:11–31.

56. Rohrich RJ, Rios JL, Smith PD et al. Neck rejuvenation revisited. *Plast Reconstr Surg* 2006; 118(5): 1251–63.

57. Cardoso de Castro C. The anatomy of the platysma muscle. *Plast Reconstr Surg* 1980; 66(5): 680–3.

58. Pogrel AM et al. Anatomic evaluation of anterior platysma muscle. *Int J Oral Maxillafac Surg* 1994; 23: 170–3.

59. Janfaza P, Nadol JB, Galla HJ et al. *Surgical Anatomy of the Head and Neck*. Philadelphia: Lipincott Williams and Wilkins; 2001.

60. Cardoso de Castro C. The changing role of platysma in face lifting. *Plast Reconstr Surg* 2000; 105: 764–75.

61. Brandt FS, Boker A. Botulinum toxin for rejuvenation of the neck. *Clin Dermatol* 2003; 21: 513–20.

62. Matarasso A, Matarasso SL, Brandt FS et al. Botulinum A exotoxin for the management of platysma bands. *Plast Reconstr Surg* 1999; 103: 645–52.

63. Brandt FS, Bellman B. Cosmetic use of botulinum A exotoxin for the aging neck. *Dermatol Surg* 1999; 24: 1232–4.

64. de Almeida ART, Romiti A, Carruthers JDA, The facial platysma and its underappreciated role in lower face dynamics and contour. *Dermatol Surg* 2017; 0:1–8.

65. Bae GY, Yun YM, Seo K et al. Botulinum toxin injection for salivary gland enlargement evaluated using computed tomographic volumetry. *Dermatol Surg* 2013; 39: 1404–07.

66. Carruthers J, Carruthers A. Botulinum toxin (BOTOX®) chemodenervation for facial rejuvenation. *Facial Plast Surg Clin N Am* 2001; 9(2): 197–204.

67. Blitzer A. Botulinum neurotoxin A for the management of lower facial lines and platysmal bands. In: Lowe, ed. *Textbook of Facial Rejuvenation: The Art of Minimally Invasive Combination Therapy.* London: Martin Dunitz; 2002.

68. Kane MAC. Nonsurgical treatment of platysmal bands with injection of botulinum toxin A. *Plast Reconstr Surg* 1999; 103(2): 656–63.

69. Kane MAC. Nonsurgical treatment of platysma bands with injection of botulinum toxin A revisited. *Plast Reconstr Surg* 2003; 112(Suppl 5): s125–s126.

70. Klein AW. Complications and adverse reactions with the use of botulinum toxin. *Sem Cut Med Surg* 2001; 20: 109–20.

71. Blitzer A, Binder WJ, Aviv JE. The management of hyperfunctional facial lines with botulinum toxin: A collaborative study of 210 injection sites in 162 patients. *Arch Otolaryngol Head Neck Surg* 1997; 123: 389–92.

72. Vartanian AJ, Dayan SH. Complications of botulinum toxin A use in facial rejuvenation. *Facial Plastic Surgery Clinics of North America: Botox* 2003; 11(4): 483–92.

73. Vartanian AJ, Dayan SH. Complication of botulinum toxin A use in facial rejuvenation. *Facial Plast Surg Clin N Am* 2005; 13: 1–10.

74. Benedetto AV. Commentary: Botulinum toxin in clinical medicine: Part II. *Clin Dermatol* 2004; 22(1):1–2.

75. Carruthers J, Fagien S, Matarasso S. Consensus recommendations on the use of botulinum toxin type A in facial aesthetics. *Plast Reconstr Surg* 2004; 114(Suppl): 15–25.

76. Isaac C, Gimenez R, Ruiz RO. Breast wrinkles (décolleté folds). In: Hexsel D, de Almeida ART (eds). *Cosmetic Use of Botulinum Toxin*. Porto Allegre, Brazil: AGE Editora; 2002, 178–81.

77. Richards A, Ritz M, Donahoe S et al. BOTOX® for contractions of pectoral muscles. *Plast Reconstr Surg* 2001; 108: 270–1.

78. Becker-Wegerich PM, Rauch L, Ruzicka T. Botulinum toxin A: Successful decollete rejuvenation. *Dermatol Surg* 2002; 28: 168–71.

79. Benedetto AV. Botulinum toxin in clinical medicine. *Clin Dermatol* 2003; 21(6): 465–8.

80. Brennan PA, Mahadevan V, Evans BT, *Clinical Head and Neck Anatomy for Surgeons*, CRC Press: Boca; 2016.

81. De Almeida ART, Romiti A, Carruthers JDA. The facial platysma and its underappreciated role in lower face dynamics and contours, *Dermatol Surg* 2017; 0:1–8.

82. Benedetto AV, Cosmetic uses of BoNTs on the lower face, neck and upper chest. In: Benedetto A, ed., *Botulinum Toxins in Clinical Aesthetic Practice*, 2nd ed, London: Informa Healthcare; 2011, 173–8.

16 The use of botulinum toxin for the breast

Francisco Pérez Atamoros and Olga Macías Martínez

INTRODUCTION

The female breast is an important feature of the development of secondary sexual characteristics, serving the dual function of an end-organ, influenced by the endocrine system, and functioning as a secondary sex organ in humans. For this reason, it is frequently modified surgically in order to enhance volume, shape, and position. In this chapter, we will focus on breast aesthetics, and on nonsurgical techniques for improving the appearance of the female breast and/or some breast-associated conditions.[1]

ANATOMY

The adult female breast lies between the second and sixth/seventh ribs, and is located on the anterior chest wall between the subcutaneous fat of the skin and the superficial fascia of the pectoralis muscle (Figure 16.1). The shape and contour of the breasts is produced by dense connective tissue bands called *Cooper's ligaments*. These bands traverse the breast tissue and anchor themselves to the underlying skin and fascia.[1–3]

The upper central and medial portions of the breast lie over the pectoralis major muscle (Figure 16.2), with the lower portions of the breast covering the anterolateral serratus anterior muscle and the upper external oblique muscle, and fascia over the upper origins of the rectus abdominis muscle inferomedially.[2]

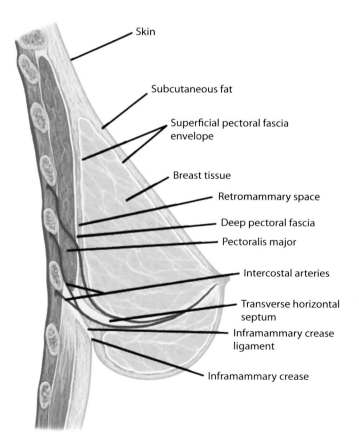

Figure 16.1 Anatomy of the breast. (With kind permission from Springer Science+Business Media: *Cosmetic Surgery: Art and Techniques*, 2013, 47–55, Prendergast P.)

Labels:
- Skin
- Subcutaneous fat
- Superficial pectoral fascia envelope
- Breast tissue
- Retromammary space
- Deep pectoral fascia
- Pectoralis major
- Intercostal arteries
- Transverse horizontal septum
- Inframammary crease ligament
- Inframammary crease

The pectoralis major is a thick, triangular-shaped muscle that covers most of the upper thoracic area, with two muscular heads, the clavicular and sternal heads that are separated by a cleft.[3]

The pectoralis minor muscle is covered by the pectoralis major muscle. This muscle is enveloped by the clavipectoral fascia that projects into the axilla to combine with the axillary fascia.[2,3]

The breast varies in shape and size depending on age, parity, body mass index, genetics, and race. They can be hemispherical, conical, teardrop-shaped, pendulous, or flattened. On profile, the aesthetically ideal female breast appears as a teardrop-shaped protuberance projecting at variable angles from the chest wall. Its ventral surface forms a line that is almost straight from the second rib to the nipple, while the lower part from the nipple to the inframammary crease is rounded. In the non-pendulous breast, the nipple is located over the fourth intercostal space. The inframammary crease represents the inferior border of the base of the breast and is an important aesthetic landmark.[4]

BREAST PTOSIS

In the normal growing phase, the breast can be considered to have a hemispheric shape, with the nipple in the middle, at the most prominent point. The breast mound and central pedicle will change position, according to gravity.

The breast mound develops a natural glide on the chest wall with age (Figure 16.3) and breast central and inferior pedicles follow the breast mound in its descending movement.[4]

Breast ptosis is one of the most common conditions treated by plastic surgeons. Despite practitioners' familiarity with the evaluation and treatment of breast ptosis, its underlying causes have not yet been clearly defined and preventative measures have not yet been discovered.[4–6]

In a 1976 review, Regnault cited glandular hormonal regression (postpartum or menopausal), weight loss, dermatochalasis, and postoperative changes as the causes of breast ptosis.[5]

In a book chapter published in 1990, Hinderer added two additional factors: weight of the breast totaling more than 400 g and ligamentous laxity. Such a list of causes, is the result of extensive experience and undoubtedly appeals to common sense, but has not been supported by scientific evidence.[5,6]

In 2010, Rinker found age, history of significant weight loss (50 lb), higher body mass index, larger brassiere cup size, number of pregnancies, and smoking history to be significant risk factors for breast ptosis. History of breast-feeding, weight gain during pregnancy, and lack of participation in regular upper body exercise were not found to be significant risk factors for ptosis.[6,7]

CLASSIFICATION OF FEMALE BREAST PTOSIS

Multiple classifications are in use, and it is important for the physician to distinguish which classification is being used. The classification of ptosis helps determine the type of treatment the patient needs.[5,6]

The standard classification for female breast ptosis has been that of Regnault from 1976 (Figure 16.4).[6,7]

- *First degree (minor ptosis)*: The nipple lies at the level of the submammary fold, above the lower contour of the gland and skin brassiere.
- *Second degree (moderate ptosis)*: The nipple lies below the level of the fold but remains above the lower contour of the breast and skin brassiere.

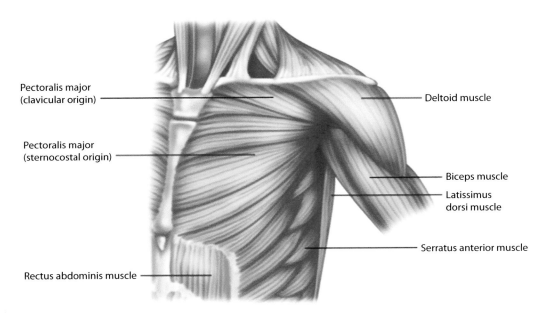

Figure 16.2 Anatomy of the breast, axilla, and chest wall. (With kind permission from Springer Science+Business Media: *Breast Disease: Conprehensive Management*, 2015, 1–22, Kalimuthu R et al.)

- *Third degree (major ptosis)*: The nipple lies below the fold level and at the lower contour of the breast and skin brassiere.
- *Pseudoptosis*: The nipple lies above the submammary fold level. The breast is not ptotic.

BOTULINUM TOXIN AND MECHANISM OF ACTION

The botulinum toxin (BoNT) molecule induces chemodenervation through its action on presynaptic neurons and inhibits acetylcholine release at the neuromuscular junction, leading to functional denervation of striated muscle for 2–6 months after injection. (See Chapter 7.)[8]

BOTULINUM TOXIN AND POSITION OF THE BREAST

Botulinum toxin could, in selected patients, produce a change in breast presentation such that the patient would obtain a breast lift nonsurgically.

In 2003, the author (FPA) conducted a study in which nearly 100 female patients between 30 and 55 years of age and with varying degrees of breast ptosis successfully achieved a noticeable elevation of the breasts (Personal communications, BOTOX®, Fillers & More, Vancouver, BC, August 2003; American Academy of Dermatology, Washington DC, February 2004, and April 2004 and *Botulinum Toxin in Clinical Dermatology*, 2006, 219–236).

The elevation of ptotic female breasts has been achieved averaging 1.1 cm with the maximum elevation being 1.8 cm. In this study, the author has noticed that the invariable distance measured between the sternal notch and the nipple does not change with the body position, thus ensuring a correct measurement of the elevation of the breast (Figure 16.5).

Muguea proposed to better define the position of the nipple-areola complex on the chest wall (Figure 16.6), that two inverted triangles be used, which are specific for the trunk as landmarks,

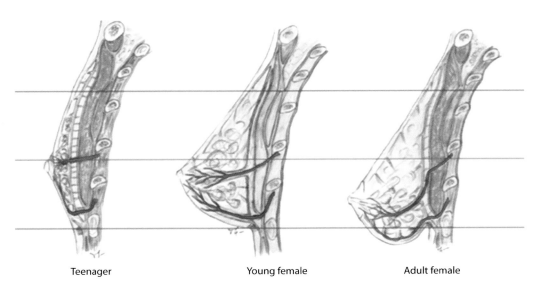

| Teenager | Young female | Adult female |

Figure 16.3 Changes in the breast mound position with age. The blue lines represent the breast mound limits and the red one the initial nipple level. (With kind permission from Springer Science+Business Media: *Aesthetic Surgery of the Breast*, 2015, 605–632, Mugea T.)

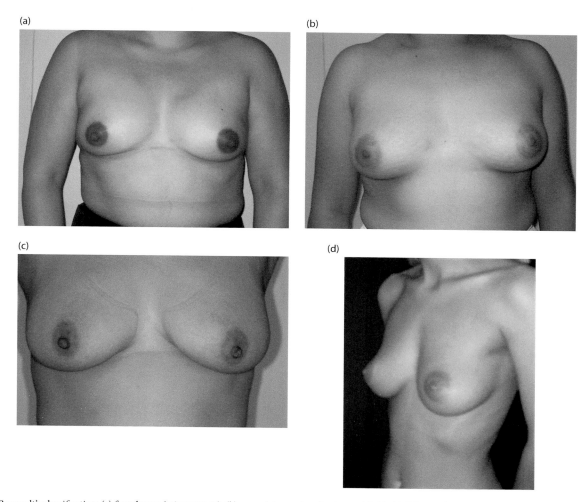

Figure 16.4 Regnault's classification: (a) first degree (minor ptosis); (b) second degree (moderate ptosis); (c) third degree (major ptosis); (d) pseudoptosis. (With kind permission from Springer Science+Business Media: *Aesthetic Surgery of the Breast*, 2015, 605–632, Mugea T.)

the acromio-pubian triangle (Ac-Pb-Ac) and the spino-manubrial triangle (Sp-Mn-Sp), which are defined by the lines between the manubrium (sternal notch) and the anterosuperior iliac spine points.[4]

Considering the natural evolution with aging, the normal nipple position is in a downward glide, on the external margins of the "inverted triangles," corresponding to a high position in young teenagers and to a low position in older female patients. The aesthetically perfect position is in the upper part of the triangles, close to the junction point of the external margins.[4]

The author (FPA) applied three injection points of 15 units of onabotulinumtoxinA/ incobotulinumtoxinA or 30 U of abobotulinumtoxinA

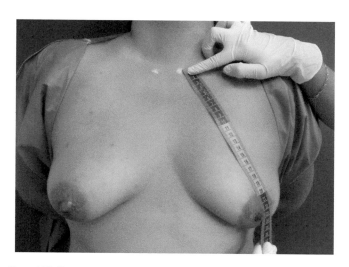

Figure 16.5 Correct measurement: distance between the sternal notch and nipple.

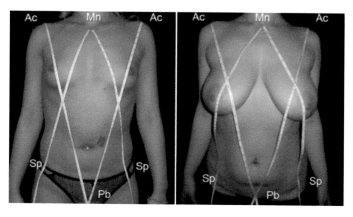

Figure 16.6 Nipple position related to the inverted triangles, acromio-pubian triangle (Ac-Pb-Ac) and the spino- manubrial triangle (Sp-Mn-Sp), in young female (a) and in mature female with breast ptosis (b). (With kind permission from Springer Science+Business Media: *Aesthetic Surgery of the Breast*, 2015, 605–632, Mugea T.)

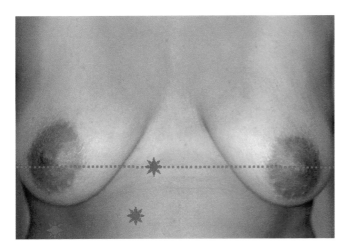

Figure 16.7 Right breast medium size "B" lift. Three injection points technique. Before treatment.

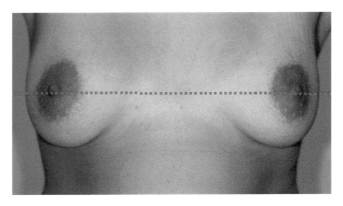

Figure 16.9 Same patient as in Figure 16.7, two weeks after left breast application and one month after right breast application of three injection points of 15 units of OnaBTX-A/IncoBTX-A or 30 U of AboBTX-A. Lift 1.8 mm.

into the inferior part of the pectoralis major which lies to the inferior part of the sternum and diaphragm (Figures 16.7 through 16.9). The total dose recommended per breast is 45–90 U of onabotulinumtoxinA (OnaBTX-A) and 90–180 U of AboBTX-A.

Each patient was injected with OnaBTX-A on only one side in this pilot study, with the contralateral side as control. Of 100 patients, 65 rated the results good to very good and 73 of the 100 patients would repeat the procedure. Five patients had pain which lasted longer than a week.

The ideal candidates for this treatment seem to be non-obese women with slightly rounded shoulders or who are slightly stooped forward, with breasts of cup size A or B. Older women, and those with larger breasts, tend to respond more slowly and to a lesser extent.

Recent refinements in the injection technique have led the author to suggest a different type of application (Figures 16.10 and 16.11) which consists of applying/injecting 10–15 U OnaBTX-A/IncoBTX-A or 20–30 U of AboBTX-A per injection at 5 points, with a total dose per breast of 50–75 ona/inco or 100–150 of AboBTX-A.

This new injection method allows the toxin to spread more readily/efficiently into the pectoralis major at the diaphragmatic and sternal union, which denervates the inferior part of the pectoralis. Without the opposing action of the inferior pectoralis muscle,

the force of the upper part of the pectoralis major is increased and moves all muscles in the direction of the shoulders, consequently lifting the breasts.

The proposed mechanism of action consists of relaxation of the inferior medial portion of the pectoralis major, which allows the superior portion to lift the ptotic breast.

We have seen in patients where this new technique is used, an increase in the average of the breast lifting, 2.5 cm with a maximum observed of 3.6 cm.

The benefits of botulinumtoxinA (BoNT-A) treatment usually develop over a period of 1–2 weeks, and persist for 3–4 months. The duration of the effect lasts somewhat longer than might be expected considering the relatively low doses of BoNT-A in proportion to the size of the muscles.

Some women have noted that there is a pleasing outward projection of their nipples which develops about a week after the OnaBTX-A treatment. The reason for this observation is not clear. However, OnaBTX-A has been shown to block the release of substance P (SP) and calcitonin gene-related peptide (CGRP) from the nerve terminal. Perhaps some of the injected BoNT-A makes its way from injection sites to the nipple-areolar complex and affects smooth muscle in the nipples by way of its effect on the release of SP and CGRP.[9]

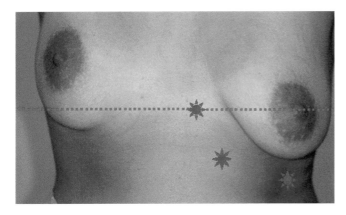

Figure 16.8 Same patient as in Figure 16.7, two weeks after treatment; right breast lifted 1.8 mm. Left breast medium size; three injection points of 15 units of OnaBTX-A/IncoBTX-A or 30 U of AboBTX-A.

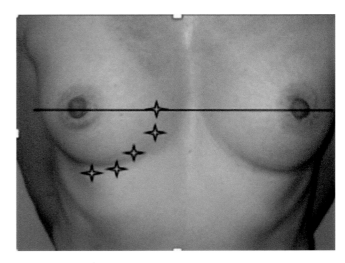

Figure 16.10 New technique proposed. 10–15 U per injection of OnaBTX-A/IncoBTX-A or 20–30 U of AboBTX-A per injection at 5 points. Before treatment.

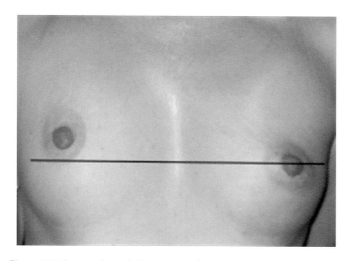

Figure 16.11 Same patient as in Figure 16.10 after treatment.

OTHER RECENT USES OF BOTULINUM TOXIN IN BREAST

Implant Stabilization and Capsular Formation

The most demanding complications involving aesthetic and reconstructive breast surgery are the malpositioning of the implant and capsular contracture. The etiology, prevention, and management remain to be fully explained. Botulinumtoxin administration has anti-inflammatory effects that can possibly decrease incidence of malrotation.[10] Sena et al. identified *in vitro* and *in vivo* negative effects of BoNT-A on capsule formation, by expression of TGF- β1 and differentiation of fibroblasts into myofibroblasts.[11]

Pectoral Muscle Spasm After Mastectomy and Post Mastectomy Pain Syndrome

In the past 10 years, reports on the use of BoNT-A for pain relief in a wide array of clinical conditions have increased tremendously. One of the most rapidly expanding indications for BoNT-A is in the treatment of various painful muscle spasms (e.g., para-vertebral muscle spasm, fibromyalgia-myofascial pain, temporomandibular joint pain, etc.). The explosion of interest in the biology and clinical applications of BoNT-A is reflected by the number of publications in the last few years on the subject.[12]

Concerning the use of botulinum toxin and its use in breast pain conditions such as post-mastectomy pain syndrome (PMPS) is a chronic pain condition, persisting for more than three months after breast surgery.[11] Pain can result from any surgical procedure, but this syndrome is more commonly associated with radical mastectomy with axillary lymphadenectomy. Although rare, in some patients, persistent spasms of the chest wall musculature develop after surgery.[12,13]

A possible etiology of the aforementioned patients' symptoms is suspected traction or manipulation of the medial pectoral nerve during reconstructive surgery, but no clear etiology has been ascertained. Neither patient had pectoral muscle spasms prior to the surgeries.[11–14]

Several studies and a systematic review[11] have been published to evaluate the effect of botulinum toxin on breast pain syndromes and pain syndromes after mammoplasty:

- A study revealed that patients who had OnaBTX-A injected into the pectoralis major before the placement of a silicone implant had less pain during recovery than those who did not receive the injection,[13]

- Three other cases reported the use of OnaBTX-A injections to treat pectoral muscle spasms after breast reconstruction or after breast implant surgery.[14,15]
- Two different cases of PMPS refractory to pain killers and intercostal nerve blocks were treated with percutaneous infiltration of OnaBTX-A under the anterior intercostal nerves. The result was the complete resolution of the syndrome.[16,17]

Pseudogynecomastia

Pseudogynecomastia is attributable to hypertrophy of the pectoralis major. This form is particularly evident in body builders, with the pectoralis major progressively enlarging due to hypertrophy of muscle fibers. In most cases, this is a desired and appreciated aspect, but it may be unpleasant for some individuals reporting a breast with a female appearance. When rapid reduction of muscular hypertrophy is desired to correct this form of pseudogynecomastia, OnaBTX-A injection represents a nonsurgical procedure for achieving it (Figures 16.12, 16.13, and 16.14).[18]

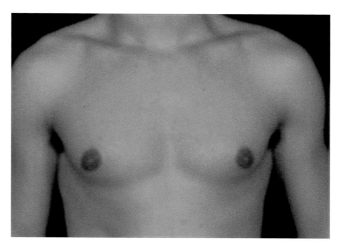

Figure 16.12 Pseudogynecomastia. Before treatment. (From Dessi L. et al. *Aesth Plast Surg* 2007; 31: 104–6, with permission.)

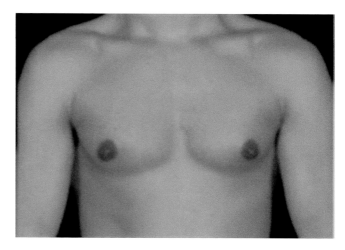

Figure 16.13 Same patient as in Figure 16.12 after treatment. (From Dessi L. et al. *Aesth Plast Surg* 2007; 31: 104–6, with permission.)

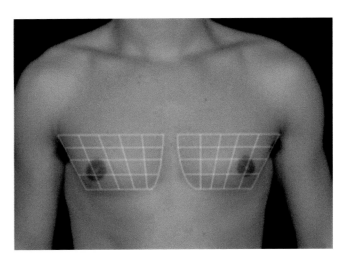

Figure 16.14 Schematic design of the OnaBTX-A injection sites in the pectoral areas (20 microinjections of 0.1 mL/2.5 U for each side). Total dose 100 U diluted with 4 mL of saline solution (From Dessi L. et al. *Aesth Plast Surg* 2007; 31: 104–6, with permission.)

CONCLUSION

The use of botulinum toxin in both aesthetic and reconstructive procedures involving the pectoralis major can be further expanded in other areas of the body. Consequently, this treatment is beneficial to female or male patients concerned with breast aesthetics (breast ptosis, pseudogynecomastia) as well as several medical conditions when other treatments have failed or are contraindicated. The effectiveness of BoNT treatments depends on the sum of mechanical forces exerted by the muscles and on the recently described analgesic, anti-inflammatory, and anti-proliferative effects of the botulinum toxin molecule.

Many patients could benefit from a temporary aesthetic improvement of the appearance of the breasts, which can be achieved with effective, safe, and non-surgical treatment with BoNT-A.

REFERENCES

1. Kalimuthu R, Yegiyants S, Brenzek C. Anatomy of the breast, axilla, and chest wall. In: *Breast Disease: Conprehensive Management*, A I Riker (ed.). Springer Science + Business Media, New York. 2015, 1–22.
2. Prendergast P. Anatomy of the breast. In: *Cosmetic Surgery: Art and Techniques*, M A Shiffman and A Di Giuseppe (eds.). Springer, Berlin. 2013, 47–55.
3. Hamdi M, Würinger E, Schlenz I, Kuzbari R. Anatomy of the breast: A clinical application. In: *Vertical Scar Mammoplasty*. Springer. 2005, 1–8.
4. Mugea T. New breast volume and ptosis classification. In: *Aesthetic Surgery of the Breast*, T Mugea and M A Shiffman (eds.). Springer Science + Business Media, New York. 2015, 605–32.
5. Regnault P. Breast ptosis, definition and treatment. *Clin Plast Surg* 1976; 3(2): 193–203.
6. Rinker B, Veneracion M, Walsh C. Breast ptosis causes and cure. *Ann Plast Surg* 2010; 64(5): 579–84.
7. Shiffman M. Classification of breast ptosis. In: *Breast Augmentation. Principles and Practice*, M A Shiffman (ed.). Springer Science + Business Media, New York. 2009, 251–255.
8. Wheeler A, Smith H. Botulinum toxins: Mechanisms of action, antinociception and clinical applications. *Toxicology*. 2013; 124–46.
9. Smith K, Pérez-Atamoros F. Other dermatologic uses of botulinum toxin. In: *Botulinum Toxin in Clinical Dermatology*, A V Benedetto (ed.). Taylor & Francis, UK. 2006, 219–36.
10. Irkoren S, Ozkan H, Ceylan E, Sivrioglu N, Tataroglu C, Durum Y. The effect of botox on the implant stabilization and capsular formation. *Ann Plast Surg* 2015; 75: 91–7.
11. Kim S, Moosang A, Piao Y, Choi D, Yi M, Shin N. Effect of botulinum toxin type A on TGF-beta/Smad pathway signaling: Implications for Silicone-induced capsule formation. *Plast Reconstr Surg* 2016; 138(5): 821e–829e.
12. Winocour S, Murad M, Bigdoli-Moghaddam M, Jacobson S, Bite U, Saint-Cyr M, Tran N, Lemaine V. A systematic review of the use of botulinum toxin type A with subpectoral breast implants. *J of Plastic, Recons Aesth Surg* 2014; 67: 34–41.
13. Gabriel A, Champaneria M, Maxwell P. The efficacy of Botulinum Toxin A in post-mastectomy breast reconstruction. A Pilot Study. *Aesth Surg J* 2015; 35(4): 402–9.
14. Cattin T. Botulinum toxin for Tethering of breast implants. *Plast Recons Surg*. Letters ahd view of points. 2005; 116(2): 687–8.
15. ÖDonnell C. Pectoral muscle spasms after mastectomy succesfully treated with botulinum toxin injections. *Phys Med and Rehab* 2011; 2011(3): 781–2.
16. Dessy L, Mazzocchi M, Scuderi N. Treatment of post Mastectomy pain syndrome after Mastopexy with botulinum toxin. *J Plast Reconstr Aesthet Surg* 2014; 67(6): 873–4.
17. de Carlos E, Cabezón A, Mosquera M, Rodríguez G, Ruiz-Soldevilla JM, Sancho B. Botulinum Toxin application for the pain control in breast cancer. *Rehabilitación (Madr)* 2012; 46(2): 112–9.
18. Dessi L, Curinga G, Mazzocchi M, Scuderi N. Treatment of muscular Pseudogynecomastia with Botulinum Toxin. Letter to the Editor. *Aesth Plast Srg* 2007; 31: 104–6.

17 Aesthetic use of botulinum toxin in Asians
Kyle K. Seo

INTRODUCTION

Individualized assessment and treatment are necessary before performing botulinum toxin injection for cosmetic use because there is significant variability among individuals in terms of facial shape and aesthetic needs. Dosages and injection points should be differentiated on the individual's muscle activity, pattern of muscle shape, and judgment of what is aesthetically appropriate in the context of the individual's overall facial shape and aesthetic needs. In such context, physicians should take a different approach when performing BoNT-A injection for Asians because there are marked ethnic differences between Asians and Caucasians. However, most publications have focused exclusively on Caucasian subjects. This chapter covers the ethnic differences between Asians and Caucasians for the aesthetic use of BoNT-A in terms of anatomy, appropriate dose, injection points, indications of BoNT-A, and aesthetic needs, thereby providing some practical guidelines for the aesthetic use of BoNT-A in Asians. However, Asia is a huge continent and Asians are not a uniform population. Therefore, this chapter does not cover ethnicities from Indian and Arab nations although these groups are often considered to be Asian in terms of their geographic location. Instead, this chapter mainly focuses on characteristics of East Asians and Southeast Asians.

Differences between Asians and Caucasians

Different Facial Shapes and Different Aesthetic Standards between Asians and Caucasians

Asians have a relatively wide, round, and flat face compared to Caucasians. Their faces tend to be wider and shorter with less anterior projection than Caucasian faces.[1] For this reason, Asians consider a smaller, narrower, and more three-dimensional face to be more attractive and so may wish to achieve this ideal using botulinum toxin. One of the most typical examples of this is treatment for masseter hypertrophy using botulinum toxin, which is not popular in western countries even though it was first developed in western countries more than 20 years ago.[2] This novel treatment helps Asians with a square-looking face to achieve a decreased facial width and "V" shape to their face in their front view. In a similar context, botulinum toxin treatment for temporalis hypertrophy and for the parotid gland enlargement, is also gaining more popularity among Asians as a method of decreasing facial width.

BoNT-A injection for widening the palpebral aperture (the eye-opening) is another typical example of the ethnic difference when considering treatment approaches between Asians and Caucasians. BoNT-A injection can remove the pretarsal bulge and slightly lower the inferior ciliary margin to widen the palpebral aperture.[3] From the viewpoint of Caucasians, this treatment may help Asians' smaller eyes to become bigger. Actually, this treatment is appealing to some Southeast Asians who regard almond shaped eyes as a beautiful hallmark because eliminating the pretarsal bulge creates more of an almond-shaped eye. However, it is important not to apply this treatment to East Asians, who consider pretarsal bulge one of the important hallmarks of female beauty.[4] The pretarsal muscular bulge is usually exaggerated when people smile by the action of the orbicularis oculi muscle. Therefore, it is called a "charming roll" in East Asians because the people with pretarsal muscular bulge when at rest look soft and friendly. Another reason for explaining the popularity of the "charming roll" in East Asians is that the "charming roll" brings the optical illusion of a "big eye" like double eyelid surgery in Asians with inherently smaller eyes. The purpose of the double eyelid surgery is

to create an upper eyelid with a crease (i.e., "double eyelid") from an eyelid that is naturally without a crease. Therefore, physicians even enhance the "charming roll" by the injection of filler in Asians. In such a context, BoNT-A injection for widening the palpebral aperture should be avoided in Asians.

Eyebrow "shaping" with BoNT-A, popular in Caucasians,[5,6] is also not recommended for East Asians, especially Koreans who consider flat eyebrows a beautiful shape for women.[7] High arched eyebrows are generally considered as tough looking in this region of Asia and are even called "Samurai eyebrows." Aesthetically high arched eyebrows may look unnatural in an Asian with wide facial shape. The "Korean look" sets a beauty standard in Asians due to the "Korean wave" influenced by Korean pop and Korean drama. Consequently, eyebrow "shaping" with BoNT-A resulting in high arched eyebrows is not recommended for Asians.

Three Asian Facial Types

Ethnic groups in East Asia and Southeast Asia can be classified into three Asian facial types as northern, intermediate, and southern type (Figure 17.1).[8] Northern facial types have a narrow palpebral fissure with no supratarsal crease, high and long nose with narrow nasal ala, prominent zygoma, well-developed mandibular angle which gives a square face or square jaw, and relatively white skin. Ethnic groups of northern type are individuals from Mongolia, Korea, and Northern China (Figure 17.1). Southern facial types have the wide palpebral fissure with a supratarsal crease, flat and short nose with wide nasal ala, less prominent zygoma, less developed bony mandibular angle which gives a narrow and oval facial shape, and relatively dark skin with a Fitzpatrick phototype of III to IV. Ethnic groups in Southern facial type are individuals from Southeast Asian countries such as the Philippines, Thailand, Indonesia, and so on. Intermediate types show intermediate characteristics between the northern type and southern type and may be seen in Southern China, Hong Kong, and Taiwan.

Of course, this classification does not cover all ethnicities in this region and mixed characteristics and variation exists even within the same ethnic group. For example, some Koreans show typical characteristics of the northern type, while others show characteristics of the southern type. In addition, it is possible for an Asian subject in one area to possess mixed characteristics of different facial types (Figure 17.2). Therefore, BoNT-A injection strategy in Asians should be guided individually and not just by facial type in their geographic region even though the Asian facial type is a good reference when planning BoNT-A injection.

Anatomic Differences between Asians and Caucasians

Asians generally tend to have a smaller muscle mass and less hyperdynamic activity compared to Caucasians. Specifically, Asians are reported to have shorter corrugator muscles than Caucasians. The smaller muscle mass of Asians seems to come not only from genetic differences[9] but also from cultural differences related to facial expression.[10] According to one paper analyzing facial expressions by videotaping, Asians tend to use their upper facial expression muscles less than Caucasians by up to 30%.[10] Moreover, Asians have fewer wrinkles, compared with Caucasians because Asians have a thicker dermis,[11] increased fat, and denser fat in comparison with Caucasians.[12] All these mean that lower doses of BoNT-A should be administered in Asians than in Caucasians.

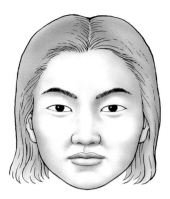 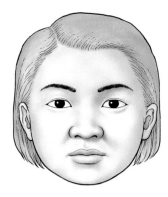 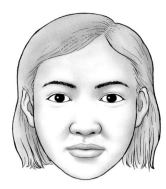

Figure 17.1 Three Asian facial types. Ethnic groups in East Asia and Southeast Asia can be simply classified into three Asian facial types as northern, intermediate, and southern types (from the left to the right). (From Sundaram H, Huang PH, Hsu NJ et al. Aesthetic applications of incobotulinumtoxinA in Asians: An international, multidisciplinary, pan-Asian consensus. *Plast Reconstr Surg Glob Open* 2016; 4(12); e872. With permission.)

Site Specific Differences

BOTOX is the only BoNT-A product used in this chapter.

Forehead Horizontal Lines

1. Asians require lower doses of BoNT-A since Asians have a smaller muscle mass and less hyperdynamic activity than Caucasians. Low initial doses from 3 U to 6 U are recommended

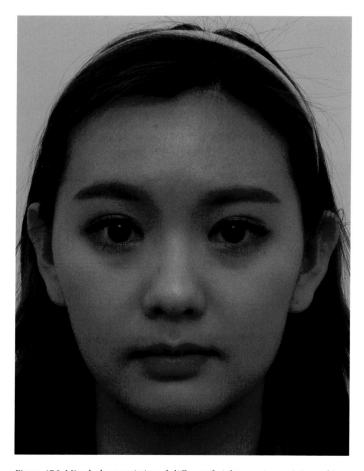

Figure 17.2 Mixed characteristics of different facial types in an Asian subject. A Korean woman shows prominent zygoma of northern facial type with round facial contour of intermediate facial type, while she has the southern characteristics such as wide palpebral fissure with a supratarsal crease and relatively short nose.

and no more than 12 U in total because of the risk of eyebrow ptosis.

2. Assessment for those at risk of eyebrow ptosis, for example, for patients with ptosis, or people who congenitally open their eyes with their frontalis, is a prerequisite because eyebrow ptosis is a more embarrassing side effect from the aesthetic viewpoint in Asians with inherently wider distance between the eyebrow and the palpebral fissure compared with Caucasians. Typical at-risk patients for eyebrow ptosis are older people, that is, in their fifties and above; these patients require a low initial dose from 2 U to 3 U.

3. *Injection points and techniques:* Generally, two rows of 6–7 injection points (IPs) are recommended (Figure 17.3a). Alternatives include three rows of injections for people with a high forehead (Figure 17.3b). Low initial doses from 3 U to 6 U are recommended and no more than 12 U in total because of the risk of eyebrow ptosis.

Glabellar Frown Lines

1. Asians require lower doses of BoNT-A since Asians have relatively shorter and narrower corrugator muscles compared to Caucasians[9] and also have less hyperdynamic activity than Caucasians.[10] Therefore, a 4-point injection pattern with injection of the medial corrugators and the procerus is generally recommended for Asian females instead of a standard 5-point pattern for Caucasians covering lateral parts of the corrugator.[13] Approximately 10–12 units (U) are usually recommended as an initial dose for glabellar frown lines. Of course, a 5-point injection pattern with 16–20 U could be appropriate for Asian subjects with greater muscle mass.

2. *Injection points and techniques*: Intramuscular injection into 4 IPs should be used (2 U of 2 IPs in the procerus and 3 U of 2 IPs in the medial part of corrugator) (Figure 17.4a). The standard Caucasian pattern for glabellar frown lines requires an additional 1–2 U at the mid-pupillary line for the lateral part of the corrugator (Figure 17.4b).

Lateral Canthal Rhytides (Crow's Feet)

1. Lower doses for lateral canthal rhytides are required in order to avoid an unnatural look since Asians with inherently smaller eye apertures look scary if they don't show any wrinkles around the eyes or their eye aperture doesn't become smaller when they smile

2. After injections of BoNT-A for the treatment of crow's feet, Asians with prominent zygomas and abundant premalar fat

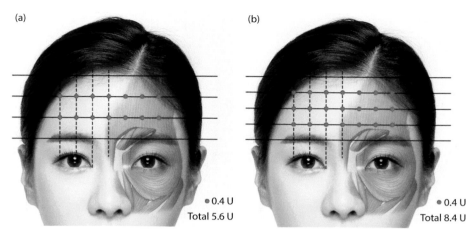

Figure 17.3 Injection points and dose of BoNT-A for forehead horizontal lines in Asians. (a) Injection points and dose of BoNT-A for two rows with 6–7 IPs per row. (b) Alternatives include three rows of injections for people with high foreheads. (Reproduced with permission from Seo K, *Botulinum Toxin for Asians*; Seoul Medical Publishing Ltd. 2014.)

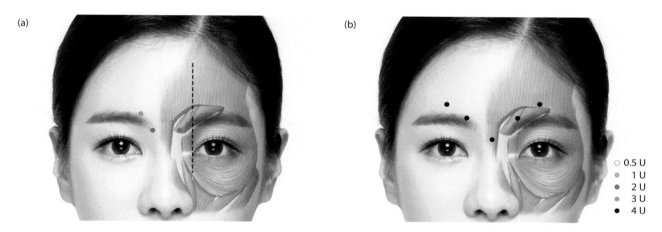

Figure 17.4 Injection points and dose of BoNT-A for glabellar frown lines. (a) Asian standard pattern with 4 IPs (2 U of 2 IP in the procerus and 3 U of 2 IP in the medial part of corrugator). (b) Standard Caucasian pattern with 5 IPs. (Reproduced with permission from Seo K, *Botulinum Toxin for Asians*; Seoul Medical Publishing Ltd. 2014.)

above the nasojugal groove tend to show more prominence of the lateral malar area when they smile because a weakened orbicularis oculi cannot elevate the lateral malar area further upward.[14] However, Asians generally hate more prominence of the lateral malar area. For those patients with a prominent zygoma and abundant premalar fat, injections at a lower part of the orbicularis oculi is unnecessary and injections in line with the lateral canthal line should be performed with a lower dose, that is, with only 0.5–1 U of BoNT-A.

3. *Injection points and techniques:* At least 3 IPs with 2 U per IP should be used, with an optional additional 1–2 IPs more and/or less than this, depending on the wrinkle pattern (Figure 17.5).

Infraorbital Wrinkles

1. It is important not to inject the pretarsal part of the orbicularis oris close to the lower ciliary margin because injections of BoNT-A into this area diminishes the pretarsal muscular bulge in Asians who consider it a hallmark of female beauty.

2. *Injection points and techniques:* IPs are usually recommended between the preseptal part and orbital part of the orbicularis oris. One row of 5–6 IP per eye, with a total of less than 2 U dose is recommended (Figure 17.5).

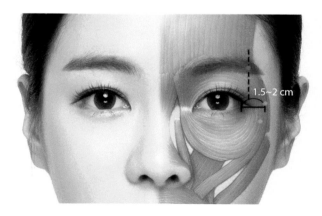

Figure 17.5 Injection points and dose of BoNT-A for lateral canthal rhytides and infraorbital wrinkles. At least 3 IPs with 2 U per IP should be used for lateral canthal rhytides, with an optional additional 1–2 IPs more and/or less than this, depending on the wrinkle pattern. One row of 5–6 IP per eye, with a total of less than 2 U dose is recommended for infraorbital wrinkle. (Reproduced with permission from Seo K, *Botulinum Toxin for Asians*; Seoul Medical Publishing Ltd. 2014.)

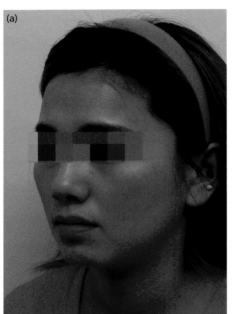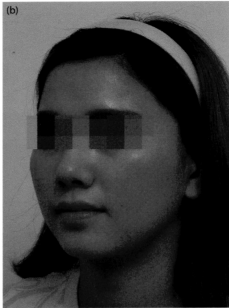

Figure 17.6 Before (a) and 2 weeks (b) after BoNT-A injection in a cobblestone chin (mentalis hyperactivity).

Cobblestone Chin

1. Asians usually tend to show stronger mentalis muscle activity than Caucasians. It is aesthetically important to reduce the mentalis activity by injections of BoNT-A since hyperactivity of the mentalis may aggravate the severity of a recessed and smaller chin in Asians (Figure 17.6).[15]

2. *Injection points and techniques:* Intramuscular injection with 4 U into 2 IPs 1 cm apart from the central line at the lower border of the chin is recommended. Two more injections with 2 U per IP above these are required subdermally (Figure 17.7).

Square jaw (Masseter Hypertrophy)

1. Botulinum toxin for masseteric hypertrophy was first reported in the Western literature in 1994.[2] However it didn't attract

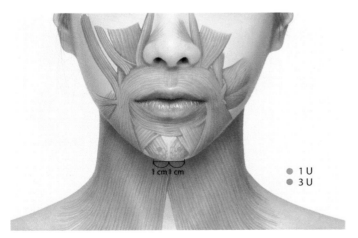

Figure 17.7 Injection points and dose of BoNT-A for cobblestone chin. Intramuscular injection with 4 U into 2 IPs 1 cm apart from the central line at the lower border of the chin is recommended. Two more injections with 2 U per IP above these are required subdermally. (Reproduced with permission from Seo K, *Botulinum Toxin for Asians*; Seoul Medical Publishing Ltd. 2014.)

much attention in western countries due to the general lack of need for its cosmetic application. In Asia, however, this novel technique has spread rapidly, owing to its advantages in terms of ensuring a quick and convenient procedure and an absence of social downtime compared to the conventional angular reduction bone surgery (Figure 17.8).

The main benefit from this novel indication for BoNT-A injections is to reduce the facial width and enhance the shape of the lower face from the frontal view. Anyone can achieve a reduced facial width to some extent by reducing the thickness of the masseter muscle since the thickness of the masseter muscle is known to be 0.8 cm in normal people and 1.3 cm in people with masseteric hypertrophy, respectively.[16]

2. The mechanism of action of BoNT-A in the treatment of masseteric hypertrophy is a type of disuse muscular atrophy. Therefore, this treatment results in a time lag both in onset and peak of action that differs from conventional treatment for wrinkles, where the onset of action begins after just 2–3 days and the peak effect is reached 1–2 weeks after injection. In clinical practice, the effect of BoNT-A for masseteric hypertrophy has an onset time of 2 weeks after injection, and the peak effect develops at 2–3 months after injection.[17,18]

3. Six months later, the muscle volume will usually have returned to some extent, and by 9–12 months postinjection, the muscle volume may approach its previous state. Therefore, repetition of BoNT-A treatment for the masseteric hypertrophy is recommended every 6 months for maintaining the best result, while 9–12 months' interval can be also possible considering the initial muscle volume as a guideline. However, the duration of the effect is variable and depends on the individual's personal habits, such as bruxism, unconscious jaw clenching, and excessive chewing of hard food.[19] There have also been many reports that the effects of BoNT-A in the treatment of masseteric hypertrophy can last for more than 1–2 years, even after only one session of injections.[20] This extended duration of the effect of BoNT-A is particularly noted in those subjects who have the acquired form of masseteric hypertrophy, as long as they avoid eating tough foods and do not have the habit of jaw clenching.

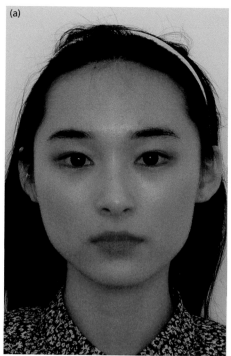 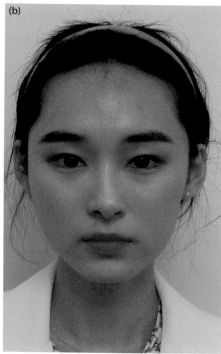

Figure 17.8 Before (a) and 3 months (b) after BoNT-A injection for a square jaw (masseter hypertrophy). (Reproduced with permission from Seo K, *Botulinum Toxin for Asians*; Seoul Medical Publishing Ltd. 2014.)

4. Proper assessment is also a prerequisite to screening at risk patients who may show unpleasing and undesirable results after BoNT-A injections for hypertrophic masseter reduction. A pre-existing sunken cheek may look more aggravated with the disappearance of the masseter muscle volume, which brings not only a fatigued and older look but also prominence of the zygoma. A pre-existing sagging jowl also tends to become more intense following this procedure because of a visual illusion. Patients at risk for such untoward results should be informed in advance of these possibilities and countermeasures with volumizing fillers for sunken cheeks and thread lifting for sagging jowls should be offered.

5. Mild temporary muscle weakness, resulting in difficulty with chewing, will occur after BoNT-A injections in a small proportion of subjects. However, this is temporary and chewing strength returns to normal within 3 months.[21]

6. For the cosmetic purpose of reshaping a lower facial contour, the lower part of the masseter under an imaginary line connecting the tragus to the corner of the mouth is the main target area for injections with BoNT-A since the lower part of the masseter is more important in lower facial contouring.

7. *Injection points and techniques:* Deep injections sufficient enough to touch the mandibular bone, rather than injections at a medium depth, are very important. Superficial injections can weaken the rizorius attached superficially to the anterior part of the masseter, causing embarrassing changes of facial expression, for example, an asymmetric unnatural smile. To reduce the risk of adverse changes of facial expression when treating masseteric hypertrophy, physicians should start by injecting at least 1 cm inside the anterior margin of the masseter muscle in addition to deep injection.

A safe and effective zone for injecting a square jaw and reducing the size of the masseter can be delineated by the upper margin being an imaginary line connecting the tragus to the corner of the mouth, the lower margin as the mandibular bony border, and the anterior and posterior margins as the anterior and posterior borders of each masseter muscle. IPs are at least 1 cm within these borders to avoid unwanted diffusion of BoNT-A into other facial muscles.

Four to six IPs of 5 U each are recommended depending on the muscle volume (Figure 17.9).

Temporalis Hypertrophy

1. While masseteric hypertrophy is an important factor for lower facial width, temporalis hypertrophy may contribute to the width of the upper face. Temporalis hypertrophy also can be improved by injections of BoNT-A producing the same disuse muscular atrophy as in masseteric hypertrophy. For Asians with wide faces, BoNT-A for temporalis hypertrophy can camouflage their congenital characteristics in terms of reducing the facial width (Figure 17.10).[22]

2. *Injection points and techniques:* Deep injections sufficient to touch the bone, rather than injections that are at medium depth, are recommended. An effective injection zone for temporalis hypertrophy can be delineated by the lower margin being an imaginary line connecting the upper margin of helix to the tail of the eyebrow and the posterior margins as an imaginary vertical line parallel to the tragus. Five to eight IPs of 5 U are recommended depending on the thickness of the muscle (Figure 17.11). Injection of BoNT-A should be focused into the muscle bulge at the superior temporal fusion line since the upper part of the temporalis is more important in upper facial contour.

3. A pre-existing temporal hollow may become aggravated with the disappearance of the temporalis fullness. However, this would be treated by filler revolumization or fat grafting. Mild, temporary muscle weakness, such as difficulty with chewing, will occur after BoNT-A injections in a

303

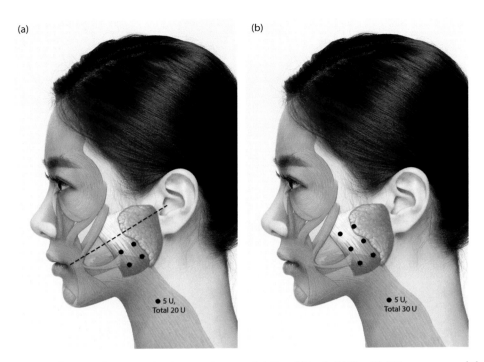

Figure 17.9 Injection points and dose of BoNT-A for a square jaw (masseter hypertrophy). Four (a) to six (b) IPs with 5 U are recommended, depending on the muscle volume. (Reproduced with permission from Seo K, *Botulinum Toxin for Asians*; Seoul Medical Publishing Ltd. 2014.)

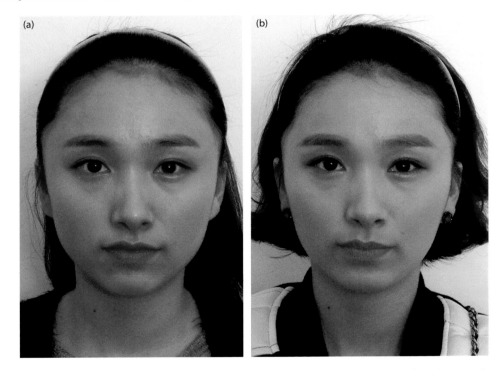

Figure 17.10 Before (a) and 3 months (b) after BoNT-A injection for temporalis hypertrophy. (Reproduced with permission from Seo K, *Botulinum Toxin for Asians*; Seoul Medical Publishing Ltd. 2014.)

small proportion of patients, especially when combined with BoNT-A injections for masseteric hypertrophy. However, this is also temporary.

Parotid Gland Enlargement

1. Enlarged parotid glands can contribute to a square-shaped lower face appearance. Because acetylcholine, the neurotransmitter in the salivary glands, can be blocked by BoNT-A, injections of BoNT-A into the parotid gland can result in atrophy of the parotid gland in humans.[23] Indeed, injection of BoNT-A into an enlarged or protruding parotid gland can reduce the width of the lower face (Figure 17.12).

2. Injecting BoNT-A into the parotid gland seldom results in dry mouth as 71% of salivary production comes from the submandibular gland.[24]

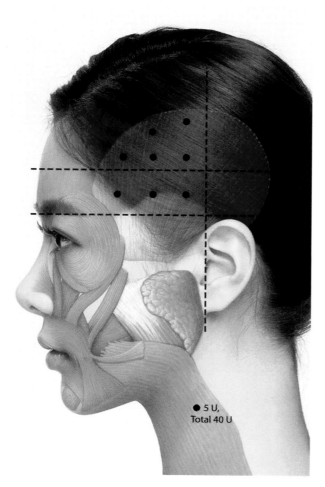

Figure 17.11 Injection points and dose of BoNT-A for temporalis hypertrophy. Five to eight IPs with 5 U are recommended depending on the muscle volume. (Reproduced with permission from Seo K, *Botulinum Toxin for Asians*; Seoul Medical Publishing Ltd. 2014.)

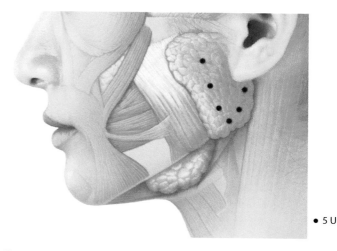

Figure 17.13 Injection points and dose of BoNT-A for parotid gland enlargement. Six to eight IPs with 5 U per injection site are recommended depending on the parotid gland volume. (Reproduced with permission from Seo K, *Botulinum Toxin for Asians*; Seoul Medical Publishing Ltd. 2014.)

3. *Injection points and techniques:* The most protruding part of the parotid gland around the mandibular angle is the most effective injection site. Deep intraglandular injections are required. Six to eight IPs with 5 U per injection site are recommended depending on the thickness of the parotid gland (Figure 17.13).

Intradermal Botulinum Toxin ("Mesobotox," "Dermotoxin," etc.)

1. Multiple intradermal injections of BoNT-A (intradermal BoNT-A) have been widely performed in Asia, under various names such as "mesobotox", "dermotoxin", or "microtoxin". The purpose of this treatment is not only for the reduction of dynamic facial wrinkles but also for the reduction of static wrinkles and pore sizes, as well as creating the so-called perceived "lifted look" or "pseudolift". Therefore, intradermal BoNT-A can be considered as a full package of antiaging effects that BTA can deliver.

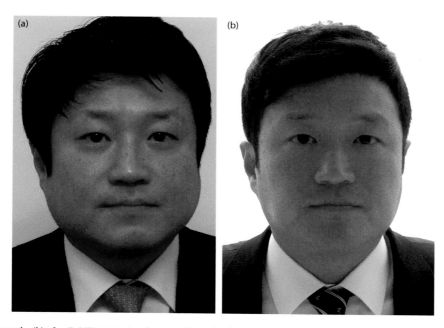

Figure 17.12 Before (a) and 3 months (b) after BoNT-A injection for parotid gland enlargement. (Reproduced with permission from Seo K, *Botulinum Toxin for Asians*; Seoul Medical Publishing Ltd. 2014.)

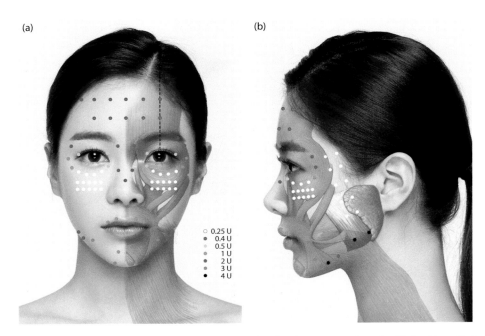

Figure 17.14 Injection points and dose of BoNT-A for intradermal BoNT-A. (Reproduced with permission from Seo K, *Botulinum Toxin for Asians*; Seoul Medical Publishing Ltd. 2014.)

2. The same dynamic wrinkle reduction as in wrinkle treatment with BoTX can also be achieved by diffusion of intradermal BoNT-A into underlying muscles of facial expression, because BoNT-A spreads in a three-dimensional manner from the dermis and because several muscles of facial expression also have intracutaneous insertions.

3. The improvement of static wrinkles and tightening of pores, which imparts a shine and a tighter look to the skin, has been already reported in conventional BoNT-A injections for the treatment of glabellar and forehead wrinkles.[25] My hypothesis

for this improvement seems to be due to dermal edema resulting from a transient and mild lymphatic insufficiency induced by underlying muscular paralysis. The same effect may happen after intradermal BoNT-A.[26]

4. Another effect of intradermal BoNT-A is the reduction of sebum production and pore size, thus improving the skin texture by giving it a smooth appearance.[27,28] This might be due to a possible humoral effect of BoNT-A reducing the activity of the sebaceous gland and the pore size since acetylcholine receptors have been reported to be present in sebaceous glands.[29] The reduction

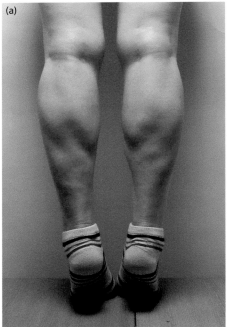
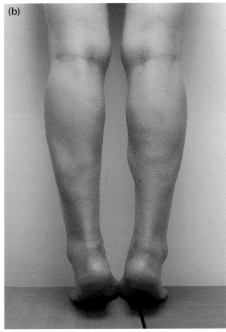

Figure 17.15 Before (a) and 2 months (b) after BoNT-A injection for calves (gastrocnemius hypertrophy). (Reproduced with permission from Seo K, *Botulinum Toxin for Asians*; Seoul Medical Publishing Ltd. 2014.)

of sebum production and pore size by intradermal BoNT-A in patients with oily skin was also objectively elucidated.[30]

5. The pseudo-lift effect is in fact not true lifting but a kind of visual illusion caused by reducing the lower part of the facial contour, and thus elevating the center of gravity upward. This effect can be achieved by narrowing the width of the lower face with reducing the volume of the masseter and giving a sharper definition to the chin line by weakening the mentalis and platysma.

6. *Injection points and techniques:* Combining multiple intradermal injections with the conventional intramuscular injection is usually recommended. Conventional intramuscular injections can be used for supplementation in areas with deep muscles such as corrugator, mentalis, and masseter. Areas for intradermal injection are forehead, periorbital, cheek, perioral, and anterior malar area (Figure 17.14).

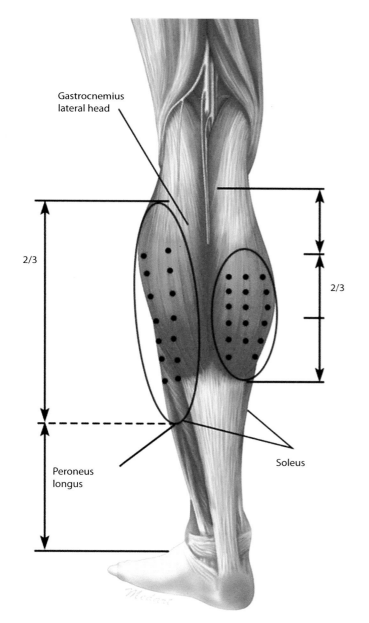

Figure 17.16 Injection points and dose of BoNT-A for calves. Approximately 50–100 U BoNTs is recommend for the head of each gastrocnemius at up to 25 injection points depending on the muscle volume. (Reproduced with permission from Seo K, *Botulinum Toxin for Asians*; Seoul Medical Publishing Ltd. 2014.)

Body Shaping (Bodytoxin)

1. The popularity of body shaping with botulinum toxin type A is rapidly increasing in Asian subjects leveraging the same mechanism of disuse atrophy as in treatment of BoNT for masseteric hypertrophy. Even though any muscles with hypertrophy can be targeted for body shaping using BoNT, the most popular site is the calves (Figure 17.15).[4,31] Asian women tend to have short legs relative to their torsos.[32] Thick calves with hypertrophied calf muscles further accentuate this disproportion in Asian women. Injection of BoNT into the calves brings about reducing muscular bulge and a slimmer lower leg line. Gastrocnemius and the lower part of the soleus muscle are target muscles for bodytoxin of the calf.

   Regarding the dose of BoNTs for bodytoxin, 50–100 U BoNTs is recommend for the head of each gastrocnemius at up to 25 IPs depending on the muscle volume[4] (Figure 17.16). Approximately 40–60 U BoNT per leg is required for the lower part of the soleus. For the cosmetic purpose of reshaping the lower leg contour, the lower two-thirds of the medial head of the gastrocnemius is the main target area for injections with BoNT-A while the upper two-thirds is the main target for the lateral head of the gastrocnemius.

2. Injection into upper body muscles, such as the deltoids and trapezius, has also been described to shape the upper arms and shoulders.[4,31] Slimming the upper arms by reducing the deltoid muscle is another novel indication of bodytoxin (Figure 17.17). Injection of BoNT-A into the upper part of the trapezius can create an elongated neck line which is useful for camouflaging women's short neck (Figure 17.18). Therefore, BoNT-A for trapezius is often called "bride toxin" and "wedding toxin" in Korea since this is helpful for brides who must wear wedding dresses revealing the shoulder and neck line. Approximately 40–50 U BoNT per side is required for the deltoid and the upper part of the trapezius, respectively (Figure 17.19).

3. Mild temporary muscle weakness would occur in some proportion of subjects. Even though this is temporary and muscle strength returns to normal within 3 months, the physician

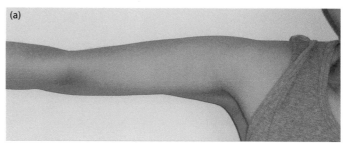
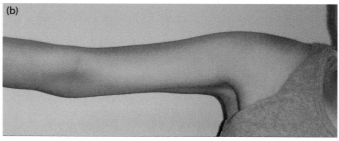

Figure 17.17 Before (a) and 2 months (b) after BoNT-A injection for arm contouring (deltoid muscle). (Reproduced with permission from Seo K, *Botulinum Toxin for Asians*; Seoul Medical Publishing Ltd. 2014.)

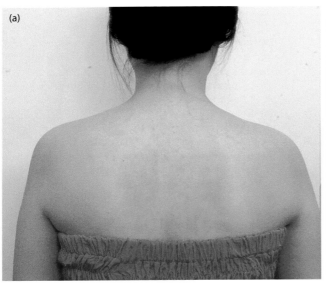
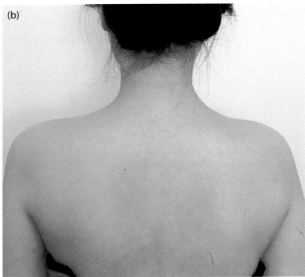

Figure 17.18 Before (a) and 2 months (b) after BoNT-A injection for shoulder contouring (trapezius muscle). (Reproduced with permission from Seo K, *Botulinum Toxin for Asians*; Seoul Medical Publishing Ltd. 2014.)

injector should pay attention to adjusting the dose of BoNT-A depending on the individual muscle volume. A two-step approach where a half dose of BoNT-A is administered at an interval of 2–3 months would be recommended in cases that require higher doses of BoNT-A.[4]

4. As is the case with treatment of masseteric hypertrophy with BoNT-A, the bodytoxin has an onset time of 2 weeks after injection, the peak effect at 2–3 months after injection, and the longevity of 6–12 months postinjection. However, the duration of the effect is variable depending on the individual's

habit to use the target muscle. Therefore, repetition of bodytoxin is recommended every 6–12 months depending on the individual's need.

REFERENCES

1. Baek SM, Chung YD, Kim SS. Reduction malarplasty. *Plast Reconstr Surg* 1991; 88(1); 53–61.
2. Smyth AG. Botulinum toxin treatment of bilateral masseteric hypertrophy. *Br J Oral Maxillofac Surg* 1994; 32: 29–33.
3. Flynn TC, Carruthers JA, Carruthers JA. Botulinum-A toxin treatment of the lower eyelid improves infraorbital rhytides and widens the eye. *Dermatol Surg* 2001; 27: 703–708.
4. Seo KK. *Botulinum Toxin for Asians*. Jeju: Seoul Medical Publishing Ltd.; 2014: 59–63.
5. Kane. Brow lifting. In: Carruthers J, Carruthers A (eds). *Procedures in Cosmetic Dermatology: Botulinum Toxin*. 3rd ed. Elsevier Saunders; 2013, 85–92.
6. Sundaram H, Kiripolsky M. Nonsurgical rejuvenation of the upper eyelid and brow. *Clin Plast Surg* 2013; 40: 55–76.
7. Seo KK. *Botulinum Toxin for Asians*. Jeju: Seoul Medical Publishing Ltd.; 2014, 116–9.
8. Sundaram H, Huang PH, Hsu NJ et al. Aesthetic applications of incobotulinumtoxinA in Asians: An international, multidisciplinary, pan-Asian consensus. *Plast Reconstr Surg Glob Open* 2016; 4(12); e872.
9. Yang HM, Kim HJ. Anatomical study of the corrugator supercilii muscle and its clinical implication with botulinum toxin A injection. *Surg Radiol Anat* 2013; 35: 817–21.
10. Tzou CH, Giovanoli P, Ploner M, Frey M. Are there ethnic differences of facial movements between Europeans and Asians? *Br J Plast Surg* 2005; 58: 183–195.
11. Lee Y, Hwang K. Skin thickness of Korean adults. *Surg Radiol Anat* 2002; 24: 183–9.
12. Sykes JM. Management of the aging face in the Asian patient. *Facial Plast Surg Clin North Am* 2007; 15: 353–60.
13. Seo KK. *Botulinum Toxin for Asians*. Jeju: Seoul Medical Publishing Ltd.; 2014: 120–32.
14. Seo KK. *Botulinum Toxin for Asians*. Jeju: Seoul Medical Publishing Ltd.; 2014: 84–97.

Neck line

2 cm

Figure 17.19 Injection points and dose of BoNT-A for trapezius. Approximately 40–50 U BoNT per side is required for the upper part of the trapezius. (Reproduced with permission from Seo K, *Botulinum Toxin for Asians*; Seoul Medical Publishing Ltd. 2014.)

15. Seo KK. *Botulinum Toxin for Asians*. Jeju: Seoul Medical Publishing Ltd.; 2014: 161–4.

16. Xu JA, Yuasa K, Yoshiura K et al. Quantitative analysis of masticatory muscles using computed tomography. *Dentomaxillofac Radiol* 1994; 23(3): 154–8.

17. Kim HJ, Yum KW, Lee SS, Heo MS, Seo K. Effects of botulinum toxin type A on bilateral masseteric hypertrophy evaluated with computed tomographic measurement. *Dermatol Surg* 2003;29: 484–9.

18. Yu CC, Chen PK, Chen YR. Botulinum toxin A for lower facial contouring: A prospective study. *Aesthetic Plast Surg* 2007; 31: 445–451; discussion 452–443.

19. Mandel L, Tharakan M. Treatment of unilateral masseteric hypertrophy with botulinum toxin: Case report. *J Oral Maxillofac Surg* 1999; 57: 1017–9.

20. Kim NH, Chung JH, Park RH, Park JB. The use of botulinum toxin type A in aesthetic mandibular contouring. *Plast Reconstr Surg* 2005; 115(3): 919–30.

21. Kim KS, Byun YS, Kim YJ, Kim ST. Muscle weakness after repeated injection of botulinum toxin type A evaluated according to bite force measurement of human masseter muscle. *Dermatol Surg* 2009; 35: 1902–6.

22. Seo KK. *Botulinum Toxin for Asians*. Jeju: Seoul Medical Publishing Ltd.; 2014: 209–11.

23. Bae GY, Yune YM, Seo K, Hwang SI. Botulinum toxin injection for salivary gland enlargement evaluated using computed tomographic volumetry. *Dermatol Surg* 2013; 39: 1404–7.

24. Elluru RG. Physiology of the salivary glands. In: Flint P, Haughey B, Lund V et al. (eds). *Cummings Otolaryngology*. Philadelphia, PA: Mosby Elsevier; 2010. Chapter 84.

25. Dessy LA, Mazzochhi M, Rubino C et al. An objective assessment of botulinum toxin A effect on superficial skin texture. *Ann Plast Surg* 2997; 58: 469–473.

26. Chang SP, Tsai HH, Chen WY, Lee WR, Chen PL, Tsai TH. The wrinkles soothing effect on the middle and lower face by intradermal injection of botulinum toxin type A. *Int J Dermatol* 2008; 47: 1287–94.

27. Rose AE, Goldberg DJ. Safety and efficacy of intradermal injection of botulinum toxin for the treatment of oily skin. *Dermatol Surg* 2013; 39: 443–8.

28. Shah AR. Use of intradermal botulinum toxin to reduce sebum production and facial pore size. *J Drugs Dermatol* 2008; 7: 847–50.

29. Kurzen H, Wessler I, Kirkpatrick CJ, Kawashima K, Grando SA. The non-neuronal cholinergic system of human skin. *Horm Metab Res* 2007; 39: 125–35.

30. Li ZJ, Park SB, Sohn KC et al. Regulation of lipid production by acetylcholine signalling in human sebaceous glands. *J Dermatol Sci* 2013;72: 116–22.

31. Seo K, Lee W. Medytoxin/Neuronox®. In: Carruthers JCA (ed). *Botulinum Toxin*. Philadelphia: Elsevier 2012, 52–8.

32. Wu WT. Facial and lower limb contouring. In: Benedetto A (ed). *Botulinum Toxins in Clinical Aesthetic Practice*. Boca Raton: CRC Press; 2011, 206–22.

APPENDIX 2 Muscles of facial expression

	Muscle	Origin	Insertion	Action	Function
I. Forehead	Frontalis (s)	Galea aponeurotica	Skin of forehead and brow	Raises eyebrow; retracts scalp	Wrinkles forehead; used in frowning and to express surprise and astonishment
II. Glabella	a. Corrugator supercilii (d)	Medial superciliary arch (nasal process of frontal bone)	Skin in the mid portion of brow	Adducts and draws brow down	Used to squint and protect eyes
	b. Orbicularis oculi, (s) i. orbital portion	Upper orbital margin, medial palpebral ligament and inferior medial orbital margin	Surrounds orbital opening as a sphincter: into eyebrow, temple and cheek skin	Shuts eyelid intentionally	Wrinkles brow to produce a frown; used to wink, squint and protect eyes
	ii. Palpebral portion (s)	Medial palpebral ligament	Lateral palpebral raphe	Shuts eye involuntarily	Produces sphincteric action of the eyelids
	iii. Lacrimal portion (d)	Lacrimal crest	Upper and lower tarsal plates	Draws eyelids posteriorly	Facilitates the lacrimal pump
	c. Depressor supercilii (s)	Nasal process of frontal bone	Skin of medial brow	Pulls down medial brow	Pulls eyebrows down, shuts eyelids, facilitates the lacrimal pump
	d. Procerus (d)	Nasal bone and transverse nasalis	Skin of forehead between eyebrows	Pulls down medial brow	Wrinkles central brow to produce frown; used to squint and shield eyes (conveys disdain or dislike)
III. Nose	a. Compressor naris (transverse nasalis) (s)	Canine eminence of maxilla	Nasal bridge aponeurosis	Compresses nasal aperture	Slows exhaled air
	b. Posterior dilator naris (alar nasalis) (s)	Maxilla above lateral incisor and alar cartilage	Nasal tip and alar skin, lateral crus cartilage and alar facial groove	Draws ala and posterior aspect of columella downward, widening nasal aperture	Prevents alar collapse in forceful breathing; flares nostrils during anger or exertion
	c. Anterior dilator naris	Lower lateral cartilage and lateral crus	Rim of the lateral alar skin and nasal spine	Stabilizes most flaccid portion of lateral nasal wall and assists in dilating nostrils	Prevents ala nasi from collapsing, especially during inspiration; maintains competency of external nasal valve
	d. Depressor septi nasi (d)	Incisive fossa of maxilla	Lower nasal septum and under surface of lower lateral alar cartilage	Draws nasal tip and alae downward	Narrows the nostrils; depresses nasal tip
IV. Mouth	a. Orbicularis oris (s & d)	Modiolus and angle of mouth; medial maxilla, mandible and many muscles that converge around mouth; deep surface of perioral skin	Mucous membrane of lips; incisive fossa of maxilla, caudal septum and anterior nasal spine	Closes lips	Forms a sphincter around mouth; closes oral aperture; protrudes, puckers and shapes lips (kissing); resists distension when blowing; inverts upper and lower lip
	b. Levator labii superioris alaeque nasi (d & s)	Frontal process of maxilla	Alar cartilage and lateral upper lip and modiolus	Dilates nares and everts and elevates lateral upper lip and elevates alae nasi	Deepens the upper nasolabial fold, dilates nasal aperture and used in scowling
	c. Levator labii superioris (d & s)	Lower margin of orbit, above infraorbital foramen on maxilla	Angle of mouth and upper lip	Elevates and everts upper lip	Used in expressing seriousness and sadness and deepens medial nasolabial fold
	d. Zygomaticus minor (d & s)	Malar surface of zygomatic bone (near maxillary suture line)	Upper lip at angle of mouth into orbicularis oris and levator labii superioris (via modiolus)	Draws mouth upward and laterally	Elevates and everts upper lip used in expressing sadness (see next above)
	e. Zygomaticus major (d & s)	Lateral surface of zygomatic bone, anterior to zygomaticotemporal suture	Modiolus and angle of mouth	Draws mouth upward and laterally	Elevates oral commissures used in laughing or smiling (bilateral); sneering and to show disdain (unilateral)
	f. Levator anguli oris (d)	Canine fossa below infraorbital foramen of maxilla	Modiolus and angle of mouth and upper lip musculature	Raises angle of mouth and lateral upper lip	Widens oral aperture to grin or grimace and used in smiling and laughing; it deepens nasolabial furrow as in contempt or disdain

(Continued)

Muscle	Origin	Insertion	Action	Function
g. Risorius (d & s)	superficial muscular aponeurotic system (SMAS), buccal skin and parotideomasseteric fascia	Modiolus and angle of mouth	Retracts angle of mouth laterally	Used in smiling and laughing when present
h. Depressor anguli oris (s)	Oblique line of mandible	Modiolus and angle of mouth, upper and lower lip	Depresses angle of mouth downward and laterally	Used in grimacing and snarling; used in expressing sadness
i. Depressor labii inferioris (d)	Between symphysis menti and mental foramen; platysma	Skin of lower lip and orbicularis oris and modiolus	Draws lower lip downward and laterally	Everts the lower lip, used in drinking, pouting and expressing irony; sorrow and doubt
j. Mentalis (d)	Incisive fossa of mandible	Skin of chin (mentolabial sulcus)	Raises and protrudes lower lip and wrinkles skin of chin	Used in pouting and to elevate skin of chin when expressing doubt or disdain
k. Buccinator (d)	Outer surface of mandible; alveolar process of maxilla and mandible; pterygomandibular raphe; buccinator crest	Modiolus and angle of mouth; upper and lower lips; interdigitates with orbicularis oris	Flattens cheek against gums; used when distending cheeks with air and compresses them to force air out of mouth	Presses cheek against molar teeth; works with tongue to keep food between occlusal surfaces and out of oral vestibule when chewing; used in sucking and to puff up cheeks and blow air out of mouth as when blowing up a balloon or playing a wind instrument
l. Platysma (s)	Pectoralis fascia of 2nd to 4th rib, deltoid fascia and subcutaneous tissue of infraclavicular and supraclavicular regions	Modiolus, angle of mouth, lower jaw, parotid fascia, skin of cheek and lower lip; orbicularis oris	Widens mouth aperture at commissures; pulls skin of lower face and neck taught	Used in expressing horror, tension and stress; assists in shaving or in relieving pressure of a tight collar; and depresses lower lip and mandible against resistance

s = superficial
d = deep

Muscles of Facial Expression in Action

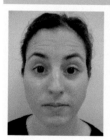

Alar part of levator labii superioris alaeque nasi and alar part of nasalis

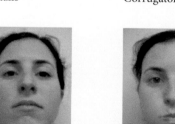

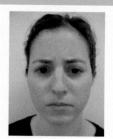

Corrugator supercilii

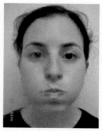

Buccinator and orbicularis oris

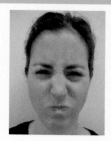

Procerus and transverse part of nasalis

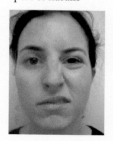

Levator labii superioris alaeque nasi

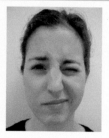

Orbicularis oculi and depressor supercilii

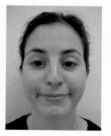

Risorius

Frontalis

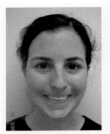

Risorius and depressor labii inferioris

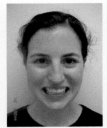

Zygomaticus major, risorius, levator anguli oris and lower lip depressors: mentalis, depressor anguli oris, and asymmetry of right depressor labii inferioris

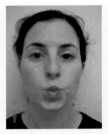

Orbicularis oris

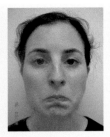

Depressor anguli oris and mentalis

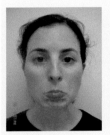

Mentalis

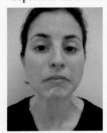

Platysma and depressor anguli oris

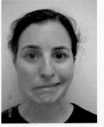

Right—platysma, pars labialis, depressor anguli oris; Left—levator labii superioris, zygomaticus major and mentalis

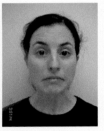

Depressor anguli oris, mentalis, and platysma

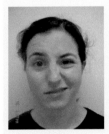

Left—levator labii superioris, levator labii superioris alaeque nasi, zygomaticus major and risorius

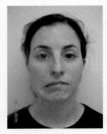

Right—depressor anguli oris, depressor labii inferioris, mentalis, and platysma labialis

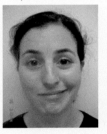

Left—zygomaticus major and minor, levator labii superioris, levator anguli oris, risorius, and mentalis

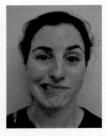

Right—zygomaticus major and minor, depressor labii inferioris, levator labii superioris, and mentalis

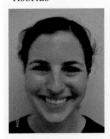

Zygomaticus major and minor, levator labii superioris, levator labii superioris alaeque nasi, levator anguli oris, risorius, depressor labii inferioris, and mentalis

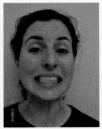

Levator labii superioris, zygomaticus minor, risorius, depressor labii inferioris, and platysma

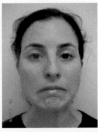

Depressor anguli oris, mentalis, and Right—depressor labii inferioris, and platysma

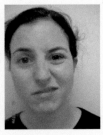

Left—levator labii superioris, levator labii superioris alaeque nasi

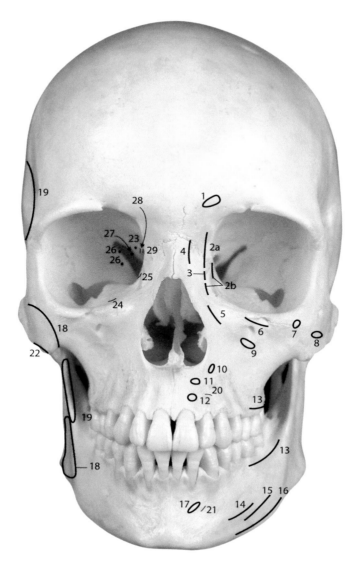

Figure A2.1 The bony origins of the muscles of facial expressions; their insertions are in soft tissue: 1, corrugator supercilli; 2, orbicularis oculi: 2a, upper orbital part; 2b, palpebral part; 3, medial palpebral ligament; 4, procerus; 5, levator labii superioris alaeque nasi; 6, levator labii superioris; 7, zygomaticus minor; 8, zygomaticus major; 9, levator anguli oris; 10, nasalis, transverse; 11, nasalis, alar; 12, depressor septi; 13, buccinator; 14, depressor labii inferioris; 15, depressor anguli oris; 16, platysma; 17, mentalis; 18, masseter; 19, temporalis; 20, incisivus labii superioris; 21, incisivus labii inferioris; 22, sternocleidomastoid; 23, levator palpebrae superioris; 24, inferior oblique; 25, inferior rectus; 26, lateral rectus; 27, superior oblique; 28, medial rectus; 29, superior oblique. (Image from Berkowitz, Moxham, *Head and Neck Anatomy: A Clinical Reference*, CRC Press, Boca Raton, FL, 2002, with permission.)

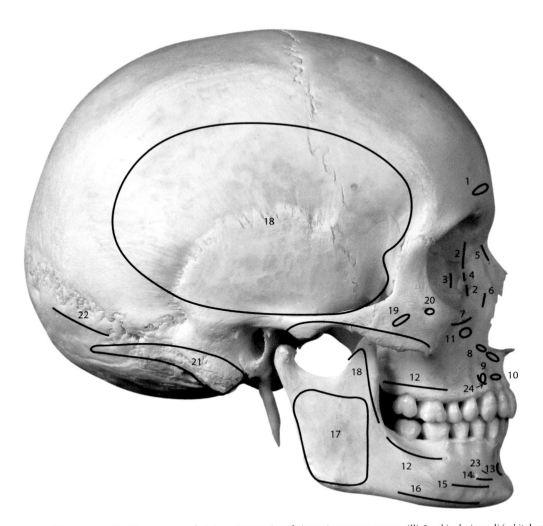

Figure A2.2 The bony origins of the muscles of facial expressions; their insertions are in soft tissue: 1, corrugator supercilli; 2, orbicularis oculi (orbital and palpebral parts); 3, orbicularis oculi (lacrimal parts); 4, medial palpebral ligament; 5, procerus; 6, levator labii superioris alaeque nasi; 7, levator labii superioris; 8, nasalis, transverse; 9, nasalis, alar; 10, depressor septi; 11, levator anguli oris; 12, buccinator; 13, mentalis; 14, depressor labii inferioris; 15, depressor anguli oris; 16, platysma; 17, masseter; 18, temporalis; 19, zygomaticus major; 20, zygomaticus minor; 21, sternocleidomastoid; 22, occipital belly of occipitofrontalis; 23, incisivus labii inferioris; 24, incisivus labii superioris. (Image from Berkowitz, Moxham, *Head and Neck Anatomy: A Clinical Reference*, CRC Press, Boca Raton, FL, 2002, with permission.)

APPENDIX 3

The preparation, handling, storage, and mode of injection of OnaBTX-A

STORAGE OF OnaBTX-A

BOTOX®/BOTOX® Cosmetic (OnaBTX-A) is a purified neurotoxin complex distributed in vials of 100 U or 50 U of sterile, vacuum-dried crystalline powder without preservative. The vials of onabotulinumtoxinA (OnaBTX-A) have a holographic film on the vial label with the name "Allergan" within the horizontal lines of rainbow color. They are shipped frozen, in insulated, styrofoam containers containing dry ice. When they reach their destination the vials of OnaBTX-A can be stored in their dry, powdered form in the refrigerator at a constant temperature of 2°C–8°C for up to 36 months for the 100 U vial and for up to 24 months for the 50 U vial.[1] Once reconstituted, the solution of OnaBTX-A can be stored again in the refrigerator at a constant temperature of 2°C–8°C. *Do not refreeze reconstituted OnaBTX-A.* Although the package insert for OnaBTX-A recommends the reconstituted product be used within 4 hours, studies have shown that after reconstitution, the potency of OnaBTX-A should remain consistent and unchanged for up to 6 weeks, and can be used without any noticeable change in clinical efficacy.[2–6] Similar results were found by Parsa et al. when they compared reconstituted OnaBTX-A frozen for up to 6 months with OnaBTX-A not frozen and used within 4 hours after reconstitution in 118 sites in the upper one third of the face in 80 patients.[7] They concluded that reconstituted OnaBTX-A may be reconstituted and refrozen, thawed, and injected without losing its potency for up to 6 months. Initially, OnaBTX-A was thought to be a fragile molecule. However, subsequent studies following anecdotal observations confirm the persistence of activity of BoNT-A in different clinical situations, confirming that BoNT-As may be sturdier and more resistant to degradation than previously understood.[8]

PREPARATION OF OnaBTX-A

The package insert for OnaBTX-A suggests that the 100 U vial be reconstituted with 2.5 mL of 0.9% non-preserved saline for a final concentration of 4 U/0.1 mL and the 50 U vial with 2.25 ml of the same.[1] The report of a consensus conference of key multispecialty physician injectors held in 2004 recommended that a 100 U vial of OnaBTX-A be reconstituted at a "dilution that minimizes the likelihood of diffusion to neighboring muscle groups," and can be anywhere from 1 to 10 mL of normal saline for each 100 U vial of product.[10] Anecdotal and published reports suggest that volume may influence duration of effect, in that the greater the volume, the shorter the duration of effect.[5] In addition, because higher dilutions can be associated with a greater risk of diffusion into untargeted sites, this also can lead to unsatisfactory results and even unexpected adverse events, along with a shorter duration of effect.[9] In a prospective, randomized, controlled study with 10 volunteers, Hsu et al. injected the forehead with 5 U of OnaBTX-A. On one side of the forehead 5 U of OnaBTX-A was injected with 0.25 mL (2 U/0.1 mL). On the other side of the forehead OnaBTX-A was injected with 5 U in 0.05 mL (2 U/0.02 mL). There was a 5-fold difference in volume injected.[9] They found that low concentration and higher-volume injections resulted in greater diffusion, affecting a larger anatomic area. They concluded that the size of the muscle and its pattern of contraction influences the pattern of toxin spread. Consequently, an ideal strategy may be to inject concentrated BoNT at a low volume to target smaller muscle groups, while using a larger volume for larger, broad muscle groups, such as the frontalis muscle. Their results show that the dilution of OnaBTX-A can have pharmacokinetic implications on the desired effect of OnaBTX-A.[9] There is

no standardized dilution for BoNT treatment of focal hyperhidrosis. Dilutions reported vary from 1 to 10 mL of saline for OnaBTX-A, with most clinicians using between 2 and 5 mL.[8]

The 2004 consensus conference report also confirmed that the majority of dermatologic and aesthetic physician injectors reconstitute OnaBTX-A with preserved normal saline instead of nonpreserved diluent and store and reuse the vials of reconstituted OnaBTX-A after more than 4 hours.[10] Preserved saline includes benzyl alcohol, which has anesthetic properties. The result of a bilateral, comparative prospective study has shown that there is less pain with injection (up to 50% reduction detected on numerical pain scales) when preserved isotonic saline is used instead of nonpreserved isotonic saline.[8,10–12] There was neither loss of efficacy nor duration of potency whether OnaBTX-A was reconstituted with preserved or unpreserved normal saline. Once reconstituted, the vial of OnaBTX-A should be clear, colorless, and free of particulate matter, regardless of diluent used.[1] There is a single report of contact dermatitis in fragrance-sensitive patients associated with reconstitution of botulinum toxin with preserved saline, but no indication of an increased risk associated with the storage or reuse of toxin.[12]

Several studies have assessed the potential risk for contamination of reconstituted botulinum toxin. In one study, 11 consecutive vials of reconstituted toxin were exposed to room air for 4 hours, then refrigerated for 3–5 days, and then cultured for possible microbial contamination; none was detected.[5,13] In another study, the routine refrigerator storage of 100 unit vials of reconstituted OnaBTX-A did not result in any microbial contamination even after serial re-extractions of the reconstituted solution from the vials by different personnel. Storage of reconstituted OnaBTX-A and subsequent multiple extractions from the same vial of botulinum toxin appears safe for clinical use for at least 7 weeks after reconstitution.[5,11,14] Up until the present, there is no evidence that any serious or nonserious adverse events have been associated with the use and reuse of vials of OnaBTX-A that have been reconstituted for more than 4 hours and reused in the treatment of multiple patients.[5] Of the 322 board-certified dermatologists who responded to a survey, 68.6% reported routinely storing toxin for more than 1 week after reconstitution and routinely using each vial for more than 1 patient. Also, 67.0% of the respondents believed that BoNT-A could be safely stored and reused for 1–4 weeks. None of the respondents, who had been in clinical practice for a median duration of 15 years, reported any local infections associated with cosmetic BoNT-A injections.[5,7,15] The consensus statement approved by the ASDS Task Force on Guidelines for the Use and Storage of Neuromodulators on March 15, 2014, and adopted as amended by the ASDS Board of Directors on May 12, 2014, reads as follows: "(1) although it is likely that reconstituted toxin can be refrigerated or refrozen for longer than 4 weeks before use, there is insufficient evidence for a strong recommendation in this regard, (2) apart from practical considerations regarding the limited volume of material available for use, there is no specific limit on the number of patients who can be treated with a single vial of reconstituted botulinum toxin."[5]

HANDLING OF OnaBTX-A

Concerns over a potential loss of potency resulting from rough handling, agitation, and foaming during reconstitution were also addressed at the 2004 consensus conference.[10] Trindade de Almeida et al. treated one side of six patients in the glabella and periocular area with OnaBTX-A that was reconstituted by agitation to the point of bubbling and foaming, and the opposite side with OnaBTX-A that was not agitated.[17] There was no difference in muscle relaxation between the two sides treated, and the duration of effect remained constant on both sides for approximately 16 weeks. In another prospective, double-blinded, randomized study by Kazim and Black, seven patients were injected with gently reconstituted OnaBTX-A at 4 sites on one side of the forehead. On the opposite side of the forehead the same seven patients were injected with vigorously reconstituted OnaBTX-A at another 4 sites that were symmetrically parallel to the contralateral side.[17] To vigorously reconstitute the vial of OnaBTX-A, it was placed on the Vortex Touch Mixer Model 232 at the maximum speed of 10 for a duration of 30 seconds. Foam was observed on the top of this vial for 1 1/2 minutes after vigorous reconstitution. Eyebrow excursion was measured in millimeters before the injections, 1 week after the injections, and every month thereafter for up to a total of 6 months. There was no statistically significant difference in eyebrow excursion between the two sides of the forehead, and the effect of OnaBTX-A was maintained and had the same duration when brow excursion was measured at every interval. This study quantitatively demonstrated that there is no change in effectiveness or duration of OnaBTX-A that is related to the speed or manner of reconstitution. Physicians administering OnaBTX-A can do so without worrying about compromising the effectiveness of the product during the reconstitution process.[17] Similar results were anecdotally confirmed by the majority of those present at the 2004 consensus conference.[10]

INJECTION TECHNIQUE OF OnaBTX-A

OnaBTX-A should be injected with sterile, plastic, single-use syringes. To minimize the pain and bruising of injection, the use of tuberculin syringes with a 30- to 32-gauge needle is recommended. For those injectors who want to reconstitute OnaBTX-A with a minimum amount of diluent (1 mL or less) and be able to control the minutest amount of solution injected, an U-100 insulin syringe with an attached 29- or 31-gauge needle can be used (Becton-Dickinson, Franklin Lakes, NJ).[18] The preattached needle is silicone-coated, which easily penetrates the skin. The needle stays sharp for approximately 4–6 punctures.[18] Insulin syringes (0.5 mL or 0.3 mL) have no potential dead space at the hub where the needle is preattached, thereby minimizing any wastage of solution.[18] Full depression of the plunger leaves less than 0.01 mL in the needle itself, a contrast with the 0.07 mL that is retained in the dead space in a commonly available 30-gauge needle attached to a Luer Lok syringe. At 100 U/mL, this means that 7 U of botulinum exotoxin A cannot be used.[18] In addition, the barrel of the syringe is scored with markings representing 0.01 mL that can be easily seen and which will correspond to 1 U of OnaBTX-A when a 100 U

vial is reconstituted with 1 mL of diluent.[18] To further reduce some of the discomfort associated with any type of intramuscular injection, the pretreatment application of either a topical anaesthetic, ice, or both on the skin surface at the injection site can help provide a more comfortable, positive experience for some patients.

Although there are no controlled studies to support certain commonly prescribed post-treatment recommendations made to prevent local spread of the OnaBTX-A beyond the injection site, many expert physician injectors still recommend the following for their patients:

1. DO NOT massage the OnaBTX-A treated areas for 2–4 hours.
2. DO contract treated muscles for 2–3 hours immediately after an OnaBTX-A treatment. This promotes the uptake of OnaBTX-A by the receptor sites at the neuromuscular junctions.
   The following recommendations have been refuted because lack of evidence:
3. DO NOT bend over (e.g., to tie shoes or pick up something from the floor) for 2–3 hours after an OnaBTX-A treatment of the upper face.
4. LIMIT heavy physical activity, and lying down or sleeping for 2–3 hours after an OnaBTX-A treatment of the upper face.[10]

Postmarketing reports indicate that the effects of OnaBTX-A and all botulinum toxin products may spread from the area of injection to produce symptoms consistent with botulinum toxin effects.[1] These symptoms have been reported hours to weeks after injection. The risk of symptoms is probably greatest in children treated for spasticity but symptoms also can occur in adults treated for spasticity and other conditions, particularly in those patients who have underlying conditions that would predispose them to these symptoms. In unapproved uses and approved indications, cases of the spread of effect have occurred at doses comparable to those used to treat cervical dystonia but not at the lower doses generally used for cosmetic purposes. Furthermore, using currently available analytical technology, it is not possible to detect OnaBTX-A in the peripheral blood following intramuscular injection at the recommended doses.[1] A thorough review and understanding of the current package insert for the brand of BoNT-A being used is recommended before treating patients.

Table A3.1 sets out specifies the recommendations and methods for preparation, handling, and storage of OnaBTX-A.

REFERENCES

1. Allergan, Inc. *Botox Cosmetic (botulinum toxin type A) purified neurotoxin complex (Package Insert)*. Irvin, California: Allergan, Inc., revised January; 2016.
2. Garcia A, Fulton JE Jr. Cosmetic denervation of the muscles of facial expression with botulinum toxin: A dose-response study. *Dermatol Surg* 1996; 22: 39–43.

Table A3.1 Current Popular Mode of Preparing, Handling, and Storing OnaBTX-A

	Popular methods	Manufacturer's recommendations[1]
Storage		
Before reconstitution	≤36 months at 2°C–8°C (100 U vial)	≤36 months at 2°C–8°C (100 U vial)
	24 months at 2°C–8°C (50 U vial)	24 months at 2°C–8°C (50 U vial)
After reconstitution	16 weeks at 2°C–8°C[3,4,10]	4 hours at 2°C–8°C
Preparation		
Diluent	Preserved normal saline (0.9% saline with 0.9% benzyl alcohol)[10,12]	Non-preserved normal saline (0.9% saline)
Concentration	Concentrations 1–10 mL/100 U vial as needed for appropriate uptake and diffusion[2,10]	2.5 mL/100 U vial
Handling	No special precautions[10,16–18]	DO NOT agitate or cause foaming
Injection technique	Insulin syringe with 30-gauge needle[18] or tuberculin syringe with 30–32-gauge needle[9]	None recommended

3. Hexsel DM, de Almeida AT, Rutowitsch M et al. Multicenter, double-blind study of the efficacy of injections with botulinum toxin type A reconstituted up to six consecutive weeks before application. 2003; 29: 523–9.

4. Hui JI, Lee WW. Efficacy of fresh versus refrigerated botulinum toxin in the treatment of lateral periorbital rhytids. *Ophthal Plast Reconstr Surg* 2007; 23(6): 433–8.

5. Alam M, Bolotin D, Carruthers J Consensus statement regarding storage and reuse of previously reconstituted euromodulators. *Dermatol Surg* 2015; 41: 321–6.

6. Yang GC, Chiu RJ, Gillman GS. Questioning the need to use Botox within 4 hours of reconstitution: A study of fresh vs. 2-week-old Botox. *Arch Facial Plast Surg* 2008; 10: 273–9.

7. Trindade de almeida AR, Cardoso Secco L, Carruthers A. Handling Botulinum toxins: An updated literature review. *Dermatol Surg* 2011; 37: 1553–65.

8. Hsu J, Dover J, Arndt K. Effect of volume and concentration on the diffusion of botulinum exotoxin A. *Arch Dermatol* 2004; 140: 1351–4.

9. Carruthers J, Fagien S, Matarasso SL. Consensus recommendations on the use of botulinum toxin type A in facial aesthetics. *Plast Reconstr Surg* 2004; 114(6 Suppl): 1S–22S.

10. Klein AW. Complications and adverse reactions with the use of botulinum toxin. *Dis Mon* 2002; 48: 336–56.

11. Alam M, Dover JS, Arndt KA. Pain associated with injection of botulinum A exotoxin reconstituted using isotonic sodium chloride with and without preservative: A double-blind, randomized controlled trial. *Arch Dermatol* 2002; 138: 510–4.

12. Amado A, Jacob SE. Letter: Benzyl alcohol preserved saline used to dilute injectables poses a risk of contact dermatitis in fragrance-sensitive patients. *Dermatol Surg* 2007; 33: 1396–7.

13. Menon J, Murray A. Microbial growth in vials of Botulinum toxin following use in clinic. *Eye (Lond)* 2007; 21: 995–7.

14. Alam M, Yoo SS, Wrone DA, et al. Sterility assessment of multiple use botulinum A exotoxin vials: A prospective simulation. *J Am Acad Dermatol* 2006; 55: 272–5.

15. Liu A, Carruthers A, Cohen JL et al. Recommendations and current practices for the reconstitution and storage of botulinum toxin type A. *J Am Acad Dermatol* 2012; 67: 373–8.

16. Trindade de Almeida AR, Kadunc BV, Di Chiacchio N, Neto DR. Foam during reconstitution does not affect the potency of botulinum toxin type A. *Dermatol Surg* 2003; 29: 530–1.

17. Kazim NA, Black EH. Botox: Shaken, not stirred. *Ophthalmic Plastic and Reconstructive Surgery* 2008; 24: 10–12.

18. Flynn TC, Carruthers A, Carruthers J. Surgical pearl: The use of the Ultra-Fine II short needle 0.3 cc insulin syringe for botulinum toxin injections. *J Am Acad Dermatol* 2002; 46: 931–3.

19. Parsa AA, Lye KD, Don Parsa F. Reconstituted botulinum type A neurotoxin: Clinical efficacy after long-term freezing before use. *Aesth Plast Surg* 2007; 31: 188–91.

20. Carruthers A, Carruthers J, Cohen J. Dilution volume of botulinum toxin type A for the treatment of glabellar rhytides: Does it matter? *Dermatol Surg* 2007; 33: S97–104.

APPENDIX 4   Patient treatment record

Doctor's name and address

INJECTION SITE TREATMENT RECORD CIRCLE ONE USED:

BOTOX (R) COSMETIC; XEOMIN (R); DYSPORT (R): (OTHER)_____

PATIENT NAME: _____

CHART #:_____

NOTES:

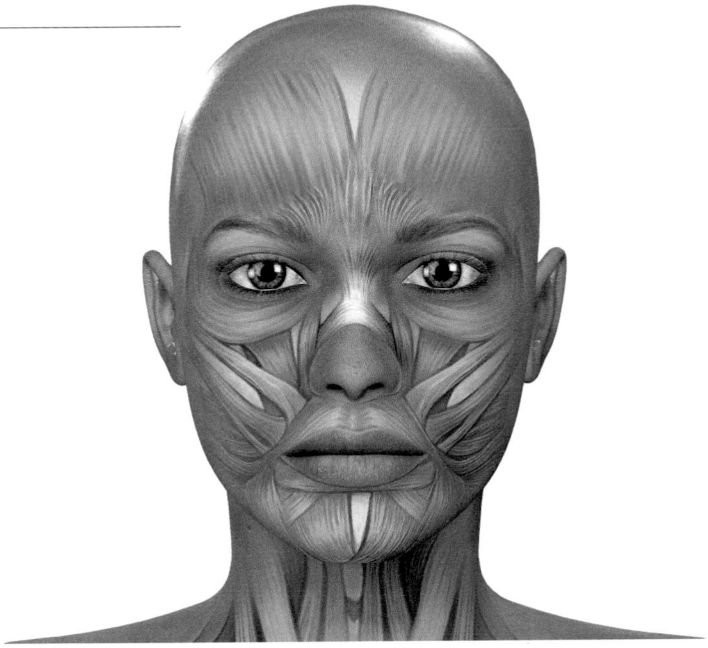

Botox Lot #: _____ Expires: _____	N. S. Lot #: _____ Expires: _____	Dilution used: ____mL/100U ____Units/0.1cc	Photos		Total Units/Site
			Pre Rx Date	Post Rx Date	
*Forehead:					
*Glabella:					
*Crow's feet:					
Eyelids: (lower); (upper)					
Nose: bunny lines					
Nose: (alar flare); (tip lift)					
Mouth corners (DAO):					
Lips: (lower); (upper)					
Lips: (Asymmetry); (Gummy smile)					
Chin: (apex)					
Neck: (Horizontal lines); (Bands)					
Mandibulocervical angle:					
MicroBoNTA:					
Décolletée:					
Breast Lift:					
Other:					
Total Units Injected					

* FDA approved.

The nature and purpose of the treatment have been explained to me and questions I had regarding the treatment have been answered to my satisfaction. I understand that only treatments for wrinkles of the forehead, central brow and crow's feet are FDA approved. Any other area of the face and neck treated with botulinum toxin is not approved by the FDA. These treatments may involve risks of complications both from known and unknown causes, and I freely assume these risks.

PATIENT'S SIGNATURE:_____   WITNESS:_____

DOCTOR'S SIGNATURE: _____   DATE:_____

APPENDIX 5
Informed consent for the treatment of facial and body wrinkles with botulinum toxin

RATIONALE

I am aware that when a small amount of purified botulinum toxin A (BoNT-A) is injected into a muscle it causes weakness of that muscle. This occurs in 3–5 days or even later, and usually lasts 3–5 months but can last for shorter or longer amounts of time, depending on which BoNT-A product is used.

Frown lines between the eyebrows are due to contraction of muscles around and between the eyebrows. Injecting BoNT-A into this area will temporarily weaken these muscles causing a reduction or disappearance of the frown lines. Similarly, crow's feet and horizontal forehead lines can be improved by injecting BoNT-A into these areas, weakening the muscles that cause the wrinkles on the forehead and around the eyes. Many other areas of the central and lower face, neck, and chest also can be treated successfully with BoNT-A, but treatment of any area other than the forehead, between the eyebrows and the crow's feet is currently **not** FDA approved and is performed off-label.

RESULTS AND AFTER TREATMENT CARE

1. I understand that I will not be able to "frown," produce crow's feet, or see certain wrinkles while the injections of BoNT-A into these areas and other areas are effective. After a period of months wrinkles will return, at which time retreatment is appropriate and needed to maintain the previously treated areas without wrinkles.
2. I understand that I must remain upright and not bend or lower my head (i.e., to tie my shoes, or pick up something from the ground), and I must not manipulate or rub the treated areas for 2–3 hours after my treatment session.
3. I understand that I might experience quicker results if I repeatedly contract and use (e.g., frown or squint) the injected muscles for the 2–3 hours after my treatment session.

RISKS AND COMPLICATIONS

The most common side effects associated with BoNT-A injections for wrinkle correction are bruising and swelling. These local reactions are temporary. Less commonly, headache, numbness, temporary drooping of one or both eyebrows or eyelids, the enlargement of skin folds under the eyelids or asymmetry can occur in 2% of those injected. Any of these side effects can last for a few hours up to 2–4 weeks and possibly longer.

In a very small number of individuals the injections may not work as completely as they do in others nor may they last as long as they do in others. Everyone responds to injections of BoNT-A in their own way. Results also may vary depending on which BoNT-A product is used. At times, a touch-up injection 2–3 weeks later can improve the initial results.

You should inform the doctor if you develop any unusual symptoms (including difficulty with swallowing, speaking, or breathing), or if any similar existing symptom worsens.

If loss of strength, muscle weakness, or impaired vision occurs, you should avoid driving a car or engaging in other potentially hazardous activities.

Adverse event information may be reported directly to Allergan Inc. by phone to 800-433-8871. In addition, adverse events may also be reported to the FDA MedWatch Reporting System by the following methods:

- Online at www.fda.gov/medwatch
- Phone at 1-800-FDA-1088

PREGNANCY, NEUROLOGIC DISEASE, AND MEDICATIONS

I am aware that BoNT-A is absolutely contraindicated in all pregnant women and must not be injected if I am not sure whether I am pregnant. If I am trying to conceive, BoNT-A should not be injected for three months prior to conception. BoNT-A should not be injected if I am breastfeeding or if I have any neurologic disease such as multiple sclerosis or myasthenia gravis. The effect of BoNT-A may be potentiated by aminoglycoside antibiotics such as spectinomycin, tobramycin, neomycin, gentamycin, kanamycin, or amikacin. Please notify the doctor or nurse if you are currently on such medications.

I am not nursing. Neither am I aware that I am pregnant nor do I have any significant neurologic disease. (_____) (initial).

Today's treatment will be performed with: (circle one used) BOTOX® Cosmetic (onabotulinumtoxinA) or DYSPORT® (abobotulinumtoxinA) or XEOMIN® (incobotulinumtoxinA) or Name other:_____.

PHOTOGRAPHS

I authorize the taking of photographs and their use for scientific and medical purposes both in publications and presentations. I understand that my identity will be protected.

PAYMENT

I understand this is a cosmetic procedure and payment is my responsibility and due at the completion of treatment.

I have read and completely understand all of the above. All of my questions have been answered satisfactorily by the doctor and nurse. I accept the risks, benefits, and potential complications of this procedure and hereby give my informed consent to be treated with: (circle one) BOTOX® Cosmetic (onabotulinumtoxinA) or DYSPORT™ (abobotulinumtoxinA) or XEOMIN® (incobotulinumtoxinA) or Name other:_____

Signed:_____Date:_____
Name:_____
Witness's name and signature:_____
Treating physician:_____

APPENDIX 6

Side effects and contraindications to injections with botulinum toxins

Physicians are instructed to have their patients read the Medication Guide that is included in every carton of onabotulinumtoxinA (OnaBTX-A) before they inject it and each time it is given to the patient. This information does not take the place of the patient talking with their physician about their medical condition(s) or their treatment. Patients are encouraged to share this information with their family members and caregivers.

OnaBTX-A (BOTOX® Cosmetic) is approved by the FDA only to treat and temporarily improve moderate to severe horizontal forehead lines, glabellar frown lines and lateral canthal lines in adults younger than 65 years of age. It is not known whether OnaBTX-A is safe or effective in patients younger than 18 years of age for the treatment of axillary hyperhidrosis, the only area on the body the FDA approved for the treatment of hyperhidrosis. OnaBTX-A is not recommended for use in patients younger than 18 years of age.

POTENTIAL SIDE EFFECTS OF OnaBTX-A INJECTIONS

1. Adverse effects of limited duration that are common, localized, and not of a serious nature:[2,3]

Distant Spread of Toxin Effect[1]

Postmarketing reports indicate that the effect of OnaBTX-A and all botulinum toxin products may spread from the area of injection to produce symptoms consistent with botulinum toxin effects. These may include asthenia, generalized muscle weakness, diplopia, blurred vision, ptosis, dysphagia, dysphonia, dysarthria, urinary incontinence, and breathing difficulties. These symptoms have been reported hours to weeks after injection. Swallowing and breathing difficulties can be life-threatening and there have been reports of death. This risk of symptoms is probably greatest in children treated for spasticity but symptoms can also occur in adults treated for spasticity and other conditions particularly in those patients who have underlying conditions that would predispose them to these symptoms. In unapproved uses, including spasticity in children and adults, and in approved indications, cases of spread of effect have occurred at doses comparable to those used to treat cervical dystonia and at lower doses.

Common with any percutaneous injection
a. Mild stinging, burning, or pain with injection
b. Edema around injection site
c. Erythema around injection site
d. Mild headache, localized and transient

Technique dependent
a. Ecchymosis lasting 3–10 days
b. Asymmetry
c. Oral incompetence and asymmetric smile
d. Lack of neck strength
e. Lack of intended cosmetic effect

Rare and idiosyncratic
a. Numbness and paresthesias, localized and transient
b. Focal tonic movements (twitching)
c. Mild nausea and occasional vomiting

d. Dizziness or syncope
e. Mild malaise and myalgias (localized and generalized)
f. Dry mouth
g. Periorbital edema

2. Adverse effects of longer duration that can be serious and are technique dependent:
a. Blepharoptosis
b. Brow ptosis
c. Diplopia
d. Blurred vision or diminished visual acuity
e. Diminished tearing and xerophthalmia with or without keratitis
f. Ectropion (can lead to xerophthalmia)
g. Lagopthalmus (can lead to exposure keratitis)
h. Dysphagia
i. Dysarthria
j. Dysphonia

3. Adverse effects of longer duration that can be serious and are not technique dependent: Immediate hypersensitivity reactions
a. Urticaria, pruritus, rash, or generalized erythema
b. Dyspnea, wheezing, or exacerbation of asthma
c. Soft tissue edema
d. Anaphylaxis

Contraindications to OnaBTX-A Injections

Patients should not be treated or otherwise treated with extreme caution who are

1. Psychologically unstable or who have questionable motives and unrealistic expectations
2. Dependent on intact facial movements and expressions for their livelihood (e.g., actors, singers, musicians, and other media personalities)
3. Afflicted with peripheral motor neuropathic disease, amyotrophic lateral sclerosis, or neuromuscular junctional disorders (e.g., myasthenia gravis or Lambert-Eaton syndrome) or allergic to any of the component ingredients of BTX-A or BTX-B (i.e., BoNT, human albumin, saline, lactose, and sodium succinate)
4. Taking certain medications that can interfere with neuromuscular impulse transmission and potentiate the effects of BoNT (e.g., aminoglycosides, penicillamine, quinine, and calcium blockers)
5. Pregnant or lactating (BoNTs are classified as pregnancy category C drugs)
6. Experiencing an active skin infection at the planned injection site

POTENTIAL BENEFICIAL EFFECTS OF BOTOX® COSMETIC INJECTIONS

1. Relief of frontal or occipital "tension headaches"
2. Relief of migraine headaches
3. Compensatory muscle strengthening of the same muscles when segmentally treated (e.g., strengthening of the lower frontalis and elevation of the eyebrows when the upper frontalis is treated or improvement of posture and projection of breasts when the lower pectoralis major or minor are treated)

4. Compensatory muscle strengthening of synergistic muscles (e.g., strengthening of the lip levators and depressors when the orbicularis oris is treated)
5. Compensatory muscle strengthening of antagonistic muscles (e.g., strengthening of the lower frontalis and medial brow lift when the medial brow depressors are treated or lateral brow lift when lateral brow depressors are treated)

RISK EVALUATION AND MITIGATION STRATEGY

In 2009 when another BoNT-A was approved by the FDA for use in the United States, Allergan, Inc. instituted a surveillance program called "Risk Evaluation and Mitigation Strategy" (REMS) to update its physician injectors on safety issues regarding the use of BOTOX®/BOTOX® Cosmetic (OnaBTX-A). The goals of the REMS program are to minimize the risks of medication errors related to the lack of interchangeability of OnaBTX-A units with those of licensed botulinum toxins of other manufacturers and to inform prescribers and patients about the potential occurrence of the spread of toxin effect beyond the injection site.

Physician injectors are advised to discuss the risks associated with OnaBTX-A therapy outlined above and in the Medication Guide for OnaBTX-A with patients and with all the health care personnel who are involved in the preparation, prescribing, and/or injection of OnaBTX-A. According to FDA regulations, a copy of the Medication Guide must be distributed directly to each patient every time he or she receives an OnaBTX-A injection. Copies of the OnaBTX-A Medication Guide can be obtained by calling 1-800-433-8871 or printing copies directly from the websites (www.botoxmedical.com or www.botoxcosmetic.com). A copy of the Medication Guide also is included in every carton of OnaBTX-A.

Because there are currently multiple marketed botulinum toxin products with different dose to potency ratios, there is a concern about medication errors such as overdosing based on incorrect unit administration from interchanging different BoNTA products.[1] It is important to understand that BOTOX®/BOTOX® Cosmetic (OnaBTX-A, Allergan, Inc.), MYOBLOC® (rimabotulinumtoxinB, Solstice), DYSPORT® (abobotulinumtoxinA, Galderma Laboratories, L.P., 14501 North Freeway, Fort Worth, TX), and XEOMIN® (incobotulinumtoxinA, Merz Pharmaceuticals, 6501 Six Forks Road, Raleigh, NC) are unique biological products that are not interchangeable with each other. The potency units of OnaBTX-A are specific to the preparation and assay method utilized by the manufacturer. Therefore, units of biological activity of OnaBTX-A cannot be compared to or converted into units of any other BoNT product assessed with any other specific assay method. Additionally, OnaBTX-A has multiple indications which all require specific dosing. Caution should be taken to ensure that the dosing, dilution, injection volume, and injection patterns are appropriate for the product and the patient.

No definitive reports of serious adverse events of distant spread of toxin effect associated with the cosmetic and dermatologic use of OnaBTX-A have been reported when the recommended labelled dose of 20 units for glabellar lines, 24 units for lateral canthal lines, or 100 units for severe primary axillary hyperhidrosis have been used.[2,3]

REFERENCES

1. Allergan, Inc. *Botox Cosmetic (botulinum toxin type A) Purified Neurotoxin Complex (Package Insert)*. Irvin, California: Allergan, Inc., revised October 2017.
2. Coté TR, Mohan AK, Polder JA, Walton MK, Bruan MM. Botulinum toxin type A injections: Adverse events reported to the US Food and Drug Administration in therapeutic and cosmetic cases. *JAAD* 2005; 53: 07–415.
3. Gershon SK, Wise RP, Braun MM. Adverse events reported with cosmetic use of Botulinum toxin A. *Pharmacoepidemiology Drug Safety* 2001; 10(Suppl): S135–6.

Index